USE OF DIETARY SUPPLEMENTS BY MILITARY PERSONNEL

Committee on Dietary Supplement Use by Military Personnel
Food and Nutrition Board

M.R.C. Greenwood and Maria Oria, *Editors*

INSTITUTE OF MEDICINE
OF THE NATIONAL ACADEMIES

THE NATIONAL ACADEMIES PRESS
Washington, D.C.
www.nap.edu

THE NATIONAL ACADEMIES PRESS 500 Fifth Street, N.W. Washington, DC 20001

NOTICE: The project that is the subject of this report was approved by the Governing Board of the National Research Council, whose members are drawn from the councils of the National Academy of Sciences, the National Academy of Engineering, and the Institute of Medicine. The members of the committee responsible for the report were chosen for their special competences and with regard for appropriate balance.

This study was supported by Contract No. W911QY-06-C-0095 between the National Academy of Sciences and the Department of Defense; Contract No. W81XWH-06-10787 between the National Academy of Sciences and the Department of the Army; Contract No. N01-OD-4-2139 TO #177 between the National Academy of Sciences and the National Institutes of Health, U.S. Department of Health and Human Services; Contract No. HHSF223200710832P between the National Academy of Sciences and the Food and Drug Administration, U.S. Department of Health and Human Services; and Letter of Agreement No. OFED-7819 between the National Academy of Sciences and Samueli Institute. Any opinions, findings, conclusions, or recommendations expressed in this publication are those of the author(s) and do not necessarily reflect the view of the organizations or agencies that provided support for this project.

International Standard Book Number-13: 978-0-309-11617-6
International Standard Book Number-10: 0-309-11617-1

Additional copies of this report are available from the National Academies Press, 500 Fifth Street, N.W., Lockbox 285, Washington, DC 20055; (800) 624-6242 or (202) 334-3313 (in the Washington metropolitan area); Internet, http://www.nap.edu.

For more information about the Institute of Medicine, visit the IOM home page at: **www.iom.edu.**

Printed in the United States of America

The serpent has been a symbol of long life, healing, and knowledge among almost all cultures and religions since the beginning of recorded history. The serpent adopted as a logotype by the Institute of Medicine is a relief carving from ancient Greece, now held by the Staatliche Museen in Berlin.

Suggested citation: IOM (Institute of Medicine). 2008. *Use of dietary supplements by military personnel.* Washington, DC: The National Academies Press.

"Knowing is not enough; we must apply.
Willing is not enough; we must do."
—Goethe

INSTITUTE OF MEDICINE
OF THE NATIONAL ACADEMIES

Advising the Nation. Improving Health.

THE NATIONAL ACADEMIES

Advisers to the Nation on Science, Engineering, and Medicine

The **National Academy of Sciences** is a private, nonprofit, self-perpetuating society of distinguished scholars engaged in scientific and engineering research, dedicated to the furtherance of science and technology and to their use for the general welfare. Upon the authority of the charter granted to it by the Congress in 1863, the Academy has a mandate that requires it to advise the federal government on scientific and technical matters. Dr. Ralph J. Cicerone is president of the National Academy of Sciences.

The **National Academy of Engineering** was established in 1964, under the charter of the National Academy of Sciences, as a parallel organization of outstanding engineers. It is autonomous in its administration and in the selection of its members, sharing with the National Academy of Sciences the responsibility for advising the federal government. The National Academy of Engineering also sponsors engineering programs aimed at meeting national needs, encourages education and research, and recognizes the superior achievements of engineers. Dr. Charles M. Vest is president of the National Academy of Engineering.

The **Institute of Medicine** was established in 1970 by the National Academy of Sciences to secure the services of eminent members of appropriate professions in the examination of policy matters pertaining to the health of the public. The Institute acts under the responsibility given to the National Academy of Sciences by its congressional charter to be an adviser to the federal government and, upon its own initiative, to identify issues of medical care, research, and education. Dr. Harvey V. Fineberg is president of the Institute of Medicine.

The **National Research Council** was organized by the National Academy of Sciences in 1916 to associate the broad community of science and technology with the Academy's purposes of furthering knowledge and advising the federal government. Functioning in accordance with general policies determined by the Academy, the Council has become the principal operating agency of both the National Academy of Sciences and the National Academy of Engineering in providing services to the government, the public, and the scientific and engineering communities. The Council is administered jointly by both Academies and the Institute of Medicine. Dr. Ralph J. Cicerone and Dr. Charles M. Vest are chair and vice chair, respectively, of the National Research Council.

www.national-academies.org

COMMITTEE ON DIETARY SUPPLEMENT USE BY MILITARY PERSONNEL

M.R.C. GREENWOOD (*Chair*), University of California, Davis
CHERYL ANDERSON, Department of Epidemiology, Johns Hopkins University, Baltimore, MD
BRUCE BISTRIAN, Harvard Medical School, Boston, MA
JOHN W. ERDMAN, Department of Food Science and Human Nutrition, University of Illinois at Urbana-Champaign
WILLIAM C. FRANKE, Center for Advanced Food Technology, Rutgers, The State University of New Jersey, New Brunswick
ELIZABETH JEFFERY, Department of Food Science and Human Nutrition, University of Illinois at Urbana-Champaign
ROBIN B. KANAREK, Department of Psychology, Tufts University, Medford, MA
CARL L. KEEN, Department of Nutrition, University of California, Davis
GAIL B. MAHADY, Clinical Pharmacognosy Laboratories, College of Pharmacy, University of Illinois at Chicago
SANFORD A. MILLER, Center for Food, Nutrition, and Agriculture Policy, University of Maryland, College Park
ESTHER F. MYERS, Research and Scientific Affairs, American Dietetic Association, Chicago, IL
JANET WALBERG RANKIN, Department of Human Nutrition, Foods, and Exercise, Virginia Polytechnic Institute and State University, Blacksburg

Consultant

DAVID F. DINGES, Division of Sleep and Chronobiology, Department of Psychiatry, University of Pennsylvania School of Medicine, Philadelphia

Staff

MARIA P. ORIA, Study Director
SHANNON L. WISHAM, Research Associate (until April 2008)
ALICE VOROSMARTI, Research Associate (from April 2008)
SANDRA AMAMOO-KAKRA, Program Associate
HILARY RAY, Editor

STANDING COMMITTEE ON MILITARY NUTRITION RESEARCH*

JOHN W. ERDMAN (*Chair*), Department of Food Science and Human Nutrition, University of Illinois at Urbana-Champaign
ELDON WAYNE ASKEW, Division of Nutrition, University of Utah, Salt Lake City
BRUCE R. BISTRIAN, Harvard Medical School, Boston, MA
JOSEPH G. CANNON, School of Allied Health Sciences Health Research, Medical College of Georgia, Augusta
JOHANNA DWYER, Frances Stern Nutrition Center, Tufts University, Office of Dietary Supplements, National Institutes of Health, Bethesda, MD
WILLIAM C. FRANKE, Center for Advanced Food Technology, Rutgers, The State University of New Jersey, New Brunswick
RONALD GLASER, Institute for Behavioral Medicine Research, The Ohio State University College of Medicine, Columbus
ROBIN B. KANAREK, Department of Psychology, Tufts University, Medford, MA
ESTHER F. MYERS, Research and Scientific Affairs, American Dietetic Association, Chicago, IL

Staff

MARIA P. ORIA, Study Director
SANDRA AMAMOO-KAKRA, Program Associate

*IOM standing committees do not review or approve individual reports and are not asked to endorse conclusions and recommendations. The responsibility for the content of the report rests with the authoring committee and the institution.

FOOD AND NUTRITION BOARD*

---

*IOM boards do not review or approve individual reports and are not asked to endorse conclusions and recommendations. The responsibility for the content of the report rests with the authoring committee and the institution.

Reviewers

This report has been reviewed in draft form by individuals chosen for their diverse perspectives and technical expertise, in accordance with procedures approved by the National Research Council's Report Review Committee. The purpose of this independent review is to provide candid and critical comments that will assist the institution in making its published report as sound as possible and to ensure that the report meets institutional standards for objectivity, evidence, and responsiveness to the study charge. The review comments and draft manuscript remain confidential to protect the integrity of the deliberative process. We wish to thank the following individuals for their review of this report:

ELDON WAYNE ASKEW, Division of Nutrition, University of Utah, Salt Lake City
DIANE BIRT, Center for Research on Dietary Botanical Supplements, Department of Food Science and Human Nutrition, Iowa State University, Ames
GRAHAM A. COLDITZ, Department of Surgery, Washington University School of Medicine, St. Louis, MO
HARRY S. FONG, Department of Medicinal Chemistry and Pharmacognosy, Professor Emeritus, University of Illinois at Chicago
DAVID W. KAUFMAN, Slone Epidemiology Center and School of Public Health, Boston University, MA
RICK KINGSTON, SafetyCall™ International and College of Pharmacy, University of Minnesota, Bloomington

MELINDA M. MANORE, Department of Nutrition, Oregon State University, Corvallis
MOHSEN MEYDANI, Vascular Biology Laboratory, Jean Mayer USDA Human Nutrition Research Center on Aging, and Dorothy R. Friedman School of Nutrition Science, Tufts University, Boston, MA
SIMIN NIKBIN MEYDANI, Nutritional Immunology Laboratory, School of Nutrition Science and Policy and Sackler Graduate School, Tufts University, Boston, MA
JOSEPH V. RODRICKS, Environ, Institute for Health Risk Sciences, Arlington VA
A. P. SMITH, Centre for Occupational and Health Psychology, Cardiff University, Cardiff, UK
JUDITH S. STERN, Department of Nutrition, University of California, Davis
MATTHEW VUKOVICH, Applied Physiology Laboratory, Department of Health, Physical Education, and Recreation, South Dakota State University, Brookings
THOMAS R. ZIEGLER, Clinical Research Center, Emory University Hospital, Atlanta, GA

Although the reviewers listed above have provided many constructive comments and suggestions, they were not asked to endorse the conclusions or recommendations nor did they see the final draft of the report before its release. The review of this report was overseen by **JOHN C. BAILAR III,** The University of Chicago, Professor Emeritus, and **ROBERT J. COUSINS,** Food Science and Human Nutrition Department, University of Florida. Appointed by the National Research Council and Institute of Medicine, they were responsible for making certain that an independent examination of this report was carried out in accordance with institutional procedures and that all review comments were carefully considered. Responsibility for the final content of this report rests entirely with the authoring committee and the institution.

Preface

This report, titled *Use of Dietary Supplements by Military Personnel*, is the product of the work of an ad hoc committee under the auspices of the Standing Committee on Military Nutrition Research (CMNR). The CMNR, a standing committee of the Food and Nutrition Board (FNB), was established in 1982 to advise the U.S. Department of Defense (DoD) on the need for and conduct of nutrition research and related issues. This report was produced in response to a request by the Military Nutrition Division of the U.S. Army Research Institute of Environmental Medicine (USARIEM) to the Institute of Medicine (IOM) to convene a committee to review the use of dietary supplements by military personnel and recommend an approach to determine which dietary supplements need active management. Initial sponsors of the study were USARIEM, the U.S. Army Medical Research and Materiel Command, the Samueli Institute, and the National Institutes of Health Office of Dietary Supplements. Their representatives helped with the formulation of the specific questions in consultation with the CMNR. As the project was initiated, the U.S. Food and Drug Administration's (FDA's) Center for Food Safety and Applied Nutrition became a sponsor of the study.

A 12-member committee was formed that had expertise in micronutrients, protein, energy balance and sports nutrition, gastroenterology, clinical medicine, food processing and technology, eating behavior and intake regulation, clinical nutrition, dietetics, and psychology. Dietary supplements are widely available through a rapidly expanding market of products that are commonly advertised as being beneficial for health, performance enhancement, and disease prevention. These claims may influence the use of dietary supplements by military personnel, given the importance and frequent evaluation of physical performance and health as criteria to join and remain in the military. The increase in use of these products has raised some concern regarding their overall and long-term efficacy and safety. The evaluation of such products is especially difficult since many contain multiple ingredients, have a changing composition over time, or are used intermittently at doses difficult to measure. Because of these difficulties, it may take a long time for the current system of voluntary adverse event reporting to detect problems. Although the vast majority of military personnel are assumed to be at the same general risk as the overall U.S. population, the specific requirements of some military personnel require that additional due diligence be exercised both with respect to possible benefits and to the possible risks when these products are used by military personnel in particular job classifications and/or environments. For special military subpopulations, relatively minor adverse effects could seriously affect the unit's ability to perform its mission. It is clear then that these subpopulations within the military are different from the general civilian population, and guidance on managing their use of dietary supplements needs to be tailored to address their specific needs.

This expert committee analyzed the patterns of dietary supplement use among military personnel, and by examining published reviews of the scientific evidence, the committee identified those dietary supplements that are beneficial and/or warrant concern due to risks to health or performance. The committee also developed a system to monitor adverse health effects and recommended a framework to identify the need for active management of dietary supplement use by military personnel. Specifically, the committee did the following:

1. It reviewed survey data and findings made available to the committee related to supplement use by military personnel to identify (a) which dietary supplements are of most prevalent use, with consideration of differences according to demographic factors such as age, rank, sex, deployment status, military occupational specialty, organization, and unit; and (b) expectations of benefits and reasons for use of dietary supplements by military personnel.
2. It identified information gaps regarding dietary supplement use by military personnel and recommended processes and designs by which current and future usage of supplements (including dosages, quality, and forms of supplement) should be monitored, surveyed, analyzed, reported, and the resultant data shared.
3. It selected a limited number of dietary supplements from those identified as commonly used. On the basis of already published reports that review the available scientific evidence, the committee identified those supplements that may be of benefit and/or pose serious hazards to the health

and/or physical and cognitive performance capability of military personnel and determined whether further examination and integrative evaluation or research on each is warranted. The committee considered potential effects of supplement withdrawal and interactions.

4. It considered existing military policies for managing dietary supplements, and assessed the applicability to a military setting of the framework outlined in the 2005 IOM report *Dietary Supplements: A Framework for Evaluating Safety* and determined how it could be modified to determine which supplements need active management by the military.

5. It proposed an approach that could be followed to monitor military personnel for adverse health effects that might indicate a concern associated with consumption of dietary supplements.

The DoD has provided many policies and regulations on nutrition for military personnel in many different settings; however, there is currently no systematic approach by which the risks and benefits of the use of dietary supplements by the military are evaluated and whereby parallel service-wide policies address their management. In the absence of those policies, the DoD relies on the monitoring of dietary supplement safety through the FDA. This approach might be adequate for the general public and for those in the military service that perform tasks similar to those of civilians; however, a different approach is needed for specific military subpopulations so that risks that might compromise the success of military operations are not overlooked, and potential benefits in performance or health from use of dietary supplements by military personnel are realized.

The committee carried out its work over 18 months and held three meetings and numerous teleconferences. The first meeting of the committee was held in conjunction with a 2-day workshop. Speakers addressed the issues related to dietary supplement use in the military and included original data on recent military survey instruments. These presentations were useful for the committee's deliberations and recommendations and are included in this report as individually authored papers in Appendix B.

The committee expresses its appreciation to Andrew Young, Chief of the Military Nutrition Division and representative from the DoD for this task, for generously giving his time and help and for being available to clarify the task of the committee. Special thanks are extended to Rebecca Costello of the Office of Dietary Supplements; Wayne B. Jonas, Joan Walter, Christine Choate, and Deborah Ader from the Samueli Institute; and Patricia Deuster from the Uniformed Services University of the Health Sciences who helped delineate the task, and to Jean Louis Belard from the Telemedicine and Advanced Technology Research Center (TATRC) for his invaluable input during the first committee meeting. In addition, the committee thanks COL Karl Friedl, Director of TATRC, who continues to support the work of the CMNR and was readily available to provide the appropriate contacts needed to gather information for the committee.

On behalf of the committee, I sincerely thank the workshop participants and speakers for addressing topics critical to the completion of the committee's work. These presentations were important reference sources for the committee. Each speaker provided an excellent presentation, prepared a manuscript of the presentation (see Appendix B), and worked with IOM staff throughout the revision process. Presenters of military surveys on dietary supplements deserve special thanks for going the extra mile in answering questions and analyzing data throughout the study at the committee's request.

Further, the committee wants to express its deepest gratitude to David Dinges for his effort and committed participation as a consultant to the committee who helped with drafts of the report and provided valuable comments. The quality of the report was significantly improved by the comments of external reviewers, and the diligent oversight of the National Research Council monitor, John Bailar and the coordinator, Robert Cousins. The committee expresses its gratitude to them as well.

The committee owes a strong debt of gratitude to the FNB staff for their professionalism and effectiveness in ensuring that our committee adhered to its task statement, for providing discipline and experience in helping to assemble the report and effectively respond to reviewers, and for providing background research support and organizing our meetings. In particular, we thank Senior Program Officer Maria Oria, who worked on numerous drafts and revisions. Ably assisting Dr. Oria in her efforts were Program Associate Sandra Amamoo-Kakra and Research Associates Shannon Wisham and Alice Vorosmarti. The committee also wants to acknowledge the excellent work of Hilary Ray who edited numerous versions of the report. The committee is also grateful to the overall guidance and continuous support of Linda Meyers, FNB Director.

And finally I want to thank the members of this committee for their diligent and collegial work. I have worked with many committees over the years, and the members of this committee will always have my deepest respect and admiration for their individual accomplishments and their ability to work as a group on these important issues. I hope our readers will find this report informative and useful.

M.R.C. Greenwood, *Chair*
Committee on Dietary Supplement Use by Military Personnel

Contents

Summary

To achieve and maintain optimal readiness and mission performance goals, the military has the responsibility of guiding its service members in making choices that best enhance their health, including nutrition. As with other sectors of the population, the use of dietary supplements to promote health has become increasingly popular among members of the military, which faces a paradox in managing their use. Supplements available to service members range from those that might impart beneficial effects to health and performance with negligible side effects to others that have uncertain benefits and might be potentially harmful to health and performance. Furthermore, the military, cognizant of the potential benefits of dietary supplements, is conducting research on some promising supplements; in these cases, the potential for adverse effects should also not be underestimated. Without appropriate guidance on their use, military service members might not only compromise their own performance or health and the success of military operations, but might also forego dietary supplements with potential to improve performance or health.

There are no servicewide military policies (e.g., education or regulations) to guide commanders in management practices for safe use of dietary supplements; furthermore, there is no formal military pathway to report adverse events potentially associated with dietary supplements. The lack of consistent policies for the safe use of dietary supplements has raised concerns owing to the vulnerabilities of some military subpopulations. Previous Institute of Medicine (IOM) reports prepared under the auspices of the Committee on Military Nutrition Research (CMNR) have found that nutritional needs of military service members differ from those of civilians, depending on the specific subpopulation, the mission, and the environmental circumstances. Thus, the effects of dietary supplements, whether beneficial or detrimental, might be different for military service members, specifically for some subpopulations facing heightened risks (e.g., Special Forces, Rangers, aviators). Perhaps more importantly, even minor detriments to health that represent simply discomfort or inconvenience to a civilian (e.g., mild dehydration or mild diarrhea) might compromise a service member's performance or health and, thus, the success of the military operation.

The regulatory responsibility of the U.S. Food and Drug Administration (FDA) for the safety of dietary supplements is designated by the 1994 Dietary Supplement Health and Education Act. Actions to restrict the availability of a dietary supplement must proceed from a demonstration by the FDA of a significant or unreasonable risk of illness or injury to consumers under conditions of recommended use. Manufacturers are responsible for ensuring the safety of the ingredient, but the FDA is not authorized by statute to require data supporting safety, as is the case for food additives or drugs. This approach may not be sufficient to ensure the safe use of dietary supplements in some military contexts, which inherently present considerable risk to individuals.

Based on the heightened risks, potential for benefits, frequency of use among military service members, the lack of consistent policies, and the absence of an internal process to report adverse events as they occur in military settings, the Department of Defense (DoD), Samueli Institute, and National Institutes of Health, with additional support from the FDA, requested that the IOM convene an ad hoc committee under the oversight of the CMNR. The Committee on Dietary Supplement Use by Military Personnel was asked to review the patterns of dietary supplement use among military personnel, to recommend a framework to identify the need for active management of dietary supplement use by military personnel, and to develop an approach system to monitor adverse health effects. The committee was further tasked with selecting a subset of dietary supplements and, by examining published reviews of the scientific evidence, identifying those that are beneficial and/or warrant concern (see full Statement of Task in Chapter 1).

The committee held a public workshop on February 12–13, 2007, in Washington, D.C., to gather results from military surveys on the use of dietary supplements, and current approaches and innovative ideas on monitoring adverse effects; this information was of primary consideration in the preparation of this report. The committee also reviewed the 2005 IOM report *Dietary Supplements: A Framework for Evaluating Safety* as a starting point for its deliberations. The 2005 IOM report framework was prepared to assist the FDA in evaluating scientific information to determine the level of concern prompted by use of a given dietary supplement.

In developing its approach, the committee considered the special demands facing military subpopulations that set them apart from the general population. The committee further recognized that the military is able to make policy decisions (e.g., prohibit the use of a dietary supplement) based on criteria related to the needs of military subpopulations and the demands of their missions. Although the development of a detailed process to establish a dietary supplement's level of efficacy was not within the scope of the current task, the committee did consider the importance of efficacy in developing policy on the use of dietary supplements in a military context. This summary presents the committee's recommendations for an approach to management by military leadership of the use of dietary supplements and identifies general areas of research needs. Because the U.S. Army Medical Research Command has the official responsibility to make decisions regarding nutrition for all military services, many of the studies or policies refer to the U.S. Army. However, the recommended approach applies to all branches of the military.

APPROACH TO MANAGE THE USE OF DIETARY SUPPLEMENTS BY MILITARY PERSONNEL

The committee's reviews of selected dietary supplements showed that use of some popular dietary supplements among military personnel might result in health and performance detriments if misused, particularly for those subpopulations facing demanding tasks. For example, *Ginkgo biloba* and garlic have anticoagulant effects, valerian and melatonin are sedative, and ephedrine-like substances may cause harmful cardiac effects. The use of multi-ingredient dietary supplements is of concern because of the unknown interactions among ingredients. Based on these factors, the committee concluded that a separate system to monitor and evaluate adverse effects is needed. This system will be one component of the committee's recommended approach to managing dietary supplements in a military context, which comprises four related components: (1) improving monitoring of the use of dietary supplements by military personnel, (2) using a framework to determine the level of concern for dietary supplements in a military context, (3) implementing a system to report adverse events associated with dietary supplements, and (4) expanding education on dietary supplements.

To demonstrate application of the framework recommended in the second component, the committee reviewed a number of dietary supplements (Chapter 4) and identified those that might pose concerns or be beneficial (Chapter 5, Table 5-3). In addition, the overall approach (i.e., recommendations for action) was applied to a subset of those dietary supplements in Appendix D. It was outside the committee's task to provide a review of all dietary supplements. These monographs and case studies should be considered examples, and determination of the specific actions to take in response to a dietary supplement review should be the prerogative of military leadership.

The committee considered organizational resources needed to follow its approach, including existing military infrastructure, policies, and organizational units and their responsibilities. For the approach to succeed, it is crucial that a military committee or entity (hereafter referred to as the designated oversight committee) has the responsibility for coordination and oversight of various dietary supplement activities (Recommendation 8). Creation of a new entity may not be feasible and, instead, the tasks of an existing one could be expanded to include the oversight of dietary supplement-related activities. The actual operational and data collection activities would rest with other existing military organizations, such as the U.S. Army Research Institute of Environmental Medicine, Center for Health Promotion and Preventive Medicine, or Office of the Assistant Secretary of Defense (Health Affairs).

Improving Monitoring of the Use of Dietary Supplements by Military Personnel

Data from these surveys on dietary supplement use are a key component of the committee's approach, serving as a signal to apply the recommended framework and determine the level of concern. For example, increased use will serve as a signal to initiate a review. The committee reviewed questionnaire designs and results from eight surveys (conducted in groups of active duty military personnel; active duty, National Guard, and reserve military personnel; U.S. Army personnel; U.S. Army personnel deployed in Germany; U.S. Army Rangers; Special Forces members; U.S. Air Force personnel; and U.S. Army physicians). The surveys provide extensive data in some areas (e.g., demographics, frequency of use) but inadequate data in others (e.g., dose, association with beneficial or adverse outcomes). Within these limitations, the committee found a high use of dietary supplements (e.g., in one survey, 60 percent of respondents reported using at least one dietary supplement), especially vitamins and minerals, but also others. Vitamins and minerals were used by about 45 percent of service members on active duty; other popular dietary supplements were "bodybuilding" supplements (21 percent), and "weight-loss products" (18 percent) (see Appendix C). Recommendations 1, 2, and 3 are meant to improve the quantity and quality of data collected.

Recommendation 1: Surveys to collect data on the use of dietary supplements need to continue. The committee recommends that the DoD continue to exploit a large, generic survey by expanding the DoD Sur-

vey of Health-Related Behaviors managed by the Office of the Assistant Secretary of Defense (Health Affairs) with questions related to adverse events and beneficial outcomes as well as the use of specific dietary supplements that might be of concern.

Recommendation 2: More comprehensive data collection is needed from select populations. The committee recommends that in-depth, anonymous surveys about dietary supplement use be administered at select military installations. These select sites would be chosen because their military populations (e.g., Special Forces or Rangers) would be more likely to use dietary supplements and face higher or unknown risks due to greater mission demands and harsher environments (e.g., high altitude, extreme temperature) than most military personnel.

For example, the in-depth surveys should capture data during intense military operations that are similar to combat (e.g., Special Forces training or situations of deployment) when data collection will not interfere with mission completion.

Recommendation 3: Data quality needs to be improved. Surveys should be designed in consultation with the proposed designated oversight committee, which could oversee many aspects of dietary supplement management including adverse event reporting, as described below.

The system of surveillance needs to be comprehensive and include the collection of data as described in Box S-1. To obtain a more complete picture of use, survey data (from self-reported questionnaires and interviews) should be complemented with information from other sources, such as electronic health records and sales data from military installations. Professional expertise should be consulted extensively in the design, administration, and use of surveys.

Using a Framework to Characterize Concern Level for Dietary Supplements in a Military Context

The committee adapted the framework developed in the 2005 IOM report *Dietary Supplement Use: A Framework for Evaluating Safety* to characterize concern levels for dietary supplements in a military context. The 2005 IOM report framework (developed to assist the FDA in determining the level of concern from using a dietary supplement) is meant for the general population, although the report recognizes that some subpopulations may have special vulnerabilities. The committee's adapted framework is intended to evaluate concerns about use of dietary supplements, specifi-

BOX S-1
Improving Survey Designs

The committee recommends that researchers implement the following additions and modifications to the surveys on dietary supplement use in order to improve their value:

- Frame appropriate questions, with unambiguous terminology (e.g., clarify terms such as *antioxidant*) and attending to the order of the questions.
- Design questions that expressly define a dietary supplement user (e.g., an individual consuming a dietary supplement at least once a week).
- Complement exposure data on dietary supplement ingredients with data from questions on consumption from other dietary sources (e.g., foods and beverages).
- Include questions that allow the analysis of associations of dietary supplement use with health and performance outcomes, whether adverse or beneficial.
- Collect data on various demographic characteristics.
- Collect data on the environment and conditions under which respondents use supplements (e.g., special operations).
- Include questions about sources of information used by military service members to determine the most effective methods of dissemination of information.

cally considering the vulnerabilities and needs of military subpopulations (Recommendations 4, 5, and 6). For example, the criteria that categorize adverse effects differ: effects that would not be considered serious in the civilian population (e.g., drowsiness) might compromise the performance of a military service member and therefore initiate a review. Also, in contrast to the IOM framework, the review of dietary supplements and corresponding management actions attends to the specific environment, missions, and military subpopulations. Furthermore, because of the military's emphasis on individual readiness and performance, management of dietary supplements needs to weigh the potential for risks against benefits, rather than predicate action solely on risk. The general steps in the adapted framework—signal detection, initial review of signals, and integrated safety evaluation—are depicted in Figure S-1.

The committee recognizes three challenges in applying its framework to determine level of concern: insufficient data on safety and efficacy, dietary supplements that contain multiple ingredients, and the presence of contaminants (Box S-2). When addressing these challenges, the military might need to apply temporary policies until a definitive conclusion is reached.

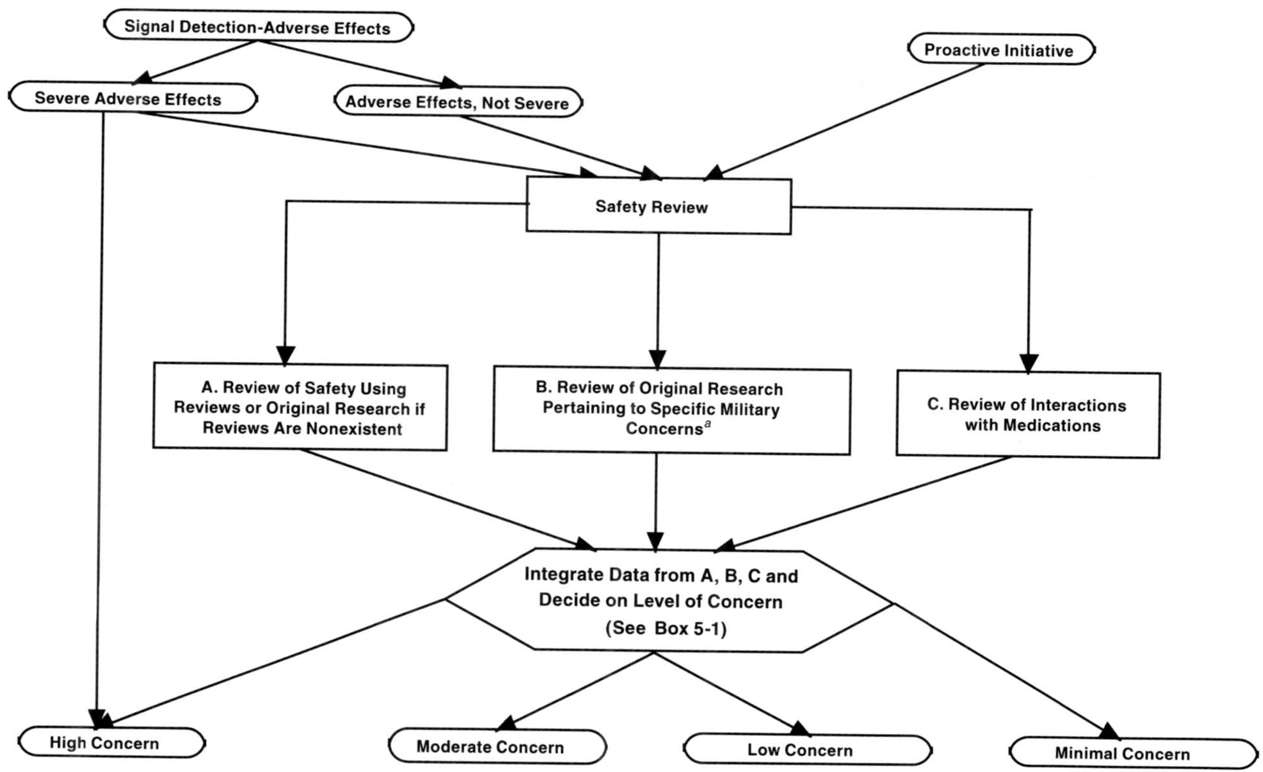

FIGURE S-1 Framework to review the safety of dietary supplements

[a]High physical activity, calorie restriction, hydration, gastrointestinal tract (diarrhea/nausea), liver health/function (xenobiotic clearance), cardiovascular health, mood/behavior altering, alertness/drowsiness, extreme heat/cold, injury/bleeding.

BOX S-2
Potential Challenges When Applying the Recommended Framework

Insufficient scientific data. Acquisition of sufficient scientific data from literature searches to support an informed decision about the safety and efficacy of a dietary supplement within the military will be a challenge. The committee emphasizes that absence of evidence of risk, a frequent reality, does not necessarily indicate that there is no risk, but might reflect inadequacy of the study design to identify risk. In areas of notable concern where significant data gaps exist, the military should perform research as recommended below.

Multi-ingredient dietary supplements. Dietary supplements commonly contain multiple ingredients, which are often reformulated with different ratios, amounts, and even constituents. Finding data on the safety of the multi-ingredient products in the market is a yet greater challenge than finding data for single-ingredient products. There are two potential approaches to determining the safety or efficacy of these products; both offer pros and cons. In one approach, the military could conduct research on the composite dietary supplement product using military subpopulations under performance environments of interest. This approach would more accurately reflect usage, but would be costly, time-consuming, and given the rapid turnover of products in the market, impractical. Another approach would be to review the safety of each individual ingredient. Here, limitations are twofold and relate not only to the possible dearth of data for the effects of the ingredients themselves, but for the interactions among ingredients. The committee concluded that these products merit special consideration and should be frequently monitored for use, sales, and adverse event reports.

Presence of contaminants. The linking of an adverse event to the use of a dietary supplement ingredient might be confounded if the product contains adulterants or contaminants. If contamination occurs, then attribution of the source of the adverse event becomes a formidable task. If enforced, the newly adopted current Good Manufacturing Practices (cGMPs) rule should minimize the potential for inclusion of adulterants or contaminants.

Recommendation 4: The decision to initiate a review of a dietary supplement should be based on two criteria: severity and number of adverse events, and prevalence of use. The selection of dietary supplements for review should consider the particular vulnerabilities of the military subpopulation, which would depend on their missions and mission environments.

Summaries of adverse events reported in military and nonmilitary settings and data on use will be evaluated by the designated oversight committee, which will provide guidance to military leadership about the need to review a dietary supplement. For example, if the surveys indicate frequent use, or if adverse events reported are of moderate concern, use of the framework by a review panel to evaluate published science-based safety reviews might be recommended. If summaries indicate serious adverse events, generating a high risk of concern, then a more immediate action might also be recommended (e.g., restriction of use) (Figure S-1). The committee recommended that the evidence (e.g., how many adverse events were associated with the dietary supplements, how strong the association, level of intake, intake of other medications/supplements, actual circumstances, characteristics of the individual) for an adverse event be reviewed and that the level of concern be determined by taking into consideration not only the the strength of the evidence but also the tasks of the specific military subpopulation and the environment in which these tasks will be conducted.

Recommendation 5: The military should use the framework (Figure S-1) to review the dietary supplements that raise safety concerns (per criteria above). The framework consists of the integrated evaluation of results from current, authoritative reviews (or, if no reviews are available, original research conducted over the previous 10 years) analyzing bioactivity and potential for drug interactions.

When evaluating the safety of a dietary supplement, the military should follow the criteria on which to determine the level of concern (i.e., high, moderate, low, and minimal) and the principles in the 2005 IOM report, but with heightened attention to optimal performance and to the risks to survivability of military service members under the environmental conditions and demands of military operations. For example, if a product significantly contributes to hypoxia, its use may be of high concern for aviators (see Chapter 1, Box 1-3). A review panel that includes nutritionists, epidemiologists, toxicologists, clinicians, and pharmacognosists should conduct the reviews and determine the level of concern.

Recommendation 6: The military's decisions on dietary supplement policy (e.g., rules, education, monitoring of use) should be based on conclusions about both safety and efficacy derived from the available published, authoritative scientific literature and considering conditions associated with a specific type of mission, location, and environment.

Determining the specific actions to take in response to a dietary supplement review should be the prerogative of military leadership. In some cases, the policies may apply to all services and therefore be established by DoD Health Affairs; in other cases, policies may be established by each service or by individual commanders who are knowledgeable about the tasks and circumstances of a particular military subpopulation.

Policy decisions based on scientific reviews should use a model similar to the risk analysis model. Determinations about the level of concern and benefit should be made by a review panel (parallel to the "risk assessment" concept in a risk analysis model), whereas the decisions about implementing military policy should be made by military leadership (e.g., DoD Health Affairs in consultation with the designated oversight committee, which has an advisory role; or military commanders in consultation with the local Medical Treatment Facilities' Pharmacy and Therapeutics [P&T] Committees and the designated oversight committee), paralleling the "risk management" concept in a risk analysis model. This model can be useful in making policy only when scientists work in consultation with military leadership, so that technical questions arising from reviews or other data and questions on the circumstances of military subpopulations can be clarified.

Implementing an Adverse Event Surveillance System

The military lacks a systematic process by which adverse events linked to dietary supplement use are reported, analyzed, and used as the basis for making management decisions. Implementing such a system is justified, especially considering the dangerous tasks and extreme environments faced by some military populations. This system, the third component of the committee's approach, will serve as a signal to initiate a review of a dietary supplement or implement policy (e.g., restrict the use of a dietary supplement). Recommendations are provided in three areas: (1) the implementation of an adverse event reporting system for military personnel (Recommendations 7, 8, and 9), (2) the establishment of a forum or coalition to share data and information related to dietary supplements (Recommendation 10), and (3) increasing the reporting of adverse events by broadening outreach activities and educational programs (Recommendations 11 and 12). To the extent possible, the adverse event reporting system currently in use for medications could be expanded to include dietary supplements.

Recommendation 7: The military should use a centralized monitoring system for reporting dietary supplement adverse events (and data on use), in which data are recorded through the integrated electronic health record system already being implemented in the military.

The DoD should ensure that future electronic health records adequately capture dietary supplement use and adverse event data by soliciting this information during medical visits. For instance, it would be appropriate during medical visits to add a standard assessment question(s) as part of the routine office check-in. In addition, future electronic health records should be capable of generating standard reports on frequency of use and adverse event data that can be aggregated for analysis; and automated alerts to signal a significant change in usage or adverse event reporting, or to signal a risk of interaction with a medication or other treatment.

Recommendation 8: The military should designate a committee or military entity to be responsible for the oversight and coordination of dietary supplement-related activities, such as overseeing the adverse event surveillance system and parallel educational components.

This designated committee will have an advisory role; it should provide input to the DoD leadership on military policies in matters addressing the safety and efficacy of dietary supplements. These include recommendations on when to initiate a safety review, where to focus research, and the design of educational programs and materials for military service members as well as for health care professionals that highlight the benefits and risks of dietary supplement use. The committee should do the following:

- Advise the DoD on the mechanisms for submission of adverse event reports and a process for provision of summaries to those with leadership or educational roles.
- Identify relevant databases and efforts related to surveillance of adverse events associated with dietary supplement use by military and nonmilitary groups.
- Participate in a coalition or forum to exchange and share data and information related to dietary supplements (Box S-3).

Recommendation 9: The responsibilities of the local Medical Treatment Facilities' Pharmacy and Therapeutics Committees should be extended to reviewing and summarizing the adverse event reports as submitted by health care providers or service members, and preparing and providing summaries via a process recommended by the designated oversight committee.

To conduct these tasks, P&T Committees should not only have appropriate scientific expertise, but should be familiar with the demands and conditions unique to military operations and be experienced in identifying serious or unexpected adverse effects, especially when relevant to military performance.

BOX S-3
Suggested Partners of a Forum or Coalition to Share Data on Dietary Supplements

- Designated military committee to oversee dietary supplements
- Registered dietitians from U.S. Air Force, U.S. Army, and U.S. Navy (DoD Nutrition Committee)
- U.S. Army Research Institute of Environmental Medicine
- Pharmacist from DoD Pharmacoeconomic Center, U.S. Air Force, U.S. Army, and U.S. Navy
- Medical representative from U.S. Air Force, U.S. Army, and U.S Navy
- FDA's Center for Food Safety and Applied Nutrition
- Federal Trade Commission
- NIH's Office of Dietary Supplements
- Army and Air Force Exchange Service, Navy Exchange Service
- Supplement sales outlets located on military installations
- Industry trade associations
- Health and Wellness and Health Promotion Centers from U.S. Air Force, U.S. Army, and U.S. Navy
- Fitness centers or unit trainers from U.S. Air Force, U.S. Army, and U.S. Navy
- Optional additional representatives

Sharing Data and Information

Recommendation 10: The committee recommends that a coalition or forum be established for the exchange of data and information related to dietary supplements, such as data from surveillance of dietary supplement use and adverse events.

The members of this forum (military and nonmilitary government organizations, nongovernmental organizations, and industry) would share data on adverse event summaries and reports as well as educational and outreach materials and activities. Members would also share data related to sales and use of dietary supplements and associated adverse events (or beneficial effects) in the military and civilian populations. Participants of the forum should include, among others, experts in toxicology and safety evaluation of natural products.

Expanding Education: Training and Outreach

The committee recognizes the importance of expanding educational programs and outreach activities to increase awareness about the effects of dietary supplements. These educational elements are key to supporting an effective, centralized adverse event monitoring system.

Recommendation 11: Military service members and commanders should be educated to recognize both the potential adverse effects and benefits from using specific dietary supplements and the importance (and the process) of reporting an adverse event.

The designated oversight committee should oversee the development of and recommend educational materials to be disseminated for this purpose (e.g., point-of-sale brochures, posters, or websites).

Recommendation 12: Health care personnel should be trained in evaluating dietary supplement use, informing and obtaining information from their patients, and appropriately reporting adverse events.

Education should be included in existing programs (e.g., Uniformed Services University of Health Sciences, internships and residencies, aerospace medicine training, independent duty medical technician training, and mandatory continuing education at medical staff meetings).

RESEARCH NEEDS

The committee was requested to select a limited number of dietary supplements to review and then determine whether further examination and integrative evaluation or research on each is warranted. Consequently, the committee did not attempt to provide an exhaustive listing of research needs and instead, presents key considerations for conducting dietary supplement research in a military context and an approach to prioritize research needs according to the special needs of military subpopulations.

Key Considerations for Conducting Military Nutrition Research

Study Designs

Studies to investigate the safety and efficacy of dietary supplements in a military context should be performed using the existing military human models that mimic the physical stresses and environments that accompany military missions and training programs (e.g., a predefined course).

The selection of subjects should take into consideration physiological differences and reflect demographic factors of the military population that might result in different effects of dietary supplement use. Research populations should particularly represent those participating in garrison training, serving in combat, or both and should be selected according to a well-designed research plan that permits generalizations to the target populations.

Access to analytical capabilities is a vital element of those studies designed to assess the identity and integrity of dietary supplement products associated with reported adverse events, possibly by contracting with appropriate research facilities.

Animal Models

Human models that simulate severe mental and emotional stresses and some toxicological tests present practical and ethical limitations. The military should continue the development of animal model systems that mimic the stresses of military personnel, particularly those facing demanding tasks and environments such as those in garrison training and combat, to allow screening for physiological effects of dietary supplements used under extreme conditions. Screening with well-designed and ethical animal studies could be followed with more focused human studies, possibly in collaboration with civilian researchers.

Approaches to Identifying Research Needs

Future studies on dietary supplement use in the military should be approached from an etiological or mechanistic perspective. To prioritize research needs, the military should include input from all the services. The designated oversight committee should be tasked with providing recommendations to the DoD on research to be pursued or funded.

Gaps in data should be identified based on the following elements of the recommended approach: (1) results of the surveillance system on the use of dietary supplements, (2) gaps identified in the reviews conducted for specific dietary supplements, and (3) occurrence of adverse events of military importance associated with the use of specific dietary supplements. In addition, research conducted in the civilian population should be monitored for potential military implications. Following a similar approach, the committee provides a list of potential, general research topics and activities in Box S-4; however, as mentioned above, to increase the value of this exercise, the identification of research gaps should include coordinated input from all military services.

Safety

The military should develop a list of adverse effects of particular concern (see Box 5-1 in Chapter 5). The military might generate requests for

BOX S-4
Potential Research Topics and Activities

- Continue to gather data on ration nutrient composition and total dietary intake of vitamins and minerals by military personnel
- Consider establishing Tolerable Upper Intake Levels (ULs) for the military in special conditions (e.g., during combat when the risk of injury is high, the intake of vitamin E [or other compounds with thrombolytic potential] might need to be restricted); follow the ULs for the general population and include them in Military Dietary Reference Intakes
- Continue collecting and analyzing data on dietary supplement use
- Monitor the frequency and severity of adverse events associated with popular or potentially beneficial dietary supplements
- Develop methodologies to assess safety (and efficacy) of multi-ingredient dietary supplements
- Study the effects of interactions with other supplements, foods, or medications
- Consider study designs that allow for identification of tolerance and withdrawal effects associated with popular or potentially beneficial dietary supplements
- Validate the recommended approach to manage dietary supplements
- Evaluate the efficacy of education methods
- Investigate the potential beneficial effects of dietary supplements to mitigate or recover from stress
- Explore the use of dietary supplements for the prevention or treatment of injuries (e.g., wound healing, traumatic brain injury, or post-traumatic stress disorder)

proposals for methods to evaluate safety in these areas, or of any classes of compounds that could be expected to cause such safety issues.

Benefit

The committee recommends that the military identify physical and mental performance areas where improvement is of interest. In addition, the military should consider a future study to develop a framework approach to determine whether a dietary supplement is efficacious. Concomitantly, the military could take an approach similar to that suggested for safety, that is, to issue requests for proposals that cover both methods for evaluation and the particular class of compound that might be expected to confer these benefits. Studies on beneficial effects should be designed so that adverse effects can be identified.

1

Introduction

For several decades, interest in optimizing performance and health in many segments of the U.S. population has increased, and the corresponding use of dietary supplements and performance-enhancing substances has grown substantially. The increase in use of these products has raised concern regarding their immediate and long-term efficacy and safety. The evaluation of such products is especially difficult as many are used intermittently at doses difficult to measure or contain multiple ingredients, and manufacturers may change their formulation. Because of these difficulties, it may take a long time for the current system of reporting adverse events to help detect problems. While the vast majority of military personnel are assumed to be at the same general risk of adverse effects as the overall U.S. population, additional diligence should be exercised both with respect to possible benefits and to the possible risks when these products are used by military personnel in particular job classifications and/or environments. For special military subpopulations, relatively minor adverse effects could seriously impair the ability of the individual or the unit to perform its mission. It is clear that these subpopulations within the military are different from the general civilian population, and guidance on managing their use of dietary supplements needs to be tailored to address their specific needs.

COMMITTEE'S TASK AND APPROACH

Statement of Task

For the reasons stated above, the Institute of Medicine (IOM) was requested to convene an ad hoc expert committee under the oversight of the Committee on Military Nutrition Research to provide recommendations on an approach to manage the use of dietary supplements by military personnel.

This expert committee analyzed the patterns of dietary supplement use among military personnel, and selected a subset of dietary supplements to evaluate; for these, by examining published reviews of the scientific evidence, the committee identified those dietary supplements that are beneficial and/or warrant concern due to risks to health or performance. The committee also developed a system to monitor adverse health effects and recommended a framework to identify the need for active management of dietary supplement use by military personnel. Specifically, the committee did the following:

1. It reviewed survey data and findings made available to the committee related to supplement use by military personnel to identify (a) which dietary supplements are of most prevalent use, with consideration of differences according to demographic factors such as age, rank, sex, deployment status, and military occupational specialty, organization, and unit; and (b) expectations of benefits and reasons for use of dietary supplements by military personnel.
2. It identified information gaps regarding dietary supplement use by military personnel and recommended processes and designs by which current and future usage of supplements (including dosages, quality, and forms of supplement) should be monitored, surveyed, analyzed, reported, and the resultant data shared.
3. It selected a limited number of dietary supplements from those identified as commonly used. On the basis of already published reports that review the available scientific evidence, the committee identified those supplements that may be of benefit and/or pose serious hazards to the health and/or physical and cognitive performance capability of military personnel and determined whether further examination and integrative evaluation or research on each is warranted. The committee considered potential effects of supplement withdrawal and interactions.
4. It considered existing military policies for managing dietary supplements, and assessed the applicability to a military setting of the framework outlined in the 2005 IOM report *Dietary Supplements: A Framework for Evaluating Safety* and determined how it could be modified to determine which supplements need active management by the military.
5. It proposed an approach to monitor military personnel for adverse health effects that might indicate a concern associated with consumption of dietary supplements.

Approach of the Committee: Definitions and Collection and Analysis of Data

The committee defined dietary supplements and reviewed the safety assessment procedures in place for those products in the United States. In particular, the committee explored the legal definitions of medications, food, food additives, and dietary supplements (Box 1-1) and mechanisms that are in place to protect the public.

The federally approved definition of a dietary supplement determines the procedures used to ensure its safety; however, in informal usage, the term *dietary supplement* applies to a broader range of products that, while not meeting the legal definition of a dietary supplement, are used in similar ways as dietary supplements and which include ingredients with similar risks and benefits. For the purposes of this report, dietary supplements included those that meet the legal definition as well as some products that are commonly perceived as nutritionally enhanced with ingredients such as botanicals, vitamins, and minerals (e.g., sports drinks and sports bars).

The first and second parts of the committee's statement of task refer to a description of the use of dietary supplements by military personnel (i.e., identifying which dietary supplements are used by whom and under what circumstances). Such usage information was identified or inferred from the results of surveys of military personnel from both published and unpublished sources. Unfortunately, many questionnaires from published sources, which are valuable because the publications have been peer reviewed, were not available to the committee. On the other hand, more recent surveys, though not peer reviewed, offer the advantage that the questionnaires themselves were available for review. Because the focus of the report was the recent military surveys (for which the committee had the actual questionnaires), the committee decided not to contact the authors of the published papers to obtain the questionnaires. The findings from the surveys provided useful background information to help the committee select the elements of a system to help ensure safety and to assess the efficacy of dietary supplements used by military personnel. Because the U.S. Army Medical Command has the official responsibility to make decisions regarding nutrition for all military services, many of the studies or policies refer to them. However, the approach of the committee applies to all branches of the military.

To develop an approach to managing the use of dietary supplements in military settings, the committee drew from experience with other consumer products. Mechanisms intended to protect the public health vary among the various categories of products (e.g., can include premarket safety and benefit assessments as well as postmarket surveillance). The main basis

BOX 1-1
Legal Definitions of Drug, Food, Food Additive, and Dietary Supplement

Drug: Section 201(g) of the Federal Food, Drug, and Cosmetic Act states: (1) The term *drug* means (A) articles recognized in the official *United States Pharmacopeia*, official *Homeopathic Pharmacopeia of the United States*, or official *National Formulary*, or any supplement to any of them; and (B) articles intended for use in the diagnosis, cure, mitigation, treatment, or prevention of disease in man or other animals; and (C) articles (other than food) intended to affect the structure or any function of the body of man or other animals; and (D) articles intended for use as a component of any articles specified in clause (A), (B), or (C). A food or dietary supplement for which a claim, subject to sections 403(r)(1)(B) and 403(r)(3) or sections 403(r)(1)(B) and 403(r)(5)(D), is made in accordance with the requirements of section 403(r) is not a drug solely because the label or the labeling contains such a claim. A food, dietary ingredient, or dietary supplement for which a truthful and not misleading statement is made in accordance with section 403(r)(6) is not a drug under clause (C) solely because the label or the labeling contains such a statement (FDA, 2004).

Food: Section 201(f) of the Federal Food, Drug, and Cosmetic Act states: the term *food* means (1) articles used for food or drink for man or other animals, (2) chewing gum, and (3) articles used for components of any such article (FDA, 2004).

Food additive: Section 201(s) of the Federal Food, Drug, and Cosmetic Act states: The term *food additive* is defined as any substance the intended use of which results or may reasonably be expected to result—directly or indirectly—in its becoming a component or otherwise affecting the characteristics of any food (FDA, 2004).

This definition includes any substance used in the production, processing, treatment, packaging, transportation, or storage of food. The purpose of the legal definition, however, is to impose a premarket approval requirement. Therefore, this definition excludes ingredients whose use is generally recognized as safe (where government approval is not needed), those ingredients approved for use by the U.S. Food and Drug Administration or the U.S. Department of Agriculture prior to the food additives provisions of law, and color additives and pesticides where other legal premarket approval requirements apply (FDA, 2004).

Dietary supplement: Section 201(ff) of the Federal Food, Drug, and Cosmetic Act defines the term *dietary supplement* as a product (other than tobacco) that is intended to supplement the diet; contains one or more dietary ingredients (including vitamins, minerals, herbs or other botanicals, amino acids, and other substances) or their constituents; is intended to be taken by mouth as a pill, capsule, tablet, or liquid; and is labeled in the front panel as being a dietary supplement (FDA, 2004).

for the differences in mechanisms appears to be differences in perceptions about the safety and expected outcome of use of each category; that is, food is perceived as natural and intended to nourish, while drugs are perceived as artificial and intended to cure or treat diseases. Society and individuals are generally willing to take higher risks (e.g., adverse neurological effects) when the potential benefits are substantial (e.g., to guard against heart disease). The underlying assumptions for each type of product inform the rationale for the protective mechanisms that have been established and were also the basis for the approach recommended by this committee. These mechanisms are further explained later in the report. As an example, medications (drugs) require extensive premarket studies in animals and humans to demonstrate their benefit as well as document the level and type of side effects that can be expected. In this way, the relative benefits and risks are both addressed prior to a product's release to the marketplace. These premarket studies also provide the scientific basis for determining an association with an unexpected adverse event as reported through a postmarket surveillance system.

Food additives are also subject to a premarket petition for a safety assessment and routinely undergo research studies that document adverse events and establish the potential for risk to public health prior to their introduction to the marketplace. There is no established postmarket surveillance system for foods or food ingredients, but the U.S. Food and Drug Administration (FDA), the federal agency responsible for regulating foods and drugs, can informally ask a manufacturer to conduct postmarket monitoring of adverse events when a new ingredient is marketed. If there are postmarket problems reported, the FDA can ask the company to recall a product and remove it from the marketplace. There is, however, no premarket assessment required for foods.

Under current law, dietary supplements are regulated as foods, not as drugs. As foods, dietary supplements are not subject to the rigorous premarket safety assessments required for drugs. Postmarket surveillance systems for dietary supplements have therefore been voluntary until now, and less well developed than for drugs. The 1994 Dietary Supplement Health and Education Act (DSHEA) amended the Federal Food, Drug, and Cosmetic Act (FFD&C Act) and established a new regulatory framework for the FDA's regulation of dietary supplements (*Dietary Supplement Health and Education Act of 1994*, Public Law 103-417, 108 Stat 4325, 103rd Congress, October 25, 1994). The 2007 Dietary Supplement and Nonprescription Drug Consumer Protection Act amended the FFD&C Act to require, among other things, the mandatory reporting by manufacturers of serious adverse events associated with the use of dietary supplements to the FDA, an improvement in the postmarket monitoring of dietary supplements (*Dietary Supplement and Nonprescription Drug Consumer Protec-*

tion Act, Public Law 109-462, 109th Congress, December 22, 2006). The act also requires the collection, documenting, and archiving of non-serious adverse events reported to the manufacturer by consumers. The general public appears to regard dietary supplements as natural alternatives to traditional Western medicines for the reduction of risk or treatment of disease or the optimization of performance. The recent increase in market sales (Figure 1-1) has generated growing concern about how to appropriately ensure the safety of dietary supplements. (Unfortunately, the source of the information does not explain if the increases in value of market sales are due to sales increases alone or also to rising prices. However, it is unlikely that the increases of more than 10 percent market sales per year are due only to rising prices, especially given the increase in prevalence of use indicated by surveys mentioned above.) Because they are a unique class of products, typically consumed to sustain health but considered neither foods nor medications, the current models for evaluation of safety or efficacy of foods or medications are not entirely appropriate for dietary supplements. Implementing DSHEA has been a challenge for various reasons; unlike regulations for medication, DSHEA mandates that the FDA itself is responsible for making the determination that a dietary supplement is unsafe. This determination is not easy to make in the absence of any requirement for premarket safety assessments. To help with this challenging implementation, the FDA asked the IOM to prepare the report *Dietary Supplements: A Framework for Evaluating Safety* (IOM, 2005), including a cost-effective approach for evaluating the safety of dietary supplements under DSHEA. This proposed framework formed the foundation of this committee's exploration options and examined potential adaptations for use by the military.

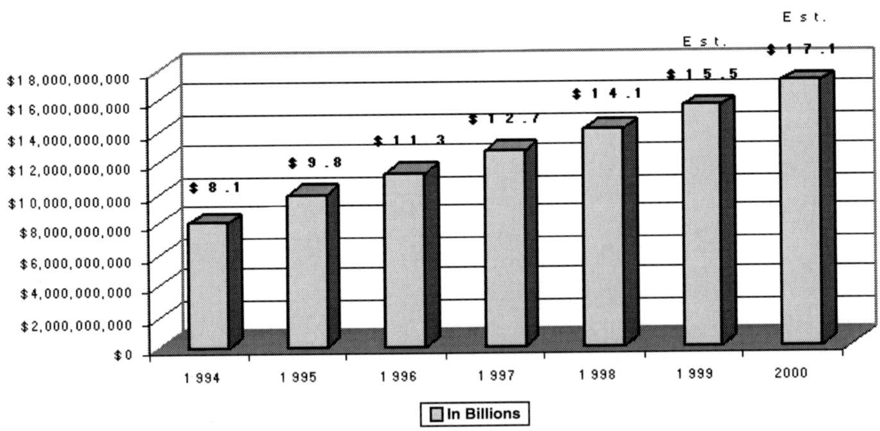

FIGURE 1-1 Dietary supplement sales, years 1994 through 2000.
NOTE: The sales figure for 2005 is estimated as $21 billion (Saldanha, 2007).
SOURCE: CFSAN, 2002.

The committee considered that for the majority of military personnel whose jobs are administrative in nature and whose work environment is otherwise similar to a civilian setting (e.g., members of Special Forces Operations constitute only about 3 percent of U.S. Army personnel [DoD, 2007a]), the risks and benefits of the use of dietary supplements would be the same as for the general population (see below for a description of the differences between the environment of the general civilian population and that of specific military subpopulations). The 2005 IOM report framework to determine the safety of dietary supplements could therefore apply for this general population. The adapted safety framework recommended by the committee for military use was based on lessons learned from implementing safety systems for drugs, foods, and dietary supplements for the general population as well as consideration of the heightened demands and risks faced by some military subpopulations, and is targeted at these military subpopulations. Although the development of a detailed process to establish a dietary supplement's level of efficacy was not within the scope of the current task and this committee was not constituted to address the question of efficacy, the committee did consider the importance of efficacy in developing policy on the use of dietary supplements in a military context. The committee also recommends specific responsibilities for military organizational units and committees; in making these recommendations, the committee considered existing military infrastructure, policy, and organizational units and their responsibilities.

ORGANIZATION OF THE REPORT

This report has been organized into the following sections: Chapter 2 describes the survey methodology to monitor the use of dietary supplements and describes the results from available surveys. Chapter 2 also describes improvements to the current surveillance methodology, that is, the addition of targeted survey designs as well as surveillance methods that may be necessary for special military populations and improvements in the questions to be used. Chapters 3 and 4 summarize current knowledge about multivitamin and mineral supplement risk and benefits (Chapter 3) and provide monographs on selected dietary supplements that are of interest to the military or in highest use as of February 2006 (Chapter 4). Although minerals and vitamins are classified as dietary supplements, they were addressed as a separate category in Chapter 3 because they are essential nutrients, and their safety as well as their necessity in the human diet have been assessed numerous times (IOM, 1997, 1998, 2000, 2001, 2002/2005, 2004). Chapter 5 describes elements of the IOM framework developed to evaluate dietary supplement safety in the general population. A modified framework that considers special military environments and performance demands is recommended; the chapter also describes when and what type of safety review would be needed and provides a decision-making rubric so that educational materials are designed for and targeted to commanders, educators, health care personnel, and physical trainers. Chapter 6 describes the current civilian adverse-event monitoring system and describes a system that would meet the need for timeliness and other special military needs. Chapter 7 presents an approach to identify research needs. Tables and appendixes provide the workshop agenda, summary data from results of current surveys of dietary supplement use, key elements from the selected safety monographs from dietary supplements of high usage, adverse event reporting forms, biographical sketches of committee members and speakers, and a glossary of terms.

USE AND MANAGEMENT OF DIETARY SUPPLEMENTS IN THE UNITED STATES

The prevalence of usage of dietary supplements has been estimated in national dietary surveys (e.g., the National Health and Nutrition Examination Surveys [NHANES] I, II, III) as well as other national and local surveys. These surveys indicate that the percentage of individuals reporting the use of dietary supplements rose from 23 percent in 1971 to 37 percent in 2002 (Gardiner, 2007; Radimer et al., 2004). There is a greater tendency to use alternative medicine, including dietary supplements, to optimize performance and health, demonstrating a shift in the public's perceptions about health self-care. The range of products in the marketplace has expanded from traditional vitamin and mineral once-daily supplements to a plethora of herbals, botanicals, and combination products with a variety of bioactive ingredients, marketed in a manner that implies they will improve some aspect of health or performance. For example, the Sloan Survey, a telephone survey of a random representative (compared with 2000 U.S. Census data) sample of the U.S. population (at least 18 years of age), reports an increase from 14.2 to 18.8 percent in the use of nonvitamin/nonmineral dietary supplements from 1998 to 2002 (Figure 1-2) (Kelly et al., 2005). As mentioned above, the increase in dietary supplement use is also shown in earlier survey results (e.g., from 23 percent to 37 percent from 1971 to 2002).

In response to this rise in dietary supplement consumption, the 1994 DSHEA was implemented to govern their safe use in the U.S. population. However, with the absence of any requirement for a premarket safety assessment, many products reach the market despite a lack of clinical studies proving their safety. In 2007, one regulation was adopted, and one Act was enacted to protect the general population from health risks before and after dietary supplements reach the consumer. The FDA issued a final rule regarding current Good Manufacturing Practices (cGMPs) for dietary supplement quality (Current Good Manufacturing Practice in

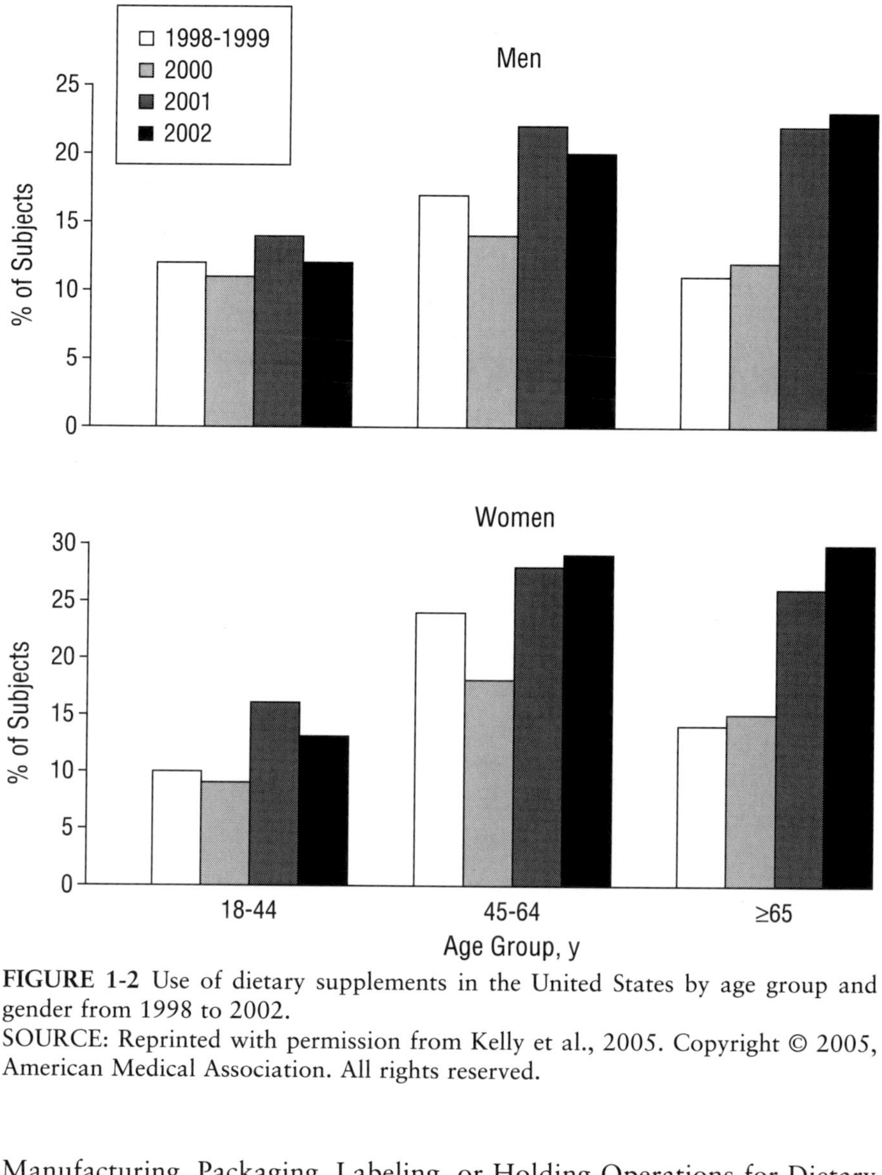

FIGURE 1-2 Use of dietary supplements in the United States by age group and gender from 1998 to 2002.
SOURCE: Reprinted with permission from Kelly et al., 2005. Copyright © 2005, American Medical Association. All rights reserved.

Manufacturing, Packaging, Labeling, or Holding Operations for Dietary Supplements, Final Rule, 21 CFR Part 111). The final rule establishes the minimum cGMPs necessary for activities related to manufacturing, packaging, labeling, or holding dietary supplements to ensure that quality standards are met. This rule will give the FDA the necessary tools to enforce rigorous manufacturing standards across the industry, which is to comply by 2008 or 2010, depending on the size of the manufacturing company. The *United States Pharmacopeia* (USP) developed voluntary dietary supplement standards that companies can use to differentiate their products from others for marketing purposes (Box 1-2). The 2007 Dietary Supplement and Nonprescription Drug Consumer Protection Act

BOX 1-2
United States Pharmacopeia's Role in Certification of Dietary Supplements

The United States Pharmacopeia (USP) is a nonprofit, standards-setting organization for foods, drugs, and dietary supplements. The USP has served as an independent, science-based public health organization since its foundation by an independent group of practitioners in 1820. Two of its principal publications, the *United States Pharmacopeia* (*USP*) and the *National Formulary* (*NF*), are recognized in the Federal Food, Drug, and Cosmetic Act (FFDCA) as official compendia of the United States (Bhattacharyya et al., 2004; Schiff et al., 2006). USP documentary standards and reference materials (RMs, also termed *official USP Reference Standards*) are recognized not only in the United States but also in approximately 130 nations worldwide. USP's voluntary standards-setting body is the Council of Experts, which has five expert committees devoted to creation of official standards for dietary supplements. These are the Dietary Supplement Information, Bioavailability, Botanicals, General Chapters, and Nonbotanicals, Nutrition, and Electrolytes expert committees (USP, 2007). Beyond USP's documentary standards and RMs, USP has established a dietary supplement verification program (DSVP), which includes audit, review, and testing components to assist manufacturers in assuring the public that they are making dietary supplements and dietary supplement ingredients of good quality (Atwater et al., 2005).

The current edition of the USP and NF (USP30-NF25) includes several quality monographs for dietary supplement ingredients. In addition, the USP provides several general chapters as guidance (such as 2021, Microbial enumeration tests; 2022, Microbiological procedures; 2030, Supplemental information for articles of botanical origin; 2040, Disintegration and dissolution of dietary supplements [USP, 2008a]). The USP general chapters includes recommended good manufacturing practices and the methods to be used in, and the facilities and controls to be used for, the manufacturing of a dietary supplement to assure that such a product meets the requirements of safety, meets the quality and purity characteristics, and has the identity and strength that it is represented to possess.

The USP's DSVP performs a comprehensive verification process on specific dietary supplements. Supplements that pass this process are given the USP verified dietary supplement mark. Manufacturers can display this mark on the label of USP-verified products. The mark indicates that USP has rigorously tested and verified the supplement to assure that all the listed ingredients are present in the declared amount; that the supplement does not contain harmful levels of contaminants; that the supplement will break down and release ingredients in the body; and that the supplement has been made under good manufacturing practices that ensure safe, sanitary, well-controlled, and well-documented manufacturing facilities (USP, 2008b).

(Dietary Supplement and Nonprescription Drug Consumer Protection Act, Public Law 109-462, 109th Congress, December 22, 2006) serves as an additional safety measure by mandating that manufacturers forward to the FDA reports of life-threatening events associated with dietary supplements that are submitted voluntarily by consumers. In addition, the FDA continues to obtain adverse event reports on a voluntary basis from consumers, health care providers, food manufacturers, and others. Prior to 2007, there was no required standardization of quality of dietary supplements, and there was no mandatory system of adverse event reporting. Further complicating the assessment of dietary supplement safety is the lack of a national or standardized database listing products and ingredients. Thus, establishing an association between an adverse event and a product or ingredient is often difficult.

Some product marketing claims have been questioned and then modified, and a few dietary supplement products have been removed from the marketplace after reports of safety issues were documented. One example of particular concern to the military was the recall of ephedra. In this case, there were reports of adverse events including a death, and public testimony on deaths that were associated with intake of ephedra by military personnel was given at a senate hearing (U.S. Senate, 2002). The FDA finalized the ban on ephedra on February 6, 2004, and the sale of dietary supplements containing ephedra became illegal on April 12, 2004 (Final Rule Declaring Dietary Supplements Containing Ephedrine Alkaloids Adulterated Because They Present an Unreasonable Risk, Final Rule, 21 CFR Part 119).

Although there has been concern over the safety of dietary supplements, there has also been considerable interest in documenting their potential benefits. The National Institutes of Health Office of Dietary Supplements (ODS) has embarked on a research agenda to address the efficacy as well as the safety of dietary supplements, and several systematic reviews have been commissioned to determine research gaps (ODS, 2007). The ODS has also established and continues to update an extensive database that documents federally funded research on dietary supplements (ODS, 2006).

MILITARY'S INTEREST IN MANAGING DIETARY SUPPLEMENT USE

Reports from the IOM's Committee on Military Nutrition Research have concluded that some military populations differ sufficiently from the general civilian population in terms of their dietary needs and health considerations to warrant special guidance or recommendations. For example, the IOM report *Nutrient Composition of Rations for Short-Term, High-Intensity Combat Operations* recommended higher protein intake for soldiers on sustained operations to ensure nitrogen balance and minimize muscle loss in situations of high energy expenditure (IOM, 2007). Also, a previous IOM report, *Military Strategies for Sustainment of Nutrition and Immune Function in the Field*, recommended that "Soldiers should be cautioned regarding the indiscriminate use of individual supplements" and stated that the preferred method of providing supplemental nutrients in the field environment was through a ration component (IOM, 1999, p. 131).

A specific framework to manage dietary supplements is warranted because of the following military demands and cultural factors (described below): (1) heightened performance requirements; (2) strict weight standards; (3) service members' perceptions of military endorsement of the safety of dietary supplement products as a result of their sale on base; (4) risks, demands, and environments faced by specific subpopulations within the military; and (5) the insufficiency of current military policies to manage dietary supplement use.

Heightened Performance Requirements

While the general civilian population has an interest in maintaining health and preventing disease, the mission of the military forces makes health a key concern of the Department of Defense (DoD) (DoD, 2007b). Protecting the health of service members and ensuring that they are medically ready for duty are important institutional concerns in the military. Therefore, the DoD emphasizes force health protection (defined as establishing, sustaining, restoring, and improving the health of the active and reserve military forces [DoD Directive 6200.04]) and readiness (defined as a healthy and fit fighting force medically ready to deploy at all times [DoD Instruction, 6025.19]). With this emphasis on readiness and optimal performance, both mental and physical, military personnel have an additional interest in using products that might extend the benefits of a healthy diet. For that reason, it is expected that dietary supplements intended to enhance performance would be much more widely used in certain segments of the military population than in the general civilian population.

Soldiers are likely to be involved in demanding physical tasks requiring strength and endurance; most require lifting and carrying heavy loads. Combat activities can include patrolling, mountaineering, attacking, ambushing, and raiding. Significant mental demands accompany the increased speed, complexity, and lethality of modern warfare; in this regard, every individual soldier may be called upon to make rapid decisions and judgment calls, may require fine psychomotor performance (e.g., marksmanship), spatial mapping ability, pattern recognition, and so on. It is also important to maintain mood and motivation as the foundation of all their exertions. In addition to physical and cognitive abilities, a fully responsive immune system is critical for protection against endemic and deliberate infectious threats that may endanger the success of a mission.

The various military services continuously seek to achieve optimal diets for the health and performance of their troops, especially for those with unique tasks (see Box 1-3). The military emphasizes human performance optimization through improved physical training regimens, acclimation techniques, and nutritional and pharmacological supplements. Products that benefit physical capacity (e.g., may help build muscle, relieve or retard fatigue, or improve endurance) or mental capacity (e.g., diminish sleep disturbance; increase memory, attention, or alertness; or decrease stress) are of special interest for the military. Because extrapolating results from the general population might not be appropriate, research is often conducted by the military services themselves. For example, the U.S. Air Force is currently testing protein powders for pilots; this dietary supplement is already very popular among military recruits, who expect that it may increase their

BOX 1-3
Military Subpopulations Whose Tasks and Risks Differ from Those of the General Population

- Military units or specialties where there are requirements for high levels of physical activity and/or prolonged periods of mental alertness may have unique needs. In the case of high physical activity, these service members may be more similar to elite athletes than to the general population.
- Military units that are deployed and need to perform their mission in extreme hot or cold environments that are unlike those of the general population.
- Military members who may need to modify their diets or have periods of limited food consumption owing to specific types of missions. Special military rations are designed for their specific needs and logistical limitations (e.g., limited volume and weight). These missions and diets may also be conducive to the temporary use of dietary supplements in response to their availability during deployments or to the availability of other types of dietary supplements from local markets that might not be found in the U.S. marketplace.
- Military members deployed in combat or peacekeeping situations are at much higher risk of injury than the general population. Thus, any dietary supplement that has an impact on the response to or recovery from injury (e.g., bleeding) would be of greater concern.
- Military aviators share some of the same characteristics as commercial airline pilots but their performance demands differ from those of civilians. For example, unique requirements to limit substances that would affect inner ear balance, cardiovascular function, and hydration are important to ensure that military aviators are capable of flying missions that may subject their bodies to significant g-forces.
- Military members who are part of the Personnel Reliability Program (i.e., those having access to nuclear weapons) also have unique requirements to ensure that they are not taking any dietary supplements that would affect their ability to perform their mission (e.g., induce mood alterations).

endurance while carrying heavy packs or at high elevations. Other supplements that are under study are the herb *Rhodiola rosea*, or roseroot, and citrulline malate. The U.S. Army, which has been developing nutritionally rich foods for years, has considered adding more protein to the troops' diet; to maintain muscle mass, it is currently considering adding more protein through beverages. Soldiers may already carry nutritional products such as First Strike energy bars, a drink known as ERGO (Energy Rich, Glucose Optimized), or caffeine-packed Stay Alert chewing gum. The U.S. Army Research Institute of Environmental Medicine (USARIEM) in Natick, Massachusetts, has been evaluating drinks rich in carbohydrates and protein similar to those used by athletes.

Strict Weight Standards

Another difference between the military and the general civilian population is the emphasis on maintaining weight within established military standards. Like the general population, the military has experienced a rise in overweight and obesity.[1] The rate of overweight within the military is 60 percent compared to 66 percent for all civilians; 12 percent of service members are obese compared to 31 percent of civilians (DoD, 2006). Because failure to maintain established weight standards (maximum allowable body fat percentage is 20 and 30 percent for 17–20-year-old males and females, respectively [U.S. Army, 2006]), can lead to discharge from the military and the end of a potential military career, there is high interest in dietary supplement products that are linked to weight control, especially those that promise faster results than a diet or exercise program. For example, the review of data from sales of dietary supplements to military personnel indicates that one of the biggest sellers (second only to multivitamin supplements) at military bases, Hydroxycut, is sold in various forms as a thermogenic weight-loss product; it contains herbal extracts (e.g., *Gymnema sylvestre* extract), caffeine, and several tea extracts among other ingredients. Ripped Fuel, another popular product among military personnel, is sold for its weight-loss effects. Its ingredients include ma huang (*Ephedra* spp.), guarana (*Paullinia cupana*) extract, and green tea leaf. One form of Xenadrine—marketed as providing energy-promoting herbs and amino acids that support the body's natural fat-burning capacity—includes a "proprietary Thermoxanthin Blend" with L-tyrosine, yerba mate (*Ilex paraguarensis*) leaf, guarana seed, green tea leaf, green coffee bean extract, and caffeine. The survey of Army health care providers about dietary supplements found that, as shown by sales data, Hydroxycut, Ripped Fuel, and Xenadrine are among the five products most frequently used, as reported to health care providers.

[1]Overweight is defined as a body mass index (BMI) of 25.0 to 29.9 kg/m^2 and obesity as a BMI $\geq$ 30.0 kg/m^2.

Perceptions About Safety of Dietary Supplement Products Sold at Installations

Dietary supplements are widely marketed and available from both civilian stores and websites and more recently have been offered for sale in military installations in independent retail outlets and in fitness centers. While the military has not specifically endorsed the use of dietary supplements other than multivitamins (usually prenatal multivitamins), the fact that there are specific dietary supplement stores on many installations, dietary supplement sections in other stores (e.g., exchanges and commissaries), as well as products being offered for sale in health promotion and fitness centers on base, may induce belief that the military leadership has evaluated and approved of their use. This impression may not be entirely logical, since the military also has policies discouraging consumption of tobacco and alcohol, yet, in response to consumer demand, still offers these products for sale on military installations. The only apparent difference between the sale of dietary supplements and the sale of tobacco and alcohol is that tobacco and alcohol have a long tradition of availability to service members, and the movement has been to reduce their negative health impact after these products have long been widely available, while selling dietary supplements other than traditional vitamins and minerals is a relatively new phenomenon, and they were introduced for sale by a standalone commercial vendor in the last decade.

Specific Subpopulations Within the Military

Within the general military population, there are subpopulations with heightened concerns for both the benefits and safety of dietary supplement use, based on special military mission requirements and possibly special nutrition needs. These subpopulations may be defined by the type of strenuous performance required as part of their mission or by the unusual environment in which routine activities must be performed. Some of the adverse effects that may not pose a serious health threat in the general civilian population may result in significant reduction in mission readiness or greater danger owing to the increased potential for impact of injury. Specifically, the committee attempted to respond to its statement of task with a focus on the needs of military subpopulations that engage in types of physical or mental performance that differ from those of the general public, and so would warrant additional considerations (Box 1-3).

A deployed service member does not have the option to retreat from a mission and wait until symptoms subside. Because of their differences from the general civilian population, guidelines to manage the use of dietary supplements need to be tailored for them. The methods to evaluate these products in the general population might not be directly applicable to the military facing special conditions (e.g., high altitude, extreme heat and cold, intense or prolonged physical activity, caloric restriction) or risks (e.g., drug interactions, dehydration, infectious disease, injury or bleeding, impaired gastrointestinal or immune function, renal health, liver health/metabolism, cardiovascular health, and changes in mood/behavior or alertness).

Current Military Policies to Manage Dietary Supplement Use

As a large organization and with a focus on health protection and readiness, many responsibilities of the DoD are dedicated to maintaining the health and well-being of the armed forces and their families; these responsibilities include policy development and education regarding dietary supplements. The Office of the Assistant Secretary of Defense (Health Affairs) (OASD[HA]) is the main policy office for dietary supplement issues. For example, there is the DoD Directive (representing the highest level of DoD policy) on Health Promotion stating that the DoD should meet *Healthy People 2010* goals and objectives, including those listed in Chapter 19, "Nutrition and Overweight," which mentions the use of dietary supplements. However, although it is "standard of care" to discuss dietary supplement use at patient encounters, there is little written policy on the use of dietary supplements. There are also campaigns to educate military populations on the use and safety of dietary supplements, but their effectiveness is not known.

While the OASD(HA) has the responsibility and authority to direct DoD policy on dietary supplements, each military service has the capacity and authority to write specific dietary supplement policies for its own members. For example, there are service-specific policies or processes addressing the use of some nonprescription dietary supplements or prescription substances in particular controlled settings, for example, pilots on extended missions. Each military service has its own medical department led by a Surgeon General (medical issues for the Marines are overseen by the Navy Surgeon General; there is also a senior Navy officer titled Medical Officer of the Marine Corps). The Surgeons General provide the medical care policies for their respective services. The DoD writes servicewide policy; the services may write policies that are even more specific or stringent. For example, when the DoD wrote a policy to ban ephedra-containing products, each of the Surgeons General advised their service secretary and defined the methodology to enact that policy for their own service (i.e., to accomplish the actual removal of the products) and educate their service members on the potential risks from these products (Lynn Pahland, personal communication, OASD[HA], October 2, 2007).

Some of the military leadership are aware of risks derived from dietary supplements because of the evidence from associated adverse effects seen in military theaters, but still there is no consensus on a roadmap or guidance that provides a more uniform, consistent management approach. Concerns within the military over safety and efficacy led to the creation of a committee (DoD Dietary Supplements and Self-Care Products Committee), whose charter is pending approval by OASD(HA). This commmittee, which includes representatives from the OASD(HA), Uniformed Services University of the Health Sciences, and the military medical departments, will have formal authority and means to gather and discuss preliminary data about dietary supplement usage and provide policy recommendations regarding the use of dietary supplements.

The USARIEM has already explored current usage as well as the benefits and adverse effects of a few dietary supplements (e.g., caffeine, tyrosine, and creatine). The DoD has also added a large bank of questions about dietary supplement use and knowledge to the Survey of Health-Related Behaviors Among Active Duty Personnel, conducted every 2 to 3 years, and to the recent Survey of Health-Related Behaviors Among Reserve Component Personnel. These two surveys provide important information on dietary supplement use and identify areas of improvement in education or monitoring. Several other DoD surveys have addressed dietary supplement use with varying levels of scientific rigor.

In summary, the DoD has provided many policies and regulations on nutrition for military personnel in different settings; however, there is currently no systematic approach to evaluate the risks and benefits of the use of dietary supplements by the military or parallel servicewide policies to address their management. In the absence of such policies, the DoD relies on the monitoring of dietary supplement safety by the FDA and its Center for Food Safety and Applied Nutrition. This approach might be adequate for the general public and for those in the military service performing tasks similar to those of civilians; however, as discussed above, a different approach is needed for specific military subpopulations (Box 1-3) so that risks that might compromise the success of military operations are not overlooked, and potential benefits in performance or health from use of dietary supplements by military personnel are realized.

REFERENCES

Atwater, J., J. Montgomery-Salguero, and D. B. Roll. 2005. The USP Dietary Supplement Verification Program: Helping pharmacists and consumers select dietary supplements. *US Pharm* 30(6):61-64.

Bhattacharyya, L., T. Cecil, R. Dabbah, D. Roll, S. Schuber, E. B. Sheinin, and R. L.Williams. 2004. The value of USP public standards for therapeutic products. *Pharm Res* 21(10): 1725-1731.

CFSAN (Center for Food Safety and Applied Nutrition). 2002. *Dietary supplement strategic plan cost out.* http://www.cfsan.fda.gov/~dms/ds-stra2.html (accessed January 31, 2008).

DoD (U.S. Department of Defense). 2006. *Department of Defense survey of health related behaviors among active duty military personnel.* http://www.ha.osd.mil/special_reports/2005_Health_Behaviors_Survey_1-07.pdf (accessed October 17, 2007).

DoD. 2007a. *Armed forces strength figures for December 31, 2007.* http://siadapp.dmdc.osd.mil/personnel/MILITARY/ms0.pdf (accessed January 31, 2008).

DoD. 2007b. *DoD 101: An introductory overview of the Department of Defense.* http://www.defenselink.mil/pubs/dod101/dod101.html#whatwedo (accessed October 17, 2007).

FDA (U.S. Food and Drug Administration). 2004. *Food ingredients and colors.* http://www.cfsan.fda.gov/~dms/foodic.html#foodadd (accessed October 29, 2007).

Gardiner, P. 2007. *Prevalence of dietary supplements in the U.S. young adult population.* Institute of Medicine Committee on Dietary Supplement Use by Military Personnel meeting, Washington, DC.

IOM (Institute of Medicine). 1997. *Dietary reference intakes for calcium, phosphorus, magnesium, vitamin D, and fluoride.* Washington, DC: National Academy Press.

IOM. 1998. *Dietary reference intakes for thiamin, riboflavin, niacin, vitamin B_6, folate, vitamin B_{12}, pantothenic acid, biotin, and choline.* Washington, DC: National Academy Press.

IOM. 1999. *Military strategies for sustainment of nutrition and immune function in the field.* Washington, DC: National Academy Press.

IOM. 2000. *Dietary reference intakes for vitamin C, vitamin E, selenium, and carotenoids.* Washington, DC: National Academy Press.

IOM. 2001. *Dietary reference intakes for vitamin A, vitamin K, arsenic, boron, chromium, copper, iodine, iron, manganese, molybdenum, nickel, silicon, vanadium, and zinc.* Washington, DC: National Academy Press.

IOM. 2002/2005. *Dietary reference intakes for energy, carbohydrate, fiber, fat, fatty acids, cholesterol, protein, and amino acids.* Washington, DC: The National Academies Press.

IOM. 2004. *Dietary reference intakes for water, potassium, sodium, chloride, and sulfate.* Washington, DC: The National Academies Press.

IOM. 2005. *Dietary supplements: A framework for evaluating safety.* Washington, DC: The National Academies Press.

IOM. 2007. *Nutrient composition of rations for short-term, high-intensity combat operations.* Washington, DC: The National Academies Press.

Kelly, J. P., D. W. Kaufman, K. Kelley, L. Rosenberg, T. E. Anderson, and A. A. Mitchell. 2005. Recent trends in use of herbal and other natural products. *Arch Intern Med* 165(3):281-286.

ODS (Office of Dietary Supplements). 2006. *Computer access to research on dietary supplements (CARDS) database.* http://dietary-supplements.info.nih.gov/Research/CARDS_Database.aspx (accessed October 31, 2007).

ODS. 2007. *About the Office of Dietary Supplements (ODS).* http://dietary-supplements.info.nih.gov/about/about_ods.aspx (accessed February 4, 2008).

Radimer, K., B. Bindewald, J. Hughes, B. Ervin, C. Swanson, and M. F. Picciano. 2004. Dietary supplement use by US adults: Data from the National Health and Nutrition Examination Survey, 1999–2000. *Am J Epidemiol* 160(4):339-349.

Saldanha, L. G. 2007. The dietary supplement marketplace: Constantly evolving. *Nutr Today* 42(2):52-54.

Schiff, P. L., Jr., V. S. Srinivasan, G. I. Giancaspro, D. B. Roll, J. Salguero, and M. H. Sharaf. 2006. The development of USP botanical dietary supplement monographs, 1995-2005. *J Nat Prod* 69(3):464-472.

U.S. Army. 2006. *Army regulation 600-9. Personnel-General. The Army Weight Control Program.* Washington, DC: Department of the Army.

USP (United States Pharmacopeia). 2007. *USP Council of Experts and expert committees.* http://www.usp.org/aboutUSP/governance/expertList.html (accessed December 13, 2007).

USP. 2008a. *General chapters status.* http://www.usp.org/USPNF/submitMonograph/generalChapterWorkplans.html (accessed February 4, 2008).

USP. 2008b. *USP verified.* http://www.usp.org/USPVerified/ (accessed February 4, 2008).

U.S. Senate, Oversight of Government Management, Restructuring, and the District of Columbia Subcommittee of the Committee on Governmental Affairs. 2002. *Ephedra: Who is protecting the American consumers?* 107th Cong., 2d Sess. October 8.

2

Recent Survey Findings and Implications for Future Surveys of Dietary Supplement Use

INTRODUCTION

Dietary supplements are widely available through a rapidly expanding market of products that are commonly advertised as being beneficial for health, performance enhancement, and disease prevention. These claims may influence the use of dietary supplements by military personnel, given the importance and frequent evaluation of physical performance and health as criteria to join and remain in the military. Given the large number and wide variety of supplements readily available, as well as a lack of scientific evidence addressing health benefits or safety, it is important to monitor the use of supplements by military personnel. One effective approach to this is the use of surveys with comprehensive data collection (e.g., well-designed questions on patterns of use). Previous reports from the Institute of Medicine (IOM) have recommended monitoring dietary intake and supplement use (IOM, 1999, 2006).

Two national surveys have recently collected data on dietary supplement use, the National Health and Nutrition Examination Survey (NHANES) and the National Health Interview Survey (NHIS), both conducted by the Centers for Disease Control and Prevention's National Center for Health Statistics (see Gardiner et al. in Appendix B). These data, collected through in-home interviews, are representative of the U.S. population. Although to conduct military surveys might be perceived as duplicative, there is ample justification for such surveys, given the differences in population, settings, and products used.

The specific characteristics of some military subpopulations (e.g.,

Rangers, Special Forces) justify the continuation and improvement of data collection from distinct dietary supplement use surveys from military personnel for the following reasons: (1) the higher physical fitness demands of some military subpopulations (e.g., Rangers, Special Forces) compared to those of the general population, (2) the lower proportion of women in these subpopulations, (3) the differences in motivation for using dietary supplements (e.g., meeting military weight standards and improving performance), and (4) differences in military culture and behavior patterns. As an example, the military imposes serious consequences for weight gain and substandard performance, which likely lead to supplement use in the military that differs from that of the civilian population. Data from civilian populations may also not provide an accurate description of the prevalence, patterns of use, and key issues of certain military populations (e.g., Rangers, Special Forces).

In general, survey research uses questionnaires or interviews in relatively large groups of people and, if appropriately planned and conducted, gathers reliable and valid data on various characteristics of the population of interest. The use of survey methodology can be effective to investigate and monitor supplement use in the military. Since it is not feasible to survey everyone, survey data can be collected from a well-defined sample of individuals and, from this, generalized to an entire group (e.g., all military personnel or all Rangers). Challenges in performing surveys include ensuring high response rates, comprehensive data collection, and the validity of the individual responses. The validity of the data from these surveys may be compromised by several factors: incorrect sample selection, unclear terminology (common usage terms versus scientifically defined terms), or survey respondents' lack of knowledge of and inability to determine total dose of or exposure to supplements or inability to remember their supplement use accurately. A low response rate can lead to a biased sample that does not represent the supplement use of the targeted military population.

The benefits of survey use include having data on the extent of the use of dietary supplement products, changes in patterns of use, and insights on specific health behaviors (e.g., reasons for use, degree of consultation with physician, views on dietary supplements). As also recommended in Chapter 5, an important application of survey data on changes in patterns of use is their utilization as a trigger to initiate a safety review of a specific dietary supplement when there is an initial signal for concern (e.g., because it chemically resembles a hazardous product or there are adverse events associated with its consumption). The outcome of this safety review should be the basis for policy-making decisions by military leadership. A systematic evaluation of patterns of use can therefore be used to develop effective educational messages for military personnel and to formulate health policy. If survey data are representative of the targeted military subpopulation, then the frequency of use can also be used to calculate the reporting proportion (adverse events associated with a particular dietary supplement divided by level of use), an estimate of the occurrence of adverse events compared to the level of use.

When using surveys to track supplement use, it is important to clearly define the term *dietary supplement*. Published literature often includes various products in the category of dietary supplement that might not conform with the legal definition.[1] These include sport drinks, bars, or gels—products not legally qualifying as dietary supplements but which include dietary supplement ingredients in their formulas. For practical purposes, however, it is justifiable to include them in the surveys as dietary supplements. In this report, the committee's deliberations about dietary supplements also included products that meet the legal definition as well as food products that are commonly perceived as nutritionally enhanced with dietary ingredients, botanicals, or vitamins and minerals (e.g., sports drinks, sports bars). Fortified foods were not included in the report because they are not generally perceived as dietary supplements.

Several surveys (published and unpublished) have been conducted on dietary supplement use by military personnel (Tables 2-1 and 2-2). Most of these surveys have been administered in the U.S. Army, with a focus on Rangers and members of Special Forces. This chapter briefly reviews the questionnaires and findings from the latest unpublished surveys on dietary supplement use conducted among various military groups and makes recommendations to improve various aspects of survey design and administration. A summary of the survey results is shown in Table C-1 (Appendix C). Table 2-1 describes the surveys' populations and focus. This chapter examines limitations of the data that decrease the value of the survey findings; it also provides recommendations for overcoming these limitations and improving the design of the surveys, including suggestions for the phrasing of specific questions and for collecting additional information. Published data from the civilian and military populations are also reviewed for comparison. For the purposes of this chapter, supplement use will be characterized by the available research (published and unpublished) in three separate general supplement categories: multivitamins, single vitamins/minerals, and ergogenic/health enhancement food supplements, including botanicals. Er-

[1]As defined by Congress in the Dietary Supplement Health and Education Act (http://www.fda.gov/opacom/laws/dshea.html#sec3), which became law in 1994, a dietary supplement is a product (other than tobacco) that is intended to supplement the diet; contains one or more dietary ingredients (defined as vitamins, minerals, herbs or other botanicals, amino acids, or other dietary substances for use by man to supplement the diet by increasing the total dietary intake, or concentrates, constituents, metabolites, extracts, or combinations of any of the aforementioned dietary ingredients); is intended to be taken by mouth as a pill, capsule, tablet, or liquid; and is labeled on the front panel as being a dietary supplement.

TABLE 2-1 Most Recent Surveys (Unpublished Data), Presented at February 2007 Workshop "Dietary Supplement Intake by Military Personnel"

Reference (see Appendix B)	Study Population and Year of Survey	Gender, Age, and Number of Respondents	Focus and Details of Survey	Sampling Method and Response Rate
Corum	Army Fiscal years 2003 to 2005	Males, n=3,789 (77%) Females, n=1,146 (23%) Mean age=25.4 y	Dietary supplement use by soldiers (frequency of use, reason for use, adverse effects, information sources, and purchasing locations), with a focus on education efforts	Center for Health Promotion and Preventive Medicine–Europe health promotion teams administered the questionnaire to soldiers as part of their in-processing at the military base. Response rate not known.
French	Military ("currently serving in the military, National Guard, or Reserve") 2005	Adults, 18+ y n=376	Military vs. nonmilitary supplement use Profile and motivations of military supplement users	Online survey. Response rate not known.
Jaghab	Army physicians and ancillary care providers	Physicians, n=573 Ancillary, n=614	Survey of Army health care providers on dietary supplement usage, supplement types, usage concerns, educational interventions for soldiers; goal was to develop educational tools for health care providers from these data sets	Electronic survey on Army Medical Department Knowledge Management website. Participants were e-mailed a link to the survey. Response rate: 15%.

continued

TABLE 2-1 Continued

Reference (see Appendix B)	Study Population and Year of Survey	Gender, Age, and Number of Respondents	Focus and Details of Survey	Sampling Method and Response Rate
Lieberman	General Army Ongoing	Males, n=444 Females, n=40 Average age= Males, 29.5 ±10.1 y Females, 28.8 ±8.2 y	Use of dietary supplements in U.S. Army populations (type and frequency of use, reasons for use, user demographics, supplement knowledge, amount spent on supplements)	A 43-question survey was used for this Army-wide assessment. At each study site, a health care professional administered the questionnaire. Response rate: 80%.
	Rangers 1999	Males, n=768 Average age=23.6 ± 4.3 y	Same as above for general Army	Response rate not known.
	Special Forces 2000	Males, n=152 Average age=31.3 ± 6.1 y	Same as above	The surveys were administered in a classroom setting by U.S. Army Research Institute of Environmental Medicine staff. Response rate not known.
	Army War College (senior-level officers) 1999–2001	Males, n=284 Females, n=31 Average age= Males, 44.0 ± 3.7 y Females, 44.7 ± 5.1 y	Same as above	This 13-question survey was one of many administered as part of a Health and Fitness Assessment at the Army War College. Response rate not known.

Marriott	Active duty military (Army, Navy, Marine Corps, Air Force) 2005	n=16,146 (Army: 3,636; Navy: 4,626; Marine Corps: 3,356; Air Force: 4,627)	Dietary supplement use by active duty military personnel (type of use, frequency of use, reasons for use, information sources); data collected as part of the 2005 DoD Survey of Health Related Behaviors Among Active Duty Military Personnel	Questions were included in the 2005 Department of Defense (DoD) Survey of Health Related Behaviors Among Active Duty Military Personnel. Military liaison officers at each installation coordinated the survey, a 50-minute questionnaire either completed in group sessions or returned by mail. Response rate: 51.8%.
Thomasos	Air Force 2006	n=11,000	Dietary supplement use by Air Force personnel (frequency of use, amount spent on supplements, where supplements were purchased, reasons for use, adverse effects, information sources)	An electronic link to the survey was sent in an e-mail invitation signed by the U.S. Air Force Surgeon General. Response rate: 24%.

TABLE 2-2 Published Surveys Used to Collect Data on Supplement Use by Military Personnel

Reference	Study Population	Age of Respondents	Focus of Survey	Sampling Method and Response Rate
Arsenault and Kennedy, 1999	U.S. Army Special Forces and Ranger training schools n=2,215 men	Average age=25 y (18–47 y)	Use of vitamins, minerals, performance or other supplements	Voluntary respondents among trainees entering the Special Forces Assessment and Selection School at Fort Bragg and the Ranger Course at Fort Benning. Response rate: 99%.
Sheppard et al., 2000	U.S. civilian and military health club users n=229 (133 military)	Average age= Civilian 33 y Military 30 y	Use of supplements	A two-page survey was placed in 12 health clubs in eastern Virginia for one month. Response rate: 40%.
McPherson and Schwenka, 2004	U.S. Army soldiers, retirees, spouses in military hospitals n=291	Average age=39 y (18–83 y)	Use of complementary and alternative medicine (CAM)	A random, anonymous, self-administered survey on the frequency of use of 18 different CAM therapies. Response rate: 73%.
McGraw et al., 2000	U.S. Army Rangers n=367	Average age=22 y	Use of supplements and associated factors	Response rate not known.
Bovill et al., 2000	U.S. Army Special Forces n=152 men	Average age=31 y	Use of supplements and nutrition knowledge	Response rate not known.
Bovill et al., 2003	U.S. Army Special Forces (SF) and support soldiers (non-SF) n=157 males (119 SF, 38 non-SF)	Average age=31 y	Use of supplements and nutrition knowledge	A questionnaire containing 54 items was administered to volunteers. Response rate: 89%.

Deuster et al., 2003	U.S. Army Rangers n=38	Average age=25 y (18–40 y)	Use of alcohol, tobacco, and supplements; diet and physical activity patterns	This survey was part of another study that examined the effects of creatine on military performance. It included measures of body weight and height, a food frequency questionnaire, a health assessment questionnaire, and a symptoms checklist questionnaire designed to assess side effects that might be associated with supplement use. Response rate: 100%.
Brasfield, 2004	U.S. Army enlisted active duty n=874 (750 males, 124 females)	Average age=24.9 y (17–49 y)	Use of supplements and motivation for use; sources of information; adverse events	The 15-question survey on dietary supplement use and demographic information was administered at 16 Army posts in the United States. Response rate: 64%.
Johnson et al., In press	U.S. Army Rangers n=294	Average age=23 y	Use of supplements, factors potentially associated: age, participation in competitive or recreational athletics, weight training; sources of information	Members of the 1st Ranger Battalion completed an anonymous, self-reported survey administered by the battalion surgeon. Response rate: 40%.

gogenic dietary supplements are those that may improve performance, remove psychological constraints that affect performance, and increase the speed of recovery from training and competition. The committee did not attempt to analyze the data collected but relied on analyses provided to them; in some instances, the committee requested that further analyses be conducted, and results were provided by military researchers. Likewise, this chapter does not provide an account of the statistical methods used; the reader is referred to excellent publications in this matter (Aday, 1996; Bernard, 1999; Converse and Presser, 1986).

PREVALENCE OF USE OF DIETARY SUPPLEMENTS BY MILITARY PERSONNEL

Overall Use and Behavioral Patterns

This section summarizes the results from surveys (published and unpublished) conducted on dietary supplement use by military personnel (Tables 2-1 and 2-2). Most of these surveys have been administered in the U.S. Army, with a focus on Rangers and members of the Special Forces. The reliability of the survey results depends strongly on the response rate. Therefore, the committee emphasizes the importance of obtaining response rates on the surveys. As Table 2-1 shows, the committee did not obtain the response rate for all surveys. The conclusions from those surveys for which response rate is not available should be drawn with this limitation in mind.

Surveys performed in the general population might not be directly applicable to military surveys because of variation in respondent demographics or differences in the questionnaires themselves. Comparison of the results can nonetheless suggest some differences in the rate of use. Gardiner et al. (2007) (see Appendix B) provides a summary of the NHANES III (1999–2002) and NHIS (2002) data on dietary supplement use for a cohort close in age to military personnel. The NHANES data from 1971–1974, 1976–1980, and 1999–2002 in response to the question, "Have you used or taken any vitamins or other dietary supplements in the last month?" indicate that the rate of dietary supplement use has increased from 23 percent to 37 percent of the U.S. population (see Gardiner et al. in Appendix B; Radimer et al., 2004). Results from NHANES I (1971–1974) showed that the prevalence rate for dietary supplement use in adults was 23 percent; NHANES II (1976–1980), 35 percent; and NHANES III (1999–2002), 37 percent (see Gardiner et al. in Appendix B; Radimer et al., 2004).

In contrast, the 2005 DoD Survey of Health Related Behaviors found that 60 percent of active duty personnel reported using a dietary supplement at least once a week over the previous 12 months (Marriott, 2007).

In the 2006 survey of active duty Air Force personnel, only 31 percent of respondents had never used a dietary supplement (Thomasos, 2007), and data published by Arsenault and Kennedy (1999) show that 85 percent of those entering Special Forces and Ranger training reported current or previous use of dietary supplements, and 64 percent reported current usage.

The patterns of dietary supplement use among athletes might be expected to be similar to those of military populations. A review of 51 studies found that among athletes participating in various sports, the overall mean prevalence of supplement use was 46 percent, and most studies reported over half the athletes used vitamins and minerals (ranging from 6 to 100 percent). Larger studies, however, found lower prevalence levels. They also found that patterns of supplement use varied by sport, with weight lifters and bodybuilders consuming the most supplements. Elite athletes were also found to use supplements more than high school and college athletes, and women used them more often than men. Only 32 of the 51 studies provided information about the types of supplements used. The most frequently used supplements, in descending order, were multivitamins/multiminerals, vitamin C, iron, B-complex vitamins, vitamin E, calcium, and vitamin A (Sobal and Marquart, 1994).

Lieberman and colleagues (2007) reported the Army-wide usage in ranges of number of supplements used per week (one or two; three or four; and five or more). Those figures showed that 30–36 percent reported using one to two different supplements per week. Among males, 12–14 percent reported using five or more supplements per week compared to 18–23 percent of females; among elite units, 41–45 percent of Special Forces and Rangers reported using one to two different supplements per week and 7–15 percent reported using more than five supplements (Lieberman et al., 2007).

Multivitamin/Multimineral Supplement Use

Vitamin and mineral supplements are often used in combination by athletes as ergogenic aids. The composition of products with vitamin and mineral combinations varies; this chapter refers to this range of supplement products as multivitamins/multiminerals (MV/MMs). National surveys report that 18–26 percent of Americans routinely take MV/MMs (see Gardiner et al. in Appendix B; French, 2007; Kaufman, 2007). The usage of MV/MM supplements by military personnel varies from 23 to 45 percent (Lieberman et al., 2007; Marriott, 2007). In a 2005 survey conducted by French (2007), 18 percent of civilians reported using MV/MMs as the only supplement versus 23 percent of those serving on active duty, in the National Guard, or in the Reserves. This contrasts with the 45 percent of active duty service members reporting such use in the 2005 DoD Survey of

Health Related Behaviors (Marriott, 2007), a difference perhaps reflecting a higher use of dietary supplements among active duty personnel compared to those in the National Guard or Reserves, although they might also be on active duty. Various smaller surveys suggest a similar level of usage among active duty military personnel. In the ongoing Army-wide survey, 30 percent of male respondents reported using MV/MM supplements (Lieberman et al., 2007). Among active duty Army personnel assigned to Europe from 2003 to 2005, 33.8 percent reported using them (Corum, 2007). Another survey found that 39 percent of active duty senior Army officers attending the U.S. Army War College in 1999–2001 used MV/MMs (Lieberman et al., 2007). Within the subpopulations of special interest—active duty Rangers and Special Forces—23 and 32 percent, respectively, were routinely taking MV/MMs (Lieberman et al., 2007).

Although perhaps a less definitive source because it requires users to have reported to a physician, 13 percent of 573 Army physicians surveyed indicated that their patients reported using MV/MM supplements and 20 percent of 614 ancillary health care personnel surveyed indicated that their patients reported using MV/MM supplements (Jaghab, 2007).

The available survey data also report usage of individual vitamin and mineral supplements (see Table 2-3); however, only one set of survey data (personal communication, Sonya Corum, U.S. Army Training and Doctrine Command, April 10, 2007) was analyzed for use of MV/MM supplements concurrent with the use of single-nutrient supplements. The single nutrients

TABLE 2-3 Percentage Ranges of Respondents Using Individual Nutrient Supplements (from military and civilian surveys)

	Military Population (%)			Civilian Population (%)
Type of Supplement	Unspecified Gender	Male	Female	Unspecified Gender
Antioxidants (unspecified)	21	6–14	23	
Vitamin E	6–9	6–22	8–32	2–20
Vitamin C	24	11–17	13–29	7
Vitamin A/Beta-carotene	13	5	16	
Calcium	6–19	5–6	15–32	3–26
Vitamin B Complex	8	6	13	1–14
Vitamin D	3–5	5	8	3–8
Vitamin B_6	12		10	
Iron	14		10	2
Folate			13	
Magnesium			13	
Potassium	12			

SOURCE: Data extracted from Table C-1, Appendix C.

most prevalently taken in conjunction with MV/MMs were vitamin C (43 percent) and calcium (38 percent).

Single Vitamin/Mineral Supplement Use

A previous IOM report (IOM, 2006) suggested that in addition to strategies to increase nutrient intake from foods, dietary supplements may be warranted for some individuals, such as iron and folate for women of childbearing age and MV/MMs for individuals restricting calorie intake for weight loss. Intake levels higher than the Tolerable Upper Intake Level might incur hazardous consequences to health. As with MV/MMs, it is likely that most users take individual vitamins or minerals to supplement their diets or with expectations of improving general health.

Table 2-3 shows the percentage of individuals (by gender, when known) of both military and civilian populations using single-nutrient supplements. In the 2005 DoD Survey of Health Related Behaviors (Marriott, 2007), 27 percent of respondents reported taking a single mineral or vitamin supplement. Based on the limited survey results reported, compared to civilians, usage by military personnel of three (i.e., vitamins E, B complex, and D) of the four single vitamin supplements appears to be similar, and usage of vitamin C and iron is slightly higher. However, the military population reported usage of single nutrients (vitamin A/beta-carotene, vitamin B_6, folate, magnesium, and potassium) not reported in the civilian surveys. Except for the 2005 DoD Survey of Health Related Behaviors (Marriott, 2007), the surveys did not define the term *antioxidant*, so it is unclear if it was understood to refer to a specific individual ingredient, a specific combination of vitamins and minerals, or botanicals. No statistical comparisons can be made between the military and civilian survey results.

Ergogenic/Health Enhancement Dietary Supplements

The third category of supplements includes single bioactive substances or combinations, other than vitamins or minerals, that are intended to enhance performance or health (e.g., creatine, ginseng). Bathalon et al. (2000) reported that 54 percent of senior officers attending the U.S. Army War College reported using "health-promoting" dietary supplements, and among Rangers, 30 percent used performance-enhancing supplements.

Analysis of data from NHANES 1999–2002 shows that dietary supplements other than vitamins and minerals are used by 7 percent of the U.S. population (see Gardiner et al. in Appendix B). Among these products, echinacea, ginseng, *Ginkgo biloba*, and garlic are the most popular. The 2005 Slone Survey reported that among Americans older than 18 years, 23 percent had taken herbals or other "natural supplements" during the week preceding the interview (Kaufman, 2007). The most commonly used herbal/natural supplements were lutein (9.4 percent), lycopene (7.8 percent), glucosamine (4.0 percent), garlic (2.6 percent), chondroitin (2.5 percent), *Ginkgo biloba* (1.6 percent), and coenzyme Q_{10} (1.5 percent). It should be noted that the most commonly used botanical supplements, lutein and lycopene, appear almost exclusively as ingredients in MV/MM supplements. The 2002 Health and Diet Survey, a national telephone survey sponsored by the U.S. Food and Drug Administration, found that 73 percent of participants (n=2,743) had consumed dietary supplements (including vitamins, minerals, MV/MMs, herbs, and/or other supplements) in the preceding 12 months. Of this number, 42 percent reported taking an herb, botanical, or other nonvitamin dietary supplement. The nonvitamin supplements most commonly reported used were echinacea (19.5 percent), garlic (16.6 percent), *Ginkgo biloba* (14.6 percent), ginseng (11.7 percent), and glucosamine (10.9 percent) (Timbo et al., 2006).

When categorized by perceived effect, the 2005 DoD Survey of Health Related Behaviors indicated that among active duty military users of dietary supplements other than vitamins and minerals, 21 percent used "bodybuilding" supplements, 18 percent used "weight-loss products," 9 percent used "joint health" products, 8 percent used "performance-enhancing" products, and 9 percent reported using other types of supplements (Marriott, 2007). Among active duty Air Force personnel, the nonvitamin, nonmineral supplements most commonly reported being used five or more times are creatine, glutamine, caffeine, protein powders, fish oils, Hydroxycut (a multi-ingredient product containing botanicals and minerals, sold to promote weight loss), chondroitin, and nitric oxide (Thomasos, 2007). The use of single bioactive substances seen in data from the surveys reviewed varies significantly, but the following examples show the percentage of respondents reporting use of androstenedione (6–13 percent); glucosamine/chondroitin (glucosamine hydrochloride and sodium chondroitin sulfate) (7–11 percent); conjugated linoleic acid (3 percent); garlic (5–7 percent); ginseng (7–21 percent); *Ginko biloba* (4–5 percent); caffeine (3–18 percent); *Ephedra*, ephedrine, or ma huang (15–21 percent); echinacea (4 percent); creatine (5–45 percent); coenzyme Q_{10} (2 percent); protein (5–16 percent); arginine (1 percent); and lycopene (2 percent) (Brasfield, 2004; Corum, 2007; French, 2007; Johnson et al., in press; Lieberman et al., 2007; Sheppard et al., 2000).

Of the 573 Army physicians surveyed, 32.5 percent listed creatine as one of the top 10 supplements used, 7.7 percent reported *Ephedra*, and 3.5 percent reported glucosamine/chondroitin. Results from other health care personnel supported these findings (Jaghab, 2007).

Consumption of caffeine—a substance included as powdered instant coffee in rations and in the form of chewing gum as a supplement to enhance performance in some specialized military rations—was reported by 18 percent of respondents (Corum, 2007). However, this level is likely underreported, since respondents might not consider caffeine a dietary supplement or might not include other dietary intake of caffeine. Only one study specifically included both dietary supplement and dietary sources of caffeine (see Lieberman et al. in Appendix B), asking respondents to indicate the serving size for each caffeinated product consumed, including various coffee beverages, sodas, and other beverages, with clear instructions on how to measure consumption. The data from these questions have not been analyzed yet.

Sports drinks and sports bars (or gels) are a broad and undefined category of dietary supplements that may contain a combination of vitamins, minerals, and other bioactive substances and essential nutrients and that are widely used. For example, 41 percent of Rangers and 36 percent of Special Forces reported using sports drinks (Lieberman et al., 2007). Within the overall Army population, 20 percent of males and 28 percent of females reported using sports drinks (Lieberman et al., 2007). Corum (2007) reported that 43 percent of active duty Army personnel assigned to Europe between 2003 and 2005 reported using sports drinks. The only military subpopulation reporting a relatively low usage of sports drinks was officers attending the Army War College, of whom only 10 percent reported routinely using sports drinks (Lieberman et al., 2007).

The use of sports bars and gels is much higher among Special Forces (15–43 percent of Special Forces use sports bars) than among Rangers (6 percent and 3 percent of Rangers reported using sports bars and sports gels, respectively). This high use is also in contrast to the lower rate (5 percent) of use among general Army personnel surveyed (Bovill et al., 2000; Lieberman et al., 2007). Those assigned to Europe had also much higher rates of use (17 percent reported use of sports bars in 2003–2005) (Corum, 2007). Some of the questionnaires (e.g., DoD Survey of Health Related Behaviors in 2005) did not have specific questions on these types of products, but reported on the use of unspecified "bodybuilding supplements" (20.5 percent) and performance-enhancing supplements (8.4 percent) (Marriott, 2007).

Protein powders are also popular dietary supplements, their use being reported by 13 percent of males and 8 percent of females in the general Army population and by as many as 18 percent of Rangers and 16–22 percent of Special Forces (Bovill et al., 2000; Lieberman et al., 2007).

Only one survey analyzed the concurrent use of other dietary supplements by MV/MM users (Personal communication, Sonya Corum, U.S. Army Training and Doctrine Command, April 10, 2007). It was found that among those taking MV/MMs , the performance enhancers most frequently reported used were creatine (13 percent), sports drinks (11 percent), and arginine (10 percent).

In general, products perceived as bodybuilders, weight-loss promoters, and performance enhancers are the most popular nonvitamin, nonmineral products. Among Special Forces and Rangers, the use of sports drinks, protein bars, and protein powders was notable, supporting one of their major reported reasons for taking supplements, that is, for increased energy intake.

Differences in Supplement Use by Demographic Factors

In the military, age and rank are closely related. Some surveys presented data categorized by rank but not age; not all of the data sets presented were analysed by demographic factors such as age or gender. Among the surveys reviewed, the greatest quantity of demographic data is available for Special Forces and Rangers, who have a distinctly higher dietary supplement use, specifically for performance-enhancing supplements (Lieberman et al., 2007).

The ongoing Army-wide survey of active duty personnel suggests that younger military members are more likely to use sports bars or gels, sports drinks, and dietary supplements believed to enhance physical performance than other products. Similarly, the 2005 DoD Survey of Health Related Behaviors indicates that dietary supplement usage is highest among the oldest survey respondents; however, bodybuilding supplements are most likely to be used by service members less than 43 years old, and weight-loss products and performance-enhancing supplements are used most frequently by service members less than 34 years old. Military members over 44 years of age are more likely to be taking multivitamins and single-ingredient dietary supplements for health enhancement, such as individual vitamins and minerals, antioxidants, and products to improve joint health (see Marriott et al. in Appendix B).

Some surveys also show differences in usage between men and women; for instance, preliminary results show that in the Army-wide survey, women appear to be more likely than men to take any dietary supplements (71 versus 58 percent) and more likely than men to take MV/MM supplements (37 versus 32 percent), but they are less likely than men to take protein supplements (10 versus 14 percent) (see Lieberman et al. in Appendix B).

Behavioral Patterns

Some questions in dietary supplement surveys are meant to elicit information on factors affecting use (e.g., consultation with health care providers, reasons for use, sources of information) to help develop effective educational programs and policies. Findings from survey questionnaires and published literature revealed that neither the general population nor military personnel typically discuss their dietary supplement usage with their health care providers. The 2002 NHIS survey showed that only about 24 percent of those who reported use of dietary supplements disclosed such use to their health care providers (see Gardiner et al. in Appendix B). Similarly, among those responding to the DoD Survey of Health Related Behaviors, 36.6 percent indicated they reported dietary supplement use to their physicians and 21.7 percent to a nurse practitioner or physician's assistant. More women (62.5 percent) than men (45.2 percent) reported usage to a health care provider. A higher percentage (47.8 percent) of service members above 35 years of age report usage to medical professionals compared to service members less than 20 years old (23.5 percent). Among all military services, approximately 50 percent of Air Force personnel report usage to health care professionals compared to 32.6 percent of Navy personnel, 31.5 percent of Army personnel, and 25.3 percent of Marines (Marriott, 2007). Even the highest percentage of those reporting usage (50 percent for Air Force personnel) is quite low, and efforts to increase reporting (e.g., educational programs) are necessary.

In response to behavioral questions about expectations of benefits and reasons for use, "health and well-being" was the top reason (given by 19 percent of respondents) to use dietary supplements in the general population (see Gardiner et al. in Appendix B). Members of the Army assigned to Europe reported different motivations for using different types of supplements. As might be expected, improvement of health and prevention of illness were more often linked with use of vitamin or mineral supplements, while performance enhancement and strength were more likely to be associated with ergogenic aids (Corum, 2007). Health improvement was consistently listed as the first or second most important reason for taking dietary supplements (Corum, 2007; Lieberman et al., 2007; Marriott, 2007; Thomasos, 2007). The ranking of other benefits was fairly consistent across surveys, as shown in Table 2-4. Other behavioral questions of interest include those related to users' sources of information or their perception of beneficial effects, because these findings may help with the design of education programs.

Adverse Events

In addition to asking questions about expectations of benefits, some surveys included questions about adverse events reported or experienced. This information is particularly valuable when obtained from the special military subpopulations facing higher risks because of demanding mental or physical tasks, and more likely to use dietary supplements. These types of survey questions are not meant to be used to draw causal inferences about dietary supplements and adverse events. Instead, they present a general view

TABLE 2-4 Reported Reasons for Taking Supplements Among Military Personnel (and, for comparison, the general U.S. population)

Study Population	Reasons Reported
Army personnel in Europe (Corum, 2007)	Health Prevent illness Performance enhancement Strength Prevent fatigue
Air Force personnel (Thomasos, 2007)	Promote health Weight loss Strength Increase lean muscle mass Stamina Fatigue reduction Cognition/alertness Memory Other
DoD Survey of Health Related Behaviors Among Active Duty Military Personnel (Marriott, 2007)	Supplement diet Improve health Improve mental health Improve cognitive function Improve physical performance Increase muscle mass Lose weight Specific health problems
Army health care personnel (Jaghab, 2007)	Performance enhancement Gain weight Lose weight Increase muscle mass, conditioning, strength Cognitive enhancement, to stay awake Supplement diet, health maintenance
General U.S. population (adults age 18 years and older) (Kelly et al., 2005)	Vitamin Supplement diet Health Physician recommended Energy Prevention, not otherwise specified Immune booster

NOTE: In order of percentage of respondents, from highest to lowest.

of the totality of adverse events in a representative sample and may signal a problem and corresponding need for action, for example, the need for focused attention during collection of data through the adverse event reporting system. Adverse events listed through the military surveys reviewed by the committee included abdominal pain, chest pain, dehydration, palpitations, numbness in extremities, and loss of consciousness. Corum (2007) reported that of 5,206 active duty Army survey respondents, 951 reported some adverse events they believed were associated with dietary supplement use (Table 2-5) and also indicated that they usually did not report these adverse events to health care personnel.

The committee inquired about additional information on potential associations between specific dietary supplements and adverse events and received one such analysis. The frequency of adverse effects across each category of dietary supplement (vitamins, performance enhancers, and herbal) frequency of use (rarely/never, 1–2× weekly, 3–4× weekly, and ≥5×

TABLE 2-5 Adverse Event Reports

Dietary Supplement Survey	Adverse Event	Rate of Adverse Event in % (number of events)
Corum	Dehydration	3 (n=148)
	Palpitations	1.8 (n=91)
	Muscle cramping	1.111 (n=54)
	Abdominal pain	0.9 (n=44)
	Diarrhea	0.3 (n=22)
	Dizziness	0.3 (n=17)
	Nausea/vomiting	0.3 (n=16)
	Numbness in extremities	0.3 (n=17)
	Tremors	0.3 (n=13)
	Chest pain	0.2 (n=8)
	Breathing difficulties	0.1 (n=7)
	Heart attack, heat stroke, or loss of consciousness	0.9 (n=1)
Thomasos	Palpitations	2.4 (n=182)
	Anxiety	2.2 (n=170)
	Nausea/vomiting	1.8 (n=137)
	Dehydration	1.5 (n=116)
	Dizziness/confusion	1.3 (n=98)
	Diarrhea	1.2 (n=92)
	Abdominal pain	1.1 (n=86)
	Tremors	1.0 (n=76)
	Muscle cramping/pain	0.6 (n=47)
	Chest pain	0.6 (n=43)
	Breathing difficulties	0.3 (n=25)
	Numbness/tingling in arms and legs	0.3 (n=25)
	Problems with heat tolerance	0.3 (n=20)
	Visual disturbances	0.3 (n=20)
	Heat exhaustion/heat injuries	0.1 (n=9)
	Blood in urine	<0.1 (n=7)
	Loss of consciousness/fainting	<0.1 (n=6)
	Heart attack	<0.1 (n=4)

SOURCES: Corum, 2007; Thomasos, 2007.

weekly) was analyzed by Corum (personal communication, Sonya Corum, U.S. Army Training and Doctrine Command, April 10, 2007). Of reported adverse events, the highest percentage, 19.4 percent, was associated with performance-enhancing supplements, compared to vitamins (5.9 percent) and herbal supplements (5.6 percent). Again, these individual incidents of association are not necessarily a cause for concern on their own, but they may signal a potential problem if the adverse event is severe or frequent and may prompt focused attention on a particular dietary supplement. With data from only one analysis, concrete conclusions about cause and effect could not be made. The committee's best conclusion is that the rate of adverse effects was higher than normal, especially for performance enhancers.

Of the approximately 11,000 service members who responded to the Air Force survey, about 8 percent reported adverse events. While these results may not be comparable to those from clinical drug trials, this rate exceeds the typical rate of adverse events resulting from placebo effects (3–5 percent). The most common adverse effects included heart palpitations, anxiety, dehydration, nausea/vomiting, chest pain, dizziness/confusion, abdominal pain, and tremors. Among those reporting adverse events, only about 15 percent reported discussing them with a health care provider. Serious adverse events were more likely to be reported to a health care provider; for example, 75 percent (3 of 4) of heart attacks were reported while only 7 percent (8 of 92) of cases of diarrhea were reported to the health care provider. Except for heart attacks, fewer than 50 percent of the perceived side effects from dietary supplements were reported to the health care provider (Thomasos, 2007). The percentage of Air Force personnel (50 percent) who indicated they discussed with their health care provider adverse effects they believed to be related to dietary supplement usage was higher than in other military services (31 and 33 percent in the Army and Navy, respectively) (Marriott, 2007).

RECOMMENDATIONS FOR CONDUCTING SURVEYS

If the military elects to use surveys for surveillance, the committee urges attention to three broad areas of survey activities: (1) planning, (2) survey administration, and (3) data processing and analysis. This chapter provides general recommendations, followed by more specific recommendations in the planning and survey administration stages. The development of a sampling plan and the data processing and analysis are beyond the scope of this chapter, but a biostatistician can provide valuable assistance in these efforts. In the planning stage, the survey objectives must be formulated, the relevant scientific literature reviewed, variables and units of analysis selected (i.e., individuals, groups, communities), a population sampling plan developed, and the survey constructed. The design of the survey involves decisions about using a structured or unstructured approach and data collection mode. Use of highly structured surveys generally results in higher quality data by minimizing measurement error between respondents. However, efforts must be made to ensure validity as respondents may interpret the same questions differently. Unstructured interviews (open-ended questions) require administration by highly trained personnel as well as complex data analysis, and are more expensive to conduct than structured surveys. There are trade-offs that need to be considered when determining whether questions should be open-ended or structured. Because of limitations with open-ended questionnaires (e.g., need for highly skilled interviewer) the committee recommends the use of a structured questionnaire with some options for open-ended questions. Obtaining additional information from participants through the use of some open-ended questions could be valuable, but such information should be obtained using a highly skilled interviewer to conduct structured prompting of survey respondents. In addition, for open-ended questions statisticians, design experts, and researchers should be engaged from the time of the planning stage, because the analysis of open-ended data requires more coding than structured questions.

In the survey administration stage, respondents are recruited, survey data are collected by interviewers or self-reported, and nonrespondents are followed up. The basis for surveillance and research questions of interest should drive data collection and analysis efforts. In addition to survey instruments, other methods to routinely monitor use may be included in the larger surveillance program, for example, extracting data from electronic health records and monitoring sales data from installation sources.

Monitoring Surveys: Overall Recommendations

Recommendation 1: Surveys to collect data on the use of dietary supplements need to continue. The committee recommends that the DoD continue to exploit a large, generic survey by expanding the DoD Survey of Health Related Behaviors managed by the Office of the Assistant Secretary of Defense (Health Affairs) with questions related to adverse events and beneficial outcomes as well as the use of specific dietary supplements that might be of concern.

Given the specific needs and challenges of military personnel, particularly of some military subpopulations, supplement use among military personnel is a special concern for the DoD. This committee recommends that the DoD continue to conduct the generic DoD Survey of Health Related Behaviors with the purpose of collecting data on use of dietary supplements. The survey should include multiple-choice questions, following the format of the current questionnaire. The value of this survey would be improved by the following:

1. Addition of a question prompting for adverse events (e.g., palpitations, seizures) experienced
2. Addition of a question prompting for beneficial outcomes (e.g., improved performance, alertness, delayed fatigue) experienced
3. Improvement of questions on frequency of use, health outcomes, and adverse events by specifying the time and circumstances surrounding the use of a product (e.g., respondent reports used creatine once a day from December through March while deployed)
4. Expansion of questions on types of dietary supplements used by adding a list of specific dietary supplements that might be of concern at the time of the survey (e.g., add entry about the use of a supplement recently suspected of causing seizures). This list must be kept up to date to reflect changes in marketing, habits of use, and occurrence of adverse events

Recommendation 2: More comprehensive data collection is needed from select populations. The committee recommends that in-depth, anonymous surveys about dietary supplement use be administered at select military installations. These select sites would be chosen because their military populations (e.g., Special Forces or Rangers) would be more likely to use dietary supplements and face higher or unknown risks due to greater mission demands and harsher environments (e.g., high altitude, extreme temperature) than most military personnel.

For example, these in-depth surveys should capture data during intense military operations that are similar to combat (e.g., Special Forces training or situations of deployment), when data collection will not interfere with the completion of the mission). Military subpopulations currently deployed in Iraq and Afghanistan could be selected to participate in surveys because of the tasks (i.e., combat service) and extreme environments they encounter. For this study, however, the committee received no data from Iraq or Afghanistan. Periodically, these surveys might also be conducted at gymnasiums and fitness centers where military service members are more likely to be using performance-enhancing dietary supplements. These in-depth surveys or interviews should incorporate the improvements for questions recommended in the section below; it is also important that questions be included about dietary supplements of particular concern.

This kind of more comprehensive survey would be expensive, especially if administered as an interview; if the less costly self-reported survey is administered, then a subset of the survey population should be recruited for in-depth probing about amount, frequency, and pattern of supplement use to verify the accuracy of the self-reported survey data. Data from surveys conducted in these select locations would complement the data collected from DoD's Survey of Health Related Behaviors Among Active Duty Military Personnel. The study designers should coordinate with the designated oversight committee (see Chapter 6) to determine specific research questions and study design. The committee believes it would be appropriate for the military to manage such surveys as separate subcontract(s) funded by DoD Health Affairs.

To develop the surveys, the military should consult with experts in the fields of nutrition, nutrition epidemiology (for survey design), pharmacognosy (for terminology used), and biostatistics (for analytical needs). Most important, it is vital that the military consult with individuals with in-depth expertise in survey design. To obtain a comprehensive description, these reports must be combined with other data, for example, data about dietary supplement use derived from electronic health records (see also Chapter 5) and sales data from military installations both on the base and at temporary duty stations (e.g., BX/PX, GNC outlets, Fitness Centers, and commissaries). Surveillance efforts should also consider monitoring of new supplements that enter the market. The DoD can develop contractual limitations for products sold on installations to require manufacturers to at least meet U.S. Pharmacopeia requirements. Contract requirements could also specify that suppliers of dietary supplements notify an appropriate health care professional when new dietary supplements in categories of interest are being introduced for sale on base. Nevertheless, electronic health records are unlikely to contain accurate information on dietary supplement use because of low report rates, while sales data do not reflect actual consumption. For example, sales data would be underestimated since they will not include purchases made off base. Thus, the best source of information on supplement use remains the results from surveys. To improve the accuracy of data on dietary supplement use in electronic health records, this committee recommends that efforts be directed to educate health care personnel (see Chapter 6).

Recommendation 3: Data quality needs to be improved. Surveys should be designed in consultation with the proposed designated oversight committee, which could oversee many aspects of dietary supplement management including adverse event reporting, as described below.

Improvement of Survey Design

The committee recommends modifications and additions to surveys to improve the design (i.e., terminology, wording, and order) and comprehensiveness of the questions. Regardless of the methodology used to administer it (i.e., self-reported questionnaires or one-on-one interviews), a comprehensive survey should include questions on dose, frequency of use, duration of use, user demographics, adverse events, motivation and expectations for use, health and performance outcomes for all dietary supplements of interest, and opportunities to review dietary supplement containers. For example, survey data that estimate total dietary exposure to a dietary supplement ingredient have been limited to sources of caffeine. As recommended above, questionnaires need to be more comprehensive, particularly when administered at installations with special subpopulations (e.g., Rangers or Special Forces). Such a comprehensive survey requires more respondent time as well as careful thought to steps from sample selection to survey design and administration.

Approaches to Increase Sample Selection and Response Rate

Sampling—the process of selecting a subset of cases that allow conclusions to be drawn about the entire population—should be designed in consultation with a survey statistician; the committee recommends that a probability sampling design be used to minimize researcher bias in selecting survey respondents. Power calculations should be conducted to ensure that the study is large enough to detect the associations for which the military is interested in testing.

Increasing the rate of response for surveys is a common challenge with population surveys. A generally acceptable range of response rate is 60–80 percent. Researchers should attempt to increase response rates by following up with people and communicating the importance of the survey, as well as providing appropriate incentives.

Obtaining Data from Longitudinal Studies Needs to Be Considered

All of the research data reviewed on dietary supplement surveys were collected from cross-sectional study designs. Patterns of behavior are likely to be affected by changes in supplement policies, and this needs to be monitored. If resources permit, the committee recommends that the military conducts surveys over an extended period of time or repeat them at certain intervals in order to evaluate time trends in supplement use. Longitudinal data would provide the opportunity to discern trends in dietary supplement use and patterns of behavior that are affected by changes in supplement policies, as well as examine relationships between dietary supplement use and health outcomes. Health- or performance-related outcomes of interest to the military would include those that are suspected of being affected by dietary supplements, such as weight loss, cardiovascular disease, palpitations, headaches, diminished alertness, or gastrointestinal disturbances. As part of the analysis of trends in use, longitudinal assessment of use of new supplements introduced into the market could be conducted. Longitudinal studies can be conducted by following up the same individual over a period of time and collecting information at prescribed times or by using a different sample each time data is collected. By following the same individuals, the variances in estimated changes in use may be lessened but other factors need to be considered, such as a higher level of dropouts. If different samples are selected, investigators need to ensure the selection of appropriate samples throughout the length of the study to minimize within-sample variance.

Planning Stage: Recommendations for Better Survey Designs

This committee believes that making a few adjustments to the surveys could remarkably improve the quality and value of the information collected. Important information gaps identified in surveys include the inability to accurately characterize respondents as users or nonusers of supplements, since frequency of use is not well characterized; and the incomplete assessment of total dose/exposure, especially of potentially important types of supplements (e.g., caffeine). Some surveys are also limited in their ability to assess prevalence of use (e.g., frequency) and difference in use by demographic factors. The surveys also, unfortunately, often used a convenience sample of respondents, making it difficult to ensure that data were adequately representative of the entire military population and decreasing the value of the data.

A common challenge in conducting surveys is ensuring the data's validity. Although complete verification of the information reported about dietary supplement use by respondents could not be attained, the validity of the questionnaires would be enhanced by greater attention to improvement of areas such as the use of defined terminology, assesing total dosage/exposure, and verifying self-reported data. This section describes overall pitfalls of the questionnaires reviewed and makes recommendations for enhancing them. Table 2-6 includes specific examples of how to improve the language and format of questions. These questions should be taken only as examples; prior to their use in questionnaires, they should be validated in the military context (i.e., in the field) so it is understood how they are interpreted and answered.

Terminology

A critical issue in using survey methods is ensuring that information is elicited in a manner that is reliable and unbiased. There is a lack of consistency in terminology used across questionnaires. If clear definitions are not

TABLE 2-6 Suggestions for Improving Survey Questions

Objective of Question/Response	Original Question	Improved Question	Considerations
Determine whether the respondent is a supplement user	Have you ever used any type of dietary supplement?	Have you used or taken any dietary supplements (i.e., vitamins, minerals, or other dietary supplements) in the past year? On the figure below, please circle the months in which you used a dietary supplement.	Important to specify time period of interest (i.e., past week, month, year), duration, and proximity of consumption period to the present time period.
		Have you used or taken any dietary supplements in the past month?	
		How many days in the past month did you use a dietary supplement?	
Assess type of supplement use	Do you use antioxidant supplements?	When you used supplements in the past month, did you use antioxidants?	Important to define supplements to ensure consistency in participant responses.
		Definition of antioxidants should be included.	Important to include specific questions about dietary supplements of concern.
Assess dose/amount of dietary supplement consumed	How much creatine do you consume during the loading phase? gm/day	Please retrieve the container for your dietary supplement before answering these questions. When you took creatine, how much did you take in one day? <500 mg, 400–499 mg, etc.	Important to have respondent retrieve the supplement container and provide information directly from it.

Provide response options to determine reasons for use of dietary supplements	Select the reasons that you use supplements: a. promote general health b. reduce fatigue c. lose weight d. prevent illness	Select the reasons that you use supplements: a. promote general health (health is defined as …) b. reduce fatigue c. lose weight d. prevent illness e. other: _______ (please explain)	Include appropriate options that are consistent with respondents' actual experiences. May be necessary to add a response such as "Other: ____ (please explain)." Response options may be obtained from open questions in preliminary interviews or pretests of the survey.
Determine whether supplement users experience adverse events when using a specific dietary supplement	Current surveys do not ask for this information.	During the time that you were using (insert supplement name here), did you experience any of the following symptoms: a. shortness of breath b. sleeplessness c. heart palpitations d. seizures e. other: _________	Response options may be composed of symptoms that are reported in civilian populations, reported through surveillance methods such as MedWatch, or obtained from open questions in preliminary interviews or pretests of the survey.
Determine whether supplement users perceive benefits when using a specific dietary supplement	Current surveys do not ask for this information.	During the time that you were using (insert supplement name here), did you experience any of the following: a. better job performance b. increased alertness c. delayed fatigue d. diminished fatigue e. weight loss f. other: _________	Response options may be obtained from product labels (i.e., health claims made by manufacturer), open questions in preliminary interviews, or pretests of the survey.

continued

TABLE 2-6 Continued

Objective of Question/Response	Original Question	Improved Question	Considerations
Determine circumstances of supplement use	Current surveys do not ask for this information.	Under what circumstances do you take dietary supplements (circle all that apply)? a. all the time b. only during deployments c. only when not deployed d. when need to do my job better e. before performance evaluations f. other: ________ Why do you take dietary supplements? a. improve job performance b. increase alertness c. delay fatigue d. diminish fatigue e. weight loss f. other: ________	

provided to respondents, simple words can be misinterpreted, which may compromise the validity of a survey. The committee reviewed some questionnaires that used ambiguous terms such as *energy* and *health*, which consumers might define differently. If left undefined, interpretation of results by analysts might be difficult. Other examples include terms such as *antioxidants*, *multivitamins/multiminerals*, or *anabolic supplements*. Antioxidants might be understood as referring to vitamins and minerals, botanicals, or some combination of both. Sports drinks, sports bars, and protein powders are highly variable in their composition and may contain any combination of vitamins, minerals, caffeine, botanicals, or other ingredients.

The committee recommends that decisions be made early in the planning stage about the appropriateness, wording, and order of questions. Ambiguous terms such as *health* and *antioxidants* should be clearly defined. To the extent possible, if ambiguous terms are necessary, they should be used in a consistent manner. To help ensure the use of accurate, clear dietary supplement terminology as well as with interpretation of data, a pharmacognosist or similar expert with in-depth knowledge of botanical and bioactive substance sources and nomenclature should be included as a member of the survey design team or as a consultant.

Ingredient Identification and Total Dosage

Questions pertaining to product dosage, composition, and frequency of use are difficult for respondents to answer. This information, however, is critical to identify signals of harm or benefit. Unfortunately, dietary supplement surveys rarely capture dosage or intake details, as questionnaires do not include entries for the number of capsules taken, weight of the product consumed, or the concentration of the active ingredients. Survey questions to establish use and determine frequency vary, as shown in Table 2-7. More attention is needed to improve accuracy in data on supplements used and quantities taken.

To complicate the exposure question, many foods and medications can contribute significantly to the total consumption of a particular substance, a factor that has not been adressed in the military dietary supplement questionnaires reviewed. This might be the case for vitamins and minerals, for example, as well as other bioactive substances such as caffeine, for which the dietary intake from several sources must be included in order to determine potential impact on military personnel. Given the broad range in caffeine content in products in the market, this is a challenging task, as shown by a recent publication that analyzed products sold in various delivery forms and found that taking the amount of product recommended on the label resulted in intake of amounts of caffeine ranging from 1 to 820 mg/day (Andrews et al., 2007). One survey (see Lieberman et al. in Appendix B)

TABLE 2-7 Examples of Questions Used in Military Surveys to Characterize Frequency of Use of Dietary Supplements

Corum (2007)	Thomasos (2007)	Marriott (2007)
Estimate how often you use each of the following vitamin and mineral supplements: • Rarely/never • 1–2 times per week • 3–4 times per week • 5 times per week or more	Do you use or have you used any type of dietary supplements? • I have never used dietary supplements. • I have in the past, but I'm not currently using dietary supplements. • I am currently using dietary supplements.	In the past 12 months, how often did you take any of the following supplements? (Note: only a few examples of each category are listed.) • Two or more times a day • Once a day • Every other day • Once a week • Once a month • Never in the past 12 months
	Estimate how often you use(d) each of the following individual vitamin supplements (pills, tablets, gel caps, etc.): • Never • Rarely • 1–2 times a week • 3–4 times a week • 5 times a week or more	In the past 12 months, what were your reasons for taking the following supplements?
		During the past 12 months, did you let any of the following conventional medical professionals know about your use of dietary supplements?

reviewed included an assessment of caffeine intake from dietary sources as well as from supplements, but the results were not available at the time of this publication. In summary, acquiring data on prevalence of use is a first step in determining the extent of dietary supplement use by military personnel; however, total dose/exposure data (e.g., from dietary supplements, food, and medication sources) is necessary to determine whether military personnel are exposed to hazardous levels of a particular dietary supplement.

Lieberman et al. (2007) (Army War College)	Lieberman et al. (2007) (Rangers)	Lieberman et al. (2007) (Special Forces)
Have you taken dietary supplements over the past year? • Yes • No Do you fairly regularly (once a week or more often) take any nutritional supplements? • Yes • No	Have you used creatine during the past 3 months? • Yes • No	Based on the past 6 months, use the table to estimate your use of each of the following supplements. Please fill in one circle for each item, then record the reason for the use and side effects.
Use the table to estimate your use of each of the following vitamin and mineral supplements during the past year. Please fill in one circle for each item for estimated use and then record the reason(s) for using the supplement. Do not fill out multivitamin/ multimineral information under the single-item section.	How frequently did you use creatine? • Seldom (less that once per week) • Occasionally (1–3 times per week) • Frequently (3–6 times per week) • Daily	How much creatine do you consume during the loading phase? How much creatine do you consume during the maintenance phase?
	What was your reason for using creatine? • Increase muscle mass, strength, and/or power • As an energy source • Promote general health • Physician directed • Other	

The committee recommends that dietary supplement surveys be complemented with questions about intake from dietary sources (foods and beverages) as well as from pills or powders. This was also supported by the IOM Committee on Mineral Requirements for Military Personnel (IOM, 2006). Special attention needs to be paid to the changing ingredients and amounts in military rations, and future determinations of total dosage and exposure should also incorporate emerging vehicles of dietary supplement ingredient delivery, such as lotions, patches, swabs, and intradermal routes.

If it is not feasible to collect data on total dose, it is important to collect descriptive data on the supplements being taken and the frequency and timing of their use.

The validity of survey responses is also compromised when the respondents are not fully aware of the ingredients of the dietary supplement product they are consuming. This lack of knowledge was evident in one ongoing Army-wide survey in which only 16.7 percent of respondents reported knowing all the ingredients in their supplements, and 9.3 percent of those taking supplements were unable to identify any of their ingredients (see Lieberman et al. in Appendix B). The majority reported knowledge of some or most of the ingredients. Some questionnaires to the general population (see Gardiner et al. in Appendix B; Kaufman, 2007) expanded this question to request that the subjects bring in containers to have the product ingredients verified, but the majority of the surveys were based on self-reporting, when verification of ingredients was unlikely. These figures demonstrate that the difficulty in acquiring dosage data on specific ingredients originates not only from the questionnaire design but also from poor consumer knowledge and lack of label accuracy. One feasible approach to address the challenge of obtaining accurate ingredient information from survey respondents would be to record detailed information about the product name and usage. The emphasis in product information collection should be on obtaining a comprehensive list and quantities of the products used so that the ingredients can be identified later. As Kaufman (2007) observes (Appendix B), when questionnaires are self-administered, as was the case with the ones reviewed, there is no control over the quality of the information received. Data quality is also easily compromised when obtaining information about dosage. Because there are many approaches to obtaining dosage information, such as open-ended questions or collection of product containers from users, it is important to establish an unbiased, practical approach to gather this information. One approach is to provide instructions on how to record product names, ingredients, and quantities.

Frequency of Use

Although none of the surveys of military populations was designed to obtain dose information, some surveys ask questions regarding frequency of use (e.g., "Are you taking it five or more times per week?"). However, the number of pills or doses per day or the amount of active component per dose was not requested. With the amount of active substance in products varying substantially, it is critical that survey respondents note the amount from the product label (though it should be noted that product labels can also be inaccurate [Andrews et al., 2007]).

In an effort to define a true "user" of supplements, the committee recommends that future surveys assess the time period of use more accurately. This would allow for consistency and clarification of prevalence of use of dietary supplements. For example, supplement use might be characterized as episodic (e.g., for short-term weight management), long-term (e.g., most of adult life), short-term (e.g., before a physical assessment), current (recently began regular use), past, or never (Table 2-6). When respondents are properly characterized by usage categories, analyses can be conducted by subgroups of users of interest (e.g., those who use only sports bars or gels) who are subsequently classified by types of dietary supplements and doses.

As mentioned above, questions on frequency should be expanded to specify the period of time and circumstances surrounding the use of a product (e.g., respondent reports used creatine once a day from December to March while deployed).

Association Between Adverse Effects and Dietary Supplement Consumed

The committee recommends enhancement of questions intended to assess associations between consumption of dietary supplements and adverse events. For example, given the common use of caffeinated products in the military and their potential synergistic effects with other stimulants, there is a need to better characterize total intake of caffeine. Several surveys included self-reported (with no adjudication) adverse effects perceived to be attributable to dietary supplements. In-depth probing about adverse events or outcomes (heart palpitations, headaches, etc.) thought to be associated with supplements should be added to the surveys. These questions are especially relevant when conducting surveys in special subpopulations, such as Rangers and Special Forces, with heightened risks and higher dietary supplement usage.

As with the data on frequency of use, questions on adverse events should be linked to information about the environment and conditions in which respondents consume the specific dietary supplement (e.g., soldiers might be taking creatine only before deployment or in between sustained missions). Questions on adverse events and beneficial outcomes should be posed prior to questions on dietary supplement use to minimize the potential for biases in responses.

Demographic Factors

Differences between U.S. military personnel and the general population (e.g., service members have higher socioeconomic status and education, different age distribution, a higher minority representation, and different levels of stress) are substantial enough to require specific military surveillance.

Available survey data on supplement use by military personnel give important clues about such use; however, they are limited in their ability to allow assessment of prevalence of use and differences in use by demographic factors across multiple studies. Surveys conducted to date do not collect this information consistently; even demographic data (e.g., age, rank, geographic area, organizational unit) collected varies among surveys. A consistent method of collecting and analyzing data by demographic characteristics would allow for a comprehensive, comparable description of dietary supplement use in various populations and across time.

Additional Questions

Questions on health and performance The committee recommends the collection of data on the association of dietary supplement use with health and performance outcomes. Data should be linked to information about the environment and conditions in which respondents consume the specific dietary supplement.

Such data would provide evidence of whether the expectations of benefit are being met under the real-life circumstances of the U.S. military. In addition, these questions help determine whether there are differences in outcomes for individuals with healthy lifestyle patterns versus those who use supplements to counter unhealthy behaviors such as smoking, drinking alcohol to excess, and eating a poor-quality diet. Such analyses may be possible if the DoD links dietary intake to dietary supplement intake. Although one survey collected self-reported Army Physical Fitness Test (APFT) results and would therefore allow correlation between dietary supplement use and APFT scores, the data to evaluate the impact of confounding factors (e.g., training regimen) are not available. Data on possible confounders are needed in the analyses of relationships between health outcomes and dietary supplement intake. Potential confounders (i.e., variables that are related to both supplement use and the health outcome of interest but are not in the causal pathway between these two variables) should be considered prior to creating surveys so that they are included in the questionnaire; it may be helpful to consult with an epidemiologist for assistance with determining confounders a priori.

Questions on effectiveness of communication The committee recommends that questions about sources of information on dietary supplements that military personnel consult be added to questionnaires as these would help determine the most effective methods to disseminate accurate information. Once strategies to disseminate information are implemented, survey questions to measure the level of outreach and effectiveness of the information strategy will also be needed.

Administration Stage: Recommendations for Data Collection

In the survey administration stage, respondents are recruited, survey data are collected by interviewers or self-report, and nonrespondents are followed up. Each survey should be pretested. Follow-up efforts may be necessary to ensure an adequate response rate. During this stage, data should also be inspected for systematic biases in response patterns and efforts made to adjust the participant demographics or account for bias in the data analysis stage.

Presurvey a Few Individuals

To validate the survey, the committee recommends that it be pretested on a small number of persons with characteristics similar to the target group of respondents. These data should also be inspected for systematic biases in response patterns. Statistical expertise should be sought prior to survey administration to prevent biases in the questions or the demographics of participants.

Verify Self-Reported Data in a Subpopulation

A choice must be made between a self-reported or personal interview survey, and the questionnaire should be designed accordingly. When validated, self-reported questionnaires provide higher quality data if designed as highly structured surveys because they minimize biases caused by misinterpretation of questions. Unstructured surveys (using open-ended questions) work better when interviews are conducted; however, they require administration by trained personnel and entail complex data analysis, resulting in higher expenses than structured surveys. Although a personal interview may be more informative than self-reported surveys, responses can be influenced by the manner, tone, and opinion of the interviewer. Thus, while personal interviews offer better survey compliance and in-depth information, interviewer training and quality control are key elements to minimize potential sources of data bias.

Surveys will likely be administered more often with self-reported questionnaires than with personal interviews due to cost considerations. Self-reported surveys present the following limitations: (1) lower response rates; (2) a higher rate of incomplete or inaccurate responses; and (3) a need for simpler, structured designs to elicit reliable responses. The committee recommends the application of strategies to overcome these limitations, which will assist with interpreting self-reported data and revising the questionnaires and, ultimately, help improve self-reported data. One strategy consists of conducting personal interviews with a smaller group of individuals, and correlating these results with self-reported data. These personal interviews allow for more controlled resposes and ensure higher accuracy and data quality. For example, to verify responses related to ingredient accuracy, this subgroup could be asked to bring in the bottles/containers of the products consumed. Lack of statistical power limits comparisons, so statistical power calculations should be conducted to ensure sufficient ability to relate findings from this group to those of the targeted military population. Another strategy to verify responses on use patterns is to compare survey results to sales data from military bases, considering both the types of products that are being purchased and the ingredients in those products.

REFERENCES

Aday, L. 1996. *Designing and conducting health surveys*. San Francisco, CA: Jossey-Bass.

Andrews, K. W., A. Schweitzer, C. Zhao, J. M. Holden, J. M. Roseland, M. Brandt, J. T. Dwyer, M. F. Picciano, L. G. Saldanha, K. D. Fisher, E. Yetley, J. M. Betz, and L. Douglass. 2007. The caffeine contents of dietary supplements commonly purchased in the U.S.: Analysis of 53 products with caffeine-containing ingredients. *Annal Bioanal Chem* 389(1):231-239.

Arsenault, J., and J. Kennedy. 1999. Dietary supplement use in U.S. Army Special Operations candidates. *Mil Med* 164(7):495-501.

Bathalon, G. P., S. M. McGraw, L. D. Hennessy, W. F. Barko, J. F. Creedon, and H. R. Lieberman. 2000. Comparison of reported nutritional supplement intake in two Army populations. *Suppl J Am Diet Assoc* 100(1):A102.

Bernard, H. R. 1999. *Social research methods: Qualitative and quantitative approaches*. Thousand Oaks, CA: Sage Publications.

Bovill, M. E., S. M. McGraw, W. J. Tharion, and H. R. Lieberman. 2000. Supplement use and nutrition knowledge in a Special Forces unit. *FASEB Journal* 15(5):A999.

Bovill, M. E., W. J. Tharion, and H. R. Lieberman. 2003. Nutrition knowledge and supplement use among elite U.S. Army soldiers. *Mil Med* 168(12):997-1000.

Brasfield, K. 2004. Dietary supplement intake in the active duty enlisted population. *U.S. Army Med Dept J* (Oct-Dec):44-56.

Converse, J. M., and S. Presser. 1986. *Survey questions: Handcrafting the standardized questionnaire*. Thousand Oaks, CA: Sage Publications.

Corum, S. J. C. 2007. *Dietary supplements questionnaire*. Institute of Medicine Committee on Dietary Supplement Use by Military Personnel meeting, Washington, DC, February 13.

Deuster, P. A., A. Sridhar, W. J. Becker, R. Coll, K. K. O'Brien, and G. Bathalon. 2003. Health assessment of U.S. Army Rangers. *Mil Med* 168(1):57-62.

French, S. 2007. *Insights into dietary supplement usage by U.S. active military personnel*. Institute of Medicine Committee on Dietary Supplement Use by Military Personnel meeting, Washington, DC, February 13.

IOM (Institute of Medicine). 1999. *Military strategies for sustainment of nutrition and immune function in the field*. Washington, DC: National Academy Press.

IOM. 2006. *Mineral requirements for military personnel: Levels needed for cognitive and physical performance during garrison training*. Washington, DC: The National Academies Press.

Jaghab, D. 2007. *Survey of Army health care providers concerning dietary supplements.* Institute of Medicine Committee on Dietary Supplement Use by Military Personnel meeting, Washington, DC, February 13.

Johnson, A. E., C. A. Haley, and J. A. Ward. In press. *Hazards of dietary supplement use.*

Kaufman, D. W. 2007. *Design and conduct of surveys on dietary supplement use.* Institute of Medicine Committee on Dietary Supplement Use by Military Personnel meeting, Washington, DC, February 12.

Kelly, J. P., D. W. Kaufman, K. Kelley, L. Rosenberg, T. E. Anderson, and A. A. Mitchell. 2005. Recent trends in use of herbal and other natural products. *Arch Intern Med* 165(3):281-286.

Lieberman, H. R., T. Stavinoha, S. McGraw, and L. Sigrist. 2007. *Use of dietary supplements in U.S. Army populations.* Institute of Medicine Committee on Dietary Supplement Use by Military Personnel meeting, Washington, DC, February 13.

Marriott, B. M. 2007. *Dietary supplement use by active duty military personnel: A world wide sample.* Institute of Medicine Committee on Dietary Supplement Use by Military Personnel meeting, Washington, DC, February 13.

McGraw, S. M., W. J. Tharion, and H. R. Lieberman. 2000. Use of nutritional supplements by U.S. Army Rangers. *FASEB Journal* 14(4):A742.

McPherson, F., and M. A. Schwenka. 2004. Use of complementary and alternative therapies among active duty soldiers, military retirees, and family members at a military hospital. *Mil Med* 169(5):354-357.

Radimer, K., B. Bindewald, J. Hughes, B. Ervin, C. Swanson, and M. F. Picciano. 2004. Dietary supplement use by U.S. adults: Data from the National Health and Nutrition Examination Survey, 1999-2000. *Am J Epidemiol* 160(4):339-349.

Sheppard, H. L., S. M. Raichada, K. M. Kouri, L. Stenson-Bar-Maor, and J. D. Branch. 2000. Use of creatine and other supplements by members of civilian and military health clubs: A cross-sectional survey. *Int J Sport Nutr Exerc Metab* 10(3):245-259.

Sobal, J., and L. F. Marquart. 1994. Vitamin/mineral supplement use among athletes: A review of the literature. *Int J Sport Nutr* 4(4):320-334.

Thomasos, C. 2007. *Assessment of Air Force dietary supplement usage by major commands.* Institute of Medicine Committee on Dietary Supplement Use by Military Personnel meeting, Washington, DC, February 13.

Timbo, B. B., M. P. Ross, P. V. McCarthy, and C. T. Lin. 2006. Dietary supplements in a national survey: Prevalence of use and reports of adverse events. *J Am Diet Assoc* 106(12):1966-1974.

3

Vitamins and Essential Minerals for Military Personnel

INTRODUCTION

Vitamins and minerals, whether taken in combination or individually, are the most frequently consumed dietary supplements among military personnel in all surveys reviewed (Chapter 2). Although levels for specific military subpopulations have been recommended in other Institute of Medicine (IOM) reports (IOM, 2005, 2006a), potential concerns with high levels of use were not addressed. This chapter includes a summary of recommendations provided in those reports and discusses safety concerns associated with the use of vitamin and mineral supplements.

Unlike other dietary supplement ingredients, vitamins and certain minerals are considered essential nutrients for which standards of adequacy are needed. These standards are developed to ensure that the nutrient needs of different populations are met. In the United States, the nutrient standards or Dietary Reference Intakes (DRIs) are compiled in various IOM reports (IOM, 1997, 1998a, 2000a,b, 2002/2005, 2004) (Table 3-1). The DRIs comprise the following four nutrient-based reference values established by gender and age group: the Estimated Average Requirement (EAR), the Recommended Dietary Allowance (RDA), the Adequate Intake (AI), and the Tolerable Upper Intake Level (UL). The IOM EARs and RDAs are the average intake levels that meet respectively the requirements of 50 and 97–98 percent of the healthy individuals in a population in a particular life stage and gender group. An RDA is the reference value—derived mathematically from the EAR population distribution—for planning individual intakes. An AI (estimated intake by a population, based on observed or

TABLE 3-1 Military Recommended Intakes for Men in Garrison Feeding, Operational, and Restricted Rations Compared to Recommended Intakes for Men Ages 19–30 Years in the General Population

Nutrient or Energy	RDA, AI, or AMDR (per day)	Military Daily Recommended Intake	Tolerable Upper Level
Energy intake (kcal)	3,600	3,250	
Protein (for an 80-kg male) (g)	56 g	91 (10–15%)	
(% of kcal)	(10–35%)		
Fat (% of kcal)	20–35%	≤35%	
PUFA (% kcal)			
n-3 as α-linolenic	0.6–1.2%		
n-6 as linoleic acid	5–10%		
Carbohydrate (g)	130	ND	
(% of kcal)	(45–65%)		
Vitamin A (μg)	900 RAE	1,000 μg RE	3,000
Vitamin C (mg)	90	90	2,000
Vitamin D (μg)	5	5	50
Vitamin E (mg)	15	15	1,000
Vitamin K (μg)	120	80	ND
Thiamin (mg)	1.2	1.2	ND
Riboflavin (mg)	1.3	1.3	ND
Niacin (mg NE)	16	16	35
Vitamin B_6 (mg)	1.3	1.3	100
Folate (μg DFE)	400	400	1,000
Vitamin B_{12} (μg)	2.4	2.4	ND
Biotin (μg)	30	ND	ND
Pantothenic acid (mg)	5	ND	ND
Calcium (mg)	1,000	1,000	2,500
Choline (mg)	550	ND	3,500
Chromium (μg)	35	ND	ND
Copper (μg)	900	ND	10,000
Fluoride (mg)	4	4	10
Iodine (μg)	150	150	1,100
Iron (mg)	8	15	45
Magnesium (mg)	400	420	350
Manganese (mg)	2.3	ND	11
Molybdenum (μg)	45	ND	2,000
Phosphorus (mg)	700	700	4,000
Potassium (mg)	4,700	3,200	ND
Selenium (μg)	55	55	400
Sodium (mg)	1,500 ≤ 2,300	5,000 (4,550–5,525)	2,300
Zinc (mg)	11	15	40

NOTE: AI = Adequate Intake; AMDR = Acceptable Macronutrient Distribution Ranges; DFE = Dietary Folate Equivalents; ND = Not Determined; NE = Niacin Equivalents; PUFA = Polyunsaturated Fatty Acids; RAE = Retinol Activity Equivalent; RDA = Recommended Dietary Allowance; RE = Retinol Equivalents.

SOURCES: IOM, 2004; U.S. Departments of the Army, Navy, and Air Force, 2001.

experimentally determined approximations of nutrient intakes) can also be used for planning individual intakes. The IOM UL is the highest intake level likely to pose no reported risk of an adverse health effect to almost all individuals. Because vitamins and minerals are required to maintain health and therefore supplementation might be needed if deficiencies occur, deliberations about their safety and benefits are fundamentally different from those about nonessential dietary supplements, which are discussed in Chapter 4. For nonessential dietary supplements, any discussion on prevention of nutrient deficiencies with dietary supplements would not apply.

The 2006 IOM report *Mineral Requirements for Military Personnel* indicates that compared to the general population, some groups in the military may require higher intakes of specific nutrients to maintain health because of sweat losses during high-intensity physical activities (IOM, 2006a). Higher nutrient intakes might also be needed to optimize military performance. Nutrient standards distinct from those for the general population have been developed for the military population: the Military Dietary Reference Intakes (MDRIs) and the nutritional standards for operational rations, which are based on MDRIs (U.S. Departments of the Army, Navy, and Air Force, 2001). The MDRIs are based on the IOM DRIs; the 2006 IOM report recommends that the MDRIs continue to reflect the IOM DRIs and that they be updated periodically by considering scientific evidence from studies on the benefits of specific nutrients (e.g., for improved cognitive function) or from studies revealing altered nutrient metabolism due to military performance (e.g., increased sweat losses) (IOM, 2006a). The committee made specific recommendations for a systematic approach to develop MDRIs for all nutrients and how to apply them. In every case, it recommended that the intake level should be lower than the UL for the age range.

The safety of vitamins and minerals therefore needs to be determined with consideration of both risks from toxicity and risks from deficiency. This chapter comments on recent recommendations made by other IOM committees on the establishment of requirements for nutrients, including vitamins and minerals, for military personnel performing high-intensity physical tasks. This committee concurs with those recommendations and provides a list of research needs.

SAFETY OF VITAMINS AND MINERALS

Risks of Vitamin and Mineral Deficiencies

Some military subpopulations engage in high-intensity physical activities while they consume low-calorie diets. Their diets might therefore be deficient in vitamins and minerals, and increasing intake might be necessary to meet nutritional requirements and maintain health. There are four basic strategies that can be applied to improve nutrient intake and nutritional status of military personnel: food-based approaches, fortification, supplementation, and complementary public health control measures (IOM, 1998b). The uses, advantages, and disadvantages of each strategy were described in the 2006 IOM report, and this section provides a summary on using supplementation as a strategy to increase intake of essential nutrients in the military.

In the 1994 Dietary Supplement Health and Education Act (*Dietary Supplement Health and Education Act of 1994*, Public Law 103-417, 108 Stat 4325, 103rd Congress, October 25, 1994), Congress defines a dietary supplement as a product (other than tobacco) that is intended to supplement the diet; that contains one or more dietary ingredients (defined as vitamins; minerals; herbs or other botanicals; amino acids; other dietary substances for use by man to supplement the diet by increasing the total dietary intake; or concentrates, constituents, metabolites, extracts, or combinations of any of the aforementioned dietary ingredients); that is intended to be taken by mouth as a pill, capsule, tablet, or liquid; and that is labeled on the front panel as being a dietary supplement. In general, the scientific community agrees that selecting a balanced diet of foods providing sufficient amounts of vitamins and minerals should be encouraged, and supplements should be used only in cases where food does not provide sufficient vitamins and minerals. If levels higher than the RDAs are necessary to achieve optimal health benefits or because of greater needs in the military subpopulations, supplementation may be the only recourse. For example, the 2006 IOM report showed that the average mineral composition of three different Meals, Ready-to-Eat rations and three different First Strike Ration menus provided by the U.S. Army Research Institute of Environmental Medicine (USARIEM) did not meet the iron requirements for women and the zinc requirements for both men and women. Since iron supplementation can be a highly effective approach to treating iron deficiency but can also be toxic, it is important to find the best means to protect women who participate in heavy training from a decrease in iron status, such as supplementation, iron fortification, dietary adjustments, or other means. When mineral sweat losses cannot be balanced with dietary intake or when there is evidence to suggest that a higher intake might benefit physical or mental function, supplementation should be considered. Supplementation might also be advisable when individuals are relying on a low-calorie diet that does not meet the RDAs or if research shows that a low-calorie diet increases micronutrient needs to higher than the RDA. For example, although confirmatory research is needed, the Committee on Mineral Requirements for Military

Personnel recommended calcium intakes of at least 1,000 mg/day and as much as 1,500–1,700 mg/day to minimize bone loss during weight-loss regimes (IOM, 2006a).

In all cases, providing such high levels of nutrients must be justified; even among the general population, the relationship between high intake levels and associated benefits or additional needs is, for many nutrients, still unclear (IOM, 2006a; Lichtenstein and Russell, 2005; Perelson and Ellenbogen, 2002), and intervention studies are needed to demonstrate conclusive nutrient–health benefit links before high levels of nutrients can be recommended.

When there are deficiencies, supplementation can generate changes in micronutrient status relatively quickly, although compared with fortification or dietary diversification, it reaches relatively small numbers of consumers and requires action on the part of many individuals. Another advantage is that, unlike other strategies mentioned, dietary supplements do not require major changes in the food supply, food processing, or distribution. Still, in general, the IOM reports have endorsed supplementation with specific nutrients only for situations in which there is clear evidence of potential harm due to dietary inadequacy.

For the military, the following factors need to be considered when selecting a strategy to increase nutrient intakes:

- The prevalence and severity of a population's nutritional inadequacy
- The consequences of failing to raise intakes to RDAs or other nutrient standard levels
- The number of nutrients in which a population is deficient
- The amount of time required to affect the health outcomes linked to the nutrient in question
- The phase, appropriateness, and feasibility of the intervention
- Other characteristics unique to the particular setting
- Other characteristics of the nutrient under consideration

In contrast, the proposition that taking a multivitamin or multimineral (MV/MM) supplement each day should be recommended is debatable, because the efficacy of using dietary supplements to alter the risk of chronic disease is not well established (Caballero, 2003), and this practice presents public health concerns if intake regularly exceeds the UL. In addition, when supplementary doses of nutrients are high, nutrient interactions tend to be accelerated. There might be harmful consequences from shifting the emphasis away from intake of nutrients from food and toward use of nutrient supplements (Caballero, 2003; Lichtenstein and Russell, 2005), in that changes in nutrient profiles might lead to alteration in absorption or metabolism of other constituents.

Upper Limits as Safety Levels for Vitamins and Minerals

As mentioned above the unique demands of some military situations suggest that nutrient requirements for the military might differ from those for the general population; however, there is no scientific basis to establish different military ULs (for chronic intake). Establishment of the DRIs (and the UL in particular) is an area of nutrition undergoing considerable changes and attracting much attention both nationally and internationally. As with previous IOM committees that have addressed questions related to the nutrient needs of military personnel, this committee recommends that the military defer to the standards established by the IOM when it evaluates the safety of vitamins and minerals (IOM, 1997, 1998a, 2000a, 2002/2005, 2004). The premises and thought process that precede the establishment of ULs are being reconsidered; as recently recognized in the IOM workshop summary *Dietary Reference Intakes Research Synthesis*, experts recognize the need for improved ULs. Much progress is needed not only in collection of data to determine ULs, but also in the establishment of clear objectives; for instance, for each particular nutrient it is critical to define the adverse effects or health end points to be used in establishing the UL. The IOM workshop summary identified data on dose–response; measures of exposure; exposure in subpopulations, especially for the upper percentiles; and long-term exposure as both critical and lacking. Finally, understanding the interactions of multiple nutrients and identifying approaches to deal with the challenges associated with human intervention studies (e.g., approaches for extrapolating conclusions from animal data) were highlighted as areas of research requiring attention (IOM, 2006b). Efforts are being made to enhance the approaches used to establish the DRIs, including models for ULs. The military leadership responsible for setting nutrition policy should closely follow current and future developments in this area.

One question that might arise during performance of military tasks is the appropriate acute intake of a mineral or vitamin. The ULs are based on chronic intakes, not acute intakes. The safety of vitamins or minerals when a large amount is consumed over a short period of time is unknown. For example, in case of injury, a patient's acute intake of doses of vitamin E lower than the UL might still be lethal because of its antithrombotic effect. On the other hand, short-term consumption of other nutrients in amounts that exceed the UL might not present a significant risk. This is an issue of concern for military personnel in combat.

Are There Safety Concerns for Vitamin and Mineral Use Among Military Populations?

Survey Data

Chapter 2 summarizes unpublished survey data on dietary supplement use that was collected during the past several years and presented during the 2007 workshop *Dietary Supplement Use by Military Personnel* and data from a small number of published surveys (Appendix C). The most recent unpublished surveys indicated that products with a combination of vitamins and minerals (MV/MM) are among the most frequently used dietary supplements in both the general active duty population (Corum, 2007; Marriott, 2007; Thomasos, 2007) and special military subpopulations (approximately 23 percent, 32 percent, and 39 percent of U.S. Army Rangers, Special Forces, and Army War College students, respectively) (Lieberman et al., 2007). The published literature also concurs with a high frequency of use of multivitamin or multimineral products or both compared to other dietary supplements among military personnel (Arsenault and Kennedy, 1999; Bovill et al., 2000; Brasfield, 2004; McGraw et al., 2000; Sheppard et al., 2000). In addition to MV/MM supplements, individual minerals or vitamins were also frequently used. A high percentage of the subjects reported "improvement of health" or "to supplement diet" as the reasons for their use of MV/MM supplements (76 percent) or individual vitamins or minerals (65 percent) (Marriott, 2007) (Chapter 2).

Data Limitations

The limitations of survey designs are presented in Chapter 2. One major limitation is that although surveys have collected partial information on frequency of use, none of the questions addressed the specific dosages or amounts of a supplement consumed, which is a critical piece of information when evaluating safety. Even with the assumption that consumers ingest one pill or tablet per day, the broad range of levels in commercially available brands would hamper any accurate estimation of consumption level. In fact, from the data available to the committee, it is not possible to determine whether the current uses of specific minerals or vitamins might be cause for concern. This state of affairs was eloquently and extensively described in the 30th National Nutrient Database Conference Report *Progress in Developing Analytical and Label-Based Dietary Supplement Databases at NIH's Office of Dietary Supplements* (Dwyer et al., 2007). This report concluded that the widespread use of dietary supplements increases the need for better data on dietary supplement composition and possible health effects. These data are critical for an accurate estimate of total intake of vitamins and minerals, including dietary. Recognizing this, the government has led several initiatives such as the development of a validated MV/MM supplement ingredient database and the update of the National Health and Nutrition Examination Survey (NHANES) dietary supplement label database as well as a study to assess the feasibility of a label database for all dietary supplements marketed in the United States. The panel at the 30th National Nutrient Database Conference concluded that the evidence was insufficient to either recommend or discourage the use of MV/MM supplements (Dwyer et al., 2007).

One factor that hinders the availability of total intake data is the lack of information on vitamin and mineral intake from food sources. For example, the 2006 IOM report *Mineral Requirements for Military Personnel* stated that the few studies available on mineral intake suggest that military servicemen's dietary intake of some minerals (i.e., magnesium and zinc) might be marginal, but the latter does not provide a clear picture of the mineral and vitamin intake from food among service members (Baker-Fulco, 2005; personal communication, Carol J. Baker-Fulco, USARIEM, April 23, 2007). This committee concurs with other IOM committees that there is an important need to collect intake data on essential minerals and vitamins from both dietary supplements and the diet.

Interactions with Other Dietary Components or Medications

Data from only two of the available surveys were analyzed to answer questions related to concomitant consumption of various dietary supplements; for example, what is the proportion of users of mineral or vitamin supplements who also consume other dietary supplements? Are some supplements taken frequently in combination? The analysis of the data from the Army-wide survey found that among multivitamin users, 21 percent take one other supplement, 22 percent take three or four other supplements, and 31 percent take five or more other supplements (Lieberman et al., 2007). The most popular "other" supplements were protein powder (taken by 29 percent of respondents), sports drinks (24 percent), vitamin C (21 percent), calcium (15 percent), other vitamins (vitamins E, D, or A) (30 percent), creatine (9 percent), or other antioxidants (9 percent). Likewise, the analysis of data from the army survey administered to active duty personnel deployed in Germany showed that among those taking multivitamins, multiminerals, or both, many also used other vitamins or minerals such as vitamin C (43 percent), calcium (38 percent), vitamin E (32 percent), or iron (30 percent); a smaller proportion were also taking performance enhancers such as creatine (13 percent), sports drinks (11 percent), and arginine; others were also taking herbal supplements such as ginseng (11 percent), garlic (8 percent), *Ginkgo biloba* (7 percent), or echinacea (6 percent); and others were also taking caffeine (5 percent) (personal communication, Sonya Corum, U.S. Army Training and Doctrine Command, April 10, 2007).

In addition to consumption of a combination of dietary supplements, there are concerns related to the use of dietary supplements while using prescription medications. Yetley (2007) briefly reviewed potential undesirable effects that may result. For instance, intake of calcium, frequently used among military personnel, may reduce absorption of some medications and reduce their efficacy. Other reported interactions include vitamin E and aspirin, with the potential for an antithrombotic effect (Yetley, 2007). Because vitamins and minerals are essential nutrients, this committee recommends that if a dietary supplement compromises the effectiveness of a medication, an alternative medication should be prescribed if possible. Similarly, if doses higher than the RDA of a specific vitamin or mineral are known to reduce the effect of medication, then advising a reduction in intake of the vitamins or minerals to the RDA level would be appropriate. As with other supplements, however, there is little research conducted on the effects of interactions between medications and vitamins or minerals.

SUMMARY

Two IOM committees have recently addressed the nutrient needs of military personnel and highlighted several areas where research is warranted, including mineral losses under high-intensity military situations; iron status and total calcium intake throughout the time served in military service; and potential beneficial effects on performance of supplementation with specific vitamins and minerals, such as iron and zinc, alone or in combination. These two IOM committees demonstrate the lack of information regarding nutrient requirements for specific subpopulations in the military as well as the lack of information on mineral or vitamin deficiencies that might result in health or performance decrements.

As suggested by the IOM Committee on Nutrient Composition of Rations for Short-Term, High-Intensity Combat Operations (IOM, 2005), nutrients should be provided in whole foods, and fortification and the use of supplementation should be limited to the extent possible owing to the potential for nutrient–nutrient interactions. To remedy deficiencies of essential vitamins or minerals, the military may find it useful to implement combined strategies that involve typical diets, fortified foods, and dietary supplements.

Whether supplement use is institutionally implemented or not, an individual might still decide to use an MV/MM dietary supplement; unfortunately, as outlined above, there is very little information on the doses and frequency of current use. In the absence of information on total dietary intake of vitamins and minerals, and assuming that individual users of

MV/MM dietary supplements take one unit (e.g., pill) per day and that the amounts of essential nutrients per unit are comparable to the military RDA, the committee concluded that the potential for adverse health effects from the use of these dietary supplements would be minimal. Acute intake beyond UL levels of some minerals and vitamins might, however, pose some risks in specific high-intensity military situations that would not be predicted by considering the ULs, which are based on chronic intake levels. Likewise, the acute intake of other minerals and vitamins beyond the UL might not pose significant risks. Thus, the recommendation to use ULs as the upper limit should be based on chronic use, as intended when the ULs were established by the IOM.

RESEARCH NEEDS

The committee recommends that research efforts for vitamins and minerals be made in the following areas:

1. Gather data on nutrient composition of rations and on total dietary intake of vitamins and minerals by military personnel. To gather these data, the military should do the following:
    a. Design and conduct surveys on dietary supplement use by military personnel following the guidance provided in Chapter 2. In particular, more accurate information about dosage and frequency needs to be gathered.
    b. Continue conducting ration composition analysis, and conduct studies to estimate the dietary intake of minerals and vitamins.
2. Participate in current government-led initiatives to construct a label database and a composition database for vitamin and mineral products.
3. Follow closely the current and future UL developments and include them in their MDRI tables. Consider establishing ULs for the military in special conditions (i.e., during combat when the risk of injury is high, when clotting medications are being used, or during wound healing when vitamin E intake might need to be restricted).
4. If surveys of use reveal that the intake of specific vitamins or minerals are approaching ULs within short periods of time, then conduct research to determine the safety of acute intakes of those minerals or vitamins under military conditions of concern. Consider establishing upper limits for acute intakes.

REFERENCES

Arsenault, J., and J. Kennedy. 1999. Dietary supplement use in U.S. Army Special Operations candidates. *Mil Med* 164(7):495-501.

Baker-Fulco, C. J. 2005. *Derivation of the military dietary reference intakes and the mineral content of military rations*. Institute of Medicine Workshop on the Mineral Requirements for Cognitive and Physical Performance of Military Personnel, Washington, DC.

Bovill, M. E., S. M. McGraw, W. J. Tharion, and H. R. Lieberman. 2000. Supplement use and nutrition knowledge in a Special Forces unit. *FASEB J* 15(5):A999.

Brasfield, K. 2004. Dietary supplement intake in the active duty enlisted population. *US Army Med Dept J* (Oct-Dec):44-56.

Caballero, B. 2003. Fortification, supplementation, and nutrient balance. *Eur J Clin Nutr* 57(Suppl 1):S76-S78.

Corum, S. J. C. 2007. *Dietary supplements questionnaire*. Institute of Medicine Committee on Dietary Supplement Use by Military Personnel meeting, Washington, DC, February 13.

Dwyer, J. T., M. F. Picciano, J. M. Betz, K. D. Fisher, L. G. Saldanha, E. A. Yetley, P. M. Coates, J. A. Milner, J. Whitted, V. Burt, K. Radimer, J. Wilger, K. E. Sharpless, J. Holden, K. Andrews, J. Roseland, C. Zhao, A. Schweitzer, J. Harnly, W. R. Wolf, and C. R. Perry. 2007. *30th National Nutrient Database Conference Report: Progress in developing analytical and label-based dietary supplement databases at NIH's Office of Dietary Supplements*. Honolulu, HI.

IOM (Institute of Medicine). 1997. *Dietary reference intakes for calcium, phosphorus, magnesium, vitamin D, and fluoride*. Washington, DC: National Academy Press.

IOM. 1998a. *Dietary reference intakes for thiamin, riboflavin, niacin, vitamin B_6, folate, vitamin B_{12}, pantothenic acid, biotin, and choline*. Washington, DC: National Academy Press.

IOM. 1998b. *Prevention of micronutrient deficiencies: Tools for policymakers and public health workers*. Washington, DC: National Academy Press.

IOM. 2000a. *Dietary reference intakes for vitamin C, vitamin E, selenium, and carotenoids*. Washington, DC: National Academy Press.

IOM. 2000b. *Dietary reference intakes for vitamin A, vitamin K, arsenic, boron, chromium, copper, iodine, iron, manganese, molybdenum, nickel, silicon, vanadium, and zinc*. Washington, DC: National Academy Press.

IOM. 2002/2005. *Dietary reference intakes for energy, carbohydrate, fiber, fat, fatty acids, cholesterol, protein, and amino acids*. Washington, DC: The National Academies Press.

IOM. 2004. *Dietary reference intakes for water, potassium, sodium, chloride, and sulfate*. Washington, DC: The National Academies Press.

IOM. 2005. *Nutrient composition of rations for short-term, high-intensity combat operations*. Washington, DC: The National Academies Press.

IOM. 2006a. *Mineral requirements for military personnel: Levels needed for cognitive and physical performance during garrison training*. Washington, DC: The National Academies Press.

IOM. 2006b. *Dietary reference intakes research synthesis: Workshop summary*. Washington, DC: The National Academies Press.

Lichtenstein, A. H., and R. M. Russell. 2005. Essential nutrients: Food or supplements? Where should the emphasis be? *JAMA* 294(3):351-358.

Lieberman, H. R., T. Stavinoha, S. McGraw, and L. Sigrist. 2007. *Use of dietary supplements in U.S. Army populations*. Institute of Medicine Committee on Dietary Supplement Use by Military Personnel meeting, Washington, DC, February 13.

Marriott, B. M. 2007. *Dietary supplement use by active duty military personnel: A worldwide sample*. Institute of Medicine Committee on Dietary Supplement Use by Military Personnel meeting, Washington, DC, February 13.

McGraw, S. M., W. J. Tharion, and H. R. Lieberman. 2000. Use of nutritional supplements by U.S. Army Rangers. *FASEB J* 14(4):A742.

Perelson, A. M., and L. Ellenbogen. 2002. Rationale for use of vitamin and mineral supplements. In *Handbook of nutrition and food*, edited by C. M. Berdanier, E. B. Feldman, W. P. Flatt, and S. T. St. Jeor. Boca Raton, FL: CRC Press. Pp. 1333-1361.

Sheppard, H. L., S. M. Raichada, K. M. Kouri, L. Stenson Bar Maor, and J. D. Branch. 2000. Use of creatine and other supplements by members of civilian and military health clubs: A cross-sectional survey. *Int J Sport Nutr Exerc Metab* 10(3):245-259.

Thomasos, C. 2007. *Assessment of Air Force dietary supplement usage by major commands.* Institute of Medicine Committee on Dietary Supplement Use by Military Personnel meeting, Washington, DC, February 13.

U.S. Departments of the Army, Navy, and Air Force. 2001. *Nutrition standards and education.* AR 40-25/BUMEDINST 10110.6/AFI 44-141. Washington, DC: U.S. Department of Defense Headquarters.

Yetley, E. A. 2007. Multivitamin and multimineral dietary supplements: Definitions, characterization, bioavailability, and drug interactions. *Amer J Clin Nutr* 85(Suppl):269S-276S.

4

Other Dietary Supplements for Military Personnel

INTRODUCTION

The committee was asked to select a limited number of dietary supplements from those identified as commonly used and, on the basis of published reports, to identify those that may be of benefit or might pose serious hazards. The committee used the information provided at the February 12–13, 2007, workshop to select dietary supplements to review based on their frequency of use, potential for adverse events, and interest for the military. This chapter includes a review of the following dietary supplements: caffeine, chromium, creatine, dehydroepiandrosterone (DHEA), *Ephedra*, garlic, *Ginkgo biloba*, ginseng, β-hydroxy-β-methylbutyrate (HMB), melatonin, quercetin, sports bars, sports drinks, tyrosine, and valerian. HMB, creatine, sports drinks and bars, garlic, *Ginkgo biloba*, and ginseng were reviewed owing to their high frequency of use (see Appendix C). A review of DHEA was conducted because the use of anabolic supplements was shown as high, it is legally considered a dietary supplement, and because DHEA is popular among athletes.

The committee also considered other factors in their selection, such as severity and number of adverse events reported for a supplement or interest of the military in a particular dietary supplement. *Ephedra* was selected for review by the committee owing to its high frequency of use by military personnel in the past, mainly to achieve weight loss and enhancement of performance, and its adverse event profile. *Ginkgo biloba* extracts were selected based on their potential to enhance mental performance. Although quercetin is not frequently used by military personnel, research evaluating its effects on performance and immune response was partially supported by the Department of Defense (DoD), indicating the level of military interest in this dietary supplement. Likewise, although the frequency of use of tyrosine was not apparent, this amino acid has been of interest to the military and the object of research investigations to counteract the decrements in cognition that are associated with stress. Because of the reported use of weight-loss products, chromium was chosen as an example of a dietary supplement ingredient that is often found in such products. The known chronobiotic effects of melatonin may justify its use to ease the effects of jet lag as well as of long or night shifts, and therefore it was included for review. Similarly, valerian could be used for its alleged sedative properties and potential to alleviate sleep disorders, common in military life especially during demanding military operations that require long periods of wakefulness or unusual working shifts.

Details about the strategies used in conducting literature searches are described in Chapter 5. In general, the committee evaluated reviews that concentrated on safety and efficacy. For some dietary supplements (e.g., *Gingko biloba*), research on use is so broad and encompasses so many areas that the committee decided to focus the review on effects that would be of interest to the military (e.g., effects on cognition). This is especially recommended for those supplements that have already been extensively studied. Reviews of safety emphasized two areas: bioactivity and interactions with other dietary supplements or medications. For the latter, a list of the medications most frequently dispensed to active duty U.S. Army personnel was obtained from the DoD Pharmacy Operations Center, as a representation of typical medications used by military personnel. Although the committee was also asked to provide information on potential withdrawal effects, and the committee recognizes their importance, caffeine is the only supplement for which such information was found. The committee did not perform an evidence-based classification of original research on each supplement. As requested in the statement of task for this study and in accordance with the primary intent to identify supplements that pose serious concerns, the committee relied, as much as possible, on existing reviews by other authors to produce the summaries for each dietary supplement. If a review was not available for the last 10 years, original research was included. In those cases, limitations were noted where appropriate (see tables in Chapter 4).

Although the committee emphasized review of safety, the management of dietary supplements for the military needs to follow an evaluation of both risks and benefits, as the recommended framework notes. The reviews therefore also include information about benefits. When reviewing safety, effects judged to be especially pertinent to specific military subpopulations because of performance demands (e.g., cognitive or physical fitness), mission environments (e.g., high altitude, extreme temperatures), or the impact of adverse events associated with the supplement (e.g., bleeding, gastrointestinal disturbances, infectious diseases) received particular attention. The committee recognizes that when trying to identify safety concerns, the fact that dietary supplements are taken in combination and also with medications is a challenge. The committee emphasizes that it is very important that interactions between dietary supplements, medications, nutrients, and other dietary supplements be considered in all elements of this framework: when conducting surveys, when applying the framework and conducting reviews, and when examining and associating adverse events with dietary supplement use. However, when conducting the reviews, it would not be feasible for this committee to address all the potential combination scenarios for dietary supplements, and only a few known and potential interactions with medications have been noted. Because new dietary supplements are being rapidly introduced into the market, information about their quantity and purity would quickly become obsolete and, therefore, it was not included in this chapter.

Although many other dietary supplements could have been reviewed, this chapter provides a selected subset as examples of monographs developed for each dietary supplement. For example, although there are risks from the misuse of growth hormones and anabolic steroids, a review of those substances is beyond the scope of this report because they are illegal, and/or there is also no evidence of use among the military. **The monographs in this chapter were developed in order to evaluate the review process outlined in Chapter 5. They present scientific reviews of safety and efficacy, but do not attempt to provide a final assessment of safety or efficacy.** Monographs are intended to serve as one key tool for making decisions about how to manage each dietary supplement. Other factors affecting the decision-making process on managing use of a specific dietary supplement relate to the characteristics of the targeted population (see Box 1-3 in Chapter 1); that is, decisions about weighing benefits and risks as well as the level of concern will have to consider the tasks (i.e., mission risks and environments) of the subpopulation. The committee recognizes that the military leadership (e.g., local commanders, or leadership at the service or DoD level) is best informed to make such assessments. Examples of how conclusions from the panel of experts could be synthesized are shown in Chapter 5, Table 5-3. This table includes summary conclusions about the level of concern and the putative benefits that will be useful in making management decisions and for developing outreach materials. Also, Appendix D shows examples of how these monographs could serve as a scientific basis for decision making and includes suggestions for management actions for DHEA, melatonin, and *Ephedra*.

A barrier to the application of the committee's framework was the lack of data from studies designed with subpopulations or circumstances similar to those of the military. Also, data from interactions with medications were infrequently found. It should be noted that the monographs are not exhaustive and present mainly data from reviews. The committee did not provide a list of research recommendations for each dietary supplement because research priorities need to be outlined within the scope of an overall research agenda for dietary supplements; such priorities are delineated in Chapter 7.

CAFFEINE

Background

Caffeine[1] [1,3,7-trimethyl-1H-purine-2,6(3H,7H)-dione] is arguably the most widely consumed psychoactive substance in the world. It is an alkaloid that occurs naturally in the leaves, seeds, and fruit of tea, coffee, cacao, kola trees, and more than 60 other plants (Reid and Sacha, 2005). It is rapidly absorbed from the gastrointestinal tract into the bloodstream. Within 1–1.5 hours following ingestion, maximum caffeine concentrations are reached in blood, and it is readily distributed throughout the body (Nawrot et al., 2003). Natural sources of caffeine generally also contain varying mixtures of other xanthine alkaloids, including the cardiac stimulants theophylline and theobromine, and other substances such as polyphenols that can form insoluble complexes with caffeine. Caffeine is metabolized in the liver by the cytochrome P450 oxidase enzyme system (1A2 isozyme) into three metabolic dimethylxanthines: (1) paraxanthine, which increases lipolysis, leading to elevated levels of glycerol and free fatty acids; (2) theobromine, the principal alkaloid in cocoa and chocolate, which dilates blood vessels and increases urine volume; and (3) theophylline, which relaxes smooth muscles of the bronchi, and is therefore used to treat asthma (but at therapeutic doses much higher than those achieved from caffeine metabolism).

Caffeine is a central nervous system (CNS) stimulant that can also have physiological effects on the autonomic nervous system as well as the cardiovascular, respiratory, and renal systems. The actions of caffeine and its metabolites on these systems are mediated by way of several mechanisms, including antagonism of adenosine receptors (caffeine and paraxanthine are nonselective antagonists for A1 and A2a receptors, but the effect of caffeine on A3 receptors is unknown). A1 receptors have been identified in many brain regions, including the hippocampus, cerebral cortex, cerebel-

[1]The monographs were developed in order to evaluate the review process outlined in Chapter 5. The monographs present scientific reviews of safety and efficacy, but do not attempt to provide a final assessment of safety or efficacy.

lar cortex, and thalamus (Porkka-Heiskanen, 1999). Other mechanistic pathways for the effects of caffeine and its metabolites include inhibition of phosphodiesterase activity, increased calcium mobilization, and antagonism of benzodiazepine receptors. Caffeine's inhibition of phosphodiesterase activity may account for its effects on both the cardiovascular and respiratory systems in that nonxanthine phosphodiesterases are cardiac stimulants as well as effective bronchiolar and tracheal relaxants (IOM, 2001).

Caffeine in Dietary Supplements

A recent review of caffeine content in common U.S. dietary supplements evaluated 53 products with caffeine-containing ingredients as part of a study initiating the development of an analytically validated Dietary Supplement Ingredient Database (Andrews et al., 2007). Selection of products for analysis was based on market share information and included those sold as tablets, caplets, or capsules and listing at least one caffeine-containing ingredient, including botanicals such as guarana, yerba mate, kola nut, and green tea extract on the label. Products were analyzed using high-pressure liquid chromatography. Caffeine intake per serving and per day was calculated using the maximum recommendations on each product label. Laboratory analyses revealed product means ranging from 1 to 829 mg caffeine per day. "For products with a label amount for comparison (n=28), 89 percent (n=25) of the products had analytically based caffeine levels per day of between –16 percent and +16 percent of the claimed levels. Lot-to-lot variability (n=2 or 3) for caffeine in most products (72 percent) was less than 10 percent" (Andrews et al., 2007). This review article also noted that caffeine can be present in supplements as a proprietary blend, but not be listed as an ingredient on the label. Less than one-third (11 of 36) of the products whose caffeine content was more than that of one cup of brewed coffee per day listed caffeine as an ingredient, although a majority of these products (27 of 36) did voluntarily list a caffeine level on the label (Andrews et al., 2007).

Changes in Caffeine Consumption Over the Past Several Decades

It appears that coffee remains the primary source of caffeine in the diets of persons in the United States. However, the Continuing Survey of Food Intakes by Individuals (CSFII) found the consumption of caffeine from soft drinks now exceeds the consumption of caffeine from tea (Frary et al., 2005). Frary et al. compared mean values of caffeine consumption as reported by the 1989 Market Research Corporation of America (MRCA) study and the CSFII study. MRCA reported a daily mean consumption value for tea of 0.54 mg/kg, and for soft drinks, 0.27 mg/kg. In contrast, the more recent CSFII study showed that soft drink consumption exceeded tea consumption, reporting mean values of 30.6 mg (16 percent of sample size) and 23.4 mg (12 percent of sample size) respectively (Frary et al., 2005).

Table 4-1 (see pages 94–95) summarizes what is known about changes in caffeine consumption over the past several decades. Most studies do not find an increase in caffeine consumption, although in 2005, Frary et al. concluded that "During the past 20 years it appears the percentage of persons consuming caffeine has increased while mean caffeine intakes may have decreased" (Frary et al., 2005). With regard to overall changes in beverage consumption, Nielsen and Popkin (2004) concluded that "Within every age group for all other beverages—including coffee and tea, alcohol, fruit drinks, and fruit juices—the changes have been minor between 1977 and 2001."

Caffeine in Energy Drinks

Energy drinks have acquired a considerable market in recent years, substantially contributing to caffeine consumption. Consumers Union recently tested 12 carbonated energy drinks and found caffeine levels ranging from 50 mg to 145 mg per 8-ounce serving (Energy drinks, 2007). Most of the drinks tested were sold in packages containing more than 8 ounces, so consumption of the entire contents could amount to intake of over 200 mg of caffeine. Furthermore, most of the energy drinks tested contained multiple stimulants, and because caffeine content is not required by law to be listed, the amount of caffeine in an energy drink (or any food for that matter) is often unknown (Energy drinks, 2007).

Although caffeine is not classified as addictive in the *Diagnostic and Statistical Manual of Mental Disorders* of the American Psychiatric Association (APA, 1994), it has been asserted in a comprehensive review of caffeine that habitual daily use of over 500 mg of caffeine (i.e., four to seven cups of coffee or seven to nine cups of tea) represents a significant health risk and may therefore be regarded as abuse (Nawrot et al., 2003). Other mental disorders such as dependence, withdrawal syndrome, and intoxication can be caused by caffeine (Pardo et al., 2007). Therefore, "depending on its use, caffeine can be considered a nutrient, a drug, or a drug of abuse" (Pardo et al., 2007, p. 225).

Update on Institute of Medicine Caffeine Report (2001)—Putative Benefits

The Institute of Medicine (IOM) Committee on Military Nutrition Research (IOM, 2001) concluded in its report on the use of caffeine for the sustainment of mental task performance for military operations that

"Research shows that caffeine in the range of 100–600 mg is effective in increasing the speed of reaction time without affecting accuracy and in improving performance on visual and audio vigilance tasks" (IOM, 2001, p. 7). The report indicated that caffeine in doses of 100–600 mg can be used to maintain cognitive performance—particularly in situations of sleep deprivation—and doses of 200–600 mg can be effective in enhancing physical endurance. Moreover, caffeine ingestion has been often associated with a increase in endurance time in physical activities of moderate intensity and long duration (IOM, 2001). Caffeine improves aerobic endurance by increasing fat oxidation and sparing muscle glycogen (IOM, 2001). Four separate reviews (Dodd et al., 1993; Graham et al., 1994; Spriet, 1995; Tarnopolsky, 1994) concluded that caffeine consistently "enhances endurance performance in a variety of activities (i.e., running, cross-country skiing, cycling), with doses from 2 to 9 mg/kg, in naïve and habituated, trained and untrained test subjects" (IOM, 2001).

Similar conclusions and recommendations regarding the effects of caffeine on cognitive performance during sleep deprivation were reached in a 2005 review of stimulants by the Sleep Deprivation and Stimulant Task Force of the American Academy of Sleep Medicine. Their review concluded that

> Caffeine is a readily available, short-acting stimulant that has been shown to reduce some of the deficits associated with sleep loss. Studies suggest that caffeine can provide improved alertness and performance at doses of 75 to 150 mg after acute restriction of sleep and at doses of 200 to 600 mg after a night or more of total sleep loss. Caffeine is unlikely to have major disruptive effects on the sleep that follows 8 hours or longer after administration. However, frequent use of caffeine can lead to tolerance and negative withdrawal effects. (Bonnet et al., 2005, p. 1168)

While caffeine consumed too close to sleep time can interfere with sleep, caffeine appears to help reverse the effects of sleep inertia (i.e., grogginess and psychomotor lethargy immediately upon awakening from deep sleep) (Van Dongen et al., 2001).

Update on IOM Caffeine Report (2001)—Safety Concerns

The safety of caffeine as a food and beverage additive has been evaluated several times (IOM, 2001). In 1987, the U.S. Food and Drug Administration (FDA) concluded that caffeine added to beverages at a level of 0.02 percent (200 mg/L) or less did not present a health risk. Another FDA review in 1992 concluded that there was no evidence that the consumption of 100 mg per day or less of caffeine in cola beverages posed a hazard to human health (but this does not imply safety at higher doses) (Bonnet et al., 2005). It was also noted in the 2001 IOM report that caffeine might be associated with a small increase of spontaneous abortion in the first trimester of pregnancy and that it can significantly increase 24-hour urine output. These effects were not seen as limitations on the military use of caffeine, although increased urine output could provide practical problems under some operational conditions. It was recommended that daily doses should not exceed 600 mg due to possible negative effects on mood and performance at higher doses.

Nawrot et al. (2003) concluded that there is ample evidence indicating that for healthy adults, there is no association between caffeine intakes of 400 mg per day and general toxicity, increase in incidence of cancer, adverse effects in the cardiovascular system, behavior, or male fertility.

However, recent data from studies at the Walter Reed Army Institute of Research (WRAIR) show that caffeine may not benefit all aspects of neurobehavioral function in sleep-deprived subjects. During military operations, the ability to make advantageous and safe decisions is vital. A 2007 WRAIR study demonstrated that after 51 continuous hours of sleep deprivation, the decision-making process was impaired under conditions of uncertainty on the Iowa Gambling Task (Killgore et al., 2007). Caffeine was reported to have no significant beneficial effects that compensated for the detriments of sleep deprivation on the performance of this risk-taking task. Even when administered caffeine, sleep-deprived study participants frequented disadvantageous high-risk scenarios as opposed to the advantageous low-risk scenarios that were learned prior to sleep deprivation (Killgore et al., 2007).

Additional effects of caffeine may be undesirable in certain environmental conditions. Among the other physiological effects of caffeine that are relevant to the military are its effects on thermoregulation. While these effects are advantageous to tolerance of cold temperatures, in a heat stress situation, the effects would be undesirable. A review of the literature found no conclusive evidence of caffeine's effect on body temperature (Armstrong et al., 2007). However, a carefully controlled study of sustained low-dose (0.3 mg/kg/hour) caffeine intake (in tablet form) by healthy adults undergoing sleep deprivation found a reliable increase in core body temperature (measured with a continuous rectal probe) (Rogers et al., 2001). It was also found that caffeine markedly increased circulating levels of noradrenaline relative to a placebo (Price et al., 2000). Research on effects of an ephedrine–caffeine mixture showed that this mixture might also have beneficial thermoregulatory effects for cold tolerance. This effect might be in part due to an 18.6 percent increase in energy expenditure compared to placebo (Vallerand et al., 1989). In a different experiment the additive effects of caffeine and cold water exposure on energy production during submaximal exercise were observed (Doubt and Hsieh, 1991). In another placebo-controlled experiment where individuals were subjected to heat stress through physical activity, Bell et al. (1999) reported that although caffeine and ephedrine treatment increased metabolic rate during moderate exercise in a hot, dry environment, there was no increase in internal body temperature; this was possibly due to heat-loss mechanisms that offset the increase in metabolic rate.

At higher dosages and/or sustained intake, caffeine can have unwanted physiological and neurobehavioral effects. In addition to the elevated core body temperature and increased plasma noradrenaline levels described by Rogers and Dinges (2005), the adverse effects of caffeine can include locomotor agitation, tachycardia, diuresis, and increased anxiety. Numerous studies of the effect of caffeine on fluid homeostasis (diuresis) have generally found a positive correlation between caffeine consumption and increased urine output (IOM, 2001). For example, Neuhäuser-Berthold et al. (1997) administered coffee containing 642 mg of caffeine to healthy volunteers over a single day and monitored fluid homeostasis in comparison with a control group given an equal amount of mineral water. The caffeine group had a highly significant increase in 24-hour urine output, corresponding to negative fluid balance and a decrease in body weight (IOM, 2001). Decreased electrolyte (sodium and potassium) levels have also been documented as a result of diuresis; however, a normal diet will restore the homeostatic balance (Armstrong et al., 2007; IOM, 2001). Moreover, fluid and food intake should be monitored under conditions of sustained military operations in hot and cold environments or at high altitudes, as these may present potential for augmented risk of dehydration (IOM, 2001).

Interactions with Other Dietary Supplements or Medications

Research has shown that caffeine interacts with other drugs in many different ways, although the magnitude of interaction is dependent on dosage. For example, diazepam (i.e., Valium) is an anxiolytic that is prescribed as a muscle relaxant, sedative-hypnotic, and anticonvulsant (Roache and Griffiths, 1987). Caffeine and diazepam produce disparate effects on the CNS through functionally opposing mechanisms. Caffeine has been demonstrated to antagonize subjects' ratings of sedation and impairment of psychomotor vigilance caused by diazepam, while diazepam countered the restlessness and subject ratings of tension, alertness, and arousal caused by caffeine (Roache and Griffiths, 1987). Less is known about the extent to which caffeine has synergistic effects with other stimulants.

Caffeine Withdrawal

The most commonly reported symptoms following withdrawal of caffeine, even at doses as low as 100 mg, are headache, irritability, increased fatigue and drowsiness, decreased alertness, difficulty concentrating, nervousness, confusion, depressed mood, and decreased energy and activity levels (Nehlig, 1999). These symptoms are typically short-lived and mild to moderate in severity. Despite the long history of use of caffeine, there have been few studies that systematically examined the nature of caffeine withdrawal (Rogers and Dinges, 2005). Depending on dosage and proximity to sleep time, caffeine can disturb sleep by lengthening sleep latency and reducing total sleep time and sleep efficiency (Rogers and Dinges, 2005). Care should therefore be taken to ensure that caffeine use by military personnel does not interfere with sleep when the latter is desirable.

Considerations Specific to the Military

Military engagements often involve extended periods of sleep restriction that are accompanied by well-documented physical and cognitive impairment (Killgore et al., 2007). Consistent with the 2001 IOM report on the military use of caffeine, studies continue to find that caffeine is an effective countermeasure to the detriments of sleep deprivation. These studies support "the recommendation for the use of caffeine to extend the period of operational effectiveness during the conduct of military operations that involve unavoidable periods of sleep loss over a three to four day period" (McLellan et al., 2007). In this 2007 study, the use of 800 mg of caffeine throughout three overnight periods maintained alertness and vigilance in comparison to a placebo group (without caffeine) (McLellan et al., 2007). However, it must also be noted that chronic frequent use of caffeine can lead to tolerance and reduce the benefits of caffeine as a countermeasure for sleep deprivation during military operations. To the extent that caffeine is being consumed in ever-larger doses via coffee, soft drinks, energy drinks, and dietary supplements or medications, the military benefits of caffeine as a cognitive and physical performance enhancer may be reduced by tolerance from such widespread consumption of caffeine (see also Chapter 2, regarding the need for obtaining ingredient identification in dietary supplement products and total dosage consumed). In addition, caffeine may not benefit all aspects of cognitive and neurobehavioral functions (e.g., risk-taking decisions), and it may produce physiological effects (e.g., heat retention, diuresis) that may compromise physical performance in certain environments (e.g., hot climates).

A summary of average daily consumption (ADC) of caffeine in the United States is shown in Table 4-1.

TABLE 4-1 Summary of Average Daily Consumption (ADC) of Caffeine in the United States

Reference	Source Data	Mean ADC
Graham, 1978	NAS[a]: Generally Recognized as Safe (GRAS) survey, 1977	Adults: 227 mg/day Children: 101 mg/day
Pao et al., 1982	USDA[b]: Nationwide Food Consumption Survey (NFCS), 1977–1978	Coffee drinkers: 3.3 mg/kg Tea drinkers: 1.1 mg/kg Cola drinkers: 0.4 mg/kg
Barone and Roberts, 1996	MRCA: National Household Menu Census Survey, 1989	Adults: 2.4 mg/kg Children: <1 mg/kg
Knight et al., 2004	NFO WorldGroup: Share of Intake Panel Survey, 1999	Adults: 1.5–2.3 mg/kg
Frary et al., 2005	USDA: CSFII, 1994, 1996, and 1998	ADC calculations in this paper are unreliable

NOTE: Average consumption numbers are based on responses from "caffeine consumers," not the entire population. The most recent paper attempting to determine average caffeine intake was published in 2004, using data from a survey taken in 1999. Thus, none of the data takes into consideration the recent surge in sales of energy drinks. In addition, the results of different

References

Andrews, K. W., A. Schweitzer, C. Zhao, J. M. Holden, J. M. Roseland, M. Brandt, J. T. Dwyer, M. F. Picciano, L. G. Saldanha, K. D. Fisher, E. Yetley, J. M. Betz, and L. Douglass. 2007. The caffeine contents of dietary supplements commonly purchased in the U.S.: Analysis of 53 products with caffeine-containing ingredients. *Annal Bioanal Chem* 389(1):231-239.

APA (American Psychiatric Association). 1994. *Diagnostic and statistical manual of mental disorders (DSM-IV)*. Arlington, VA: APA.

Armstrong, L. E., D. J. Casa, C. M. Maresh, and M. S. Ganio. 2007. Caffeine, fluid-electrolyte balance, temperature regulation, and exercise-heat tolerance. *Exerc Sport Sci Rev* 35(3): 135-140.

Barone, J. J., and H. R. Roberts. 1996. Caffeine consumption. *Food Chem Toxicol* 34(1): 119-129.

Bell, D. G., I. Jacobs, T. M. McLellan, M. Miyazaki, and C. M. Sabiston. 1999. Thermal regulation in the heat during exercise after caffeine and ephedrine ingestion. *Aviat Space Environ Med* 70(6):583-588.

Bonnet, M. H., T. J. Balkin, D. F. Dinges, T. Roehrs, N. L. Rogers, N. J. Wesensten, and Sleep Deprivation and Stimulant Task Force of the American Academy of Sleep Medicine. 2005. The use of stimulants to modify performance during sleep loss: A review by the Sleep Deprivation and Stimulant Task Force of the American Academy of Sleep Medicine. *Sleep* 28(9):1163-1187.

Dodd, S. L., R. A. Herb, and S. K. Powers. 1993. Caffeine and exercise performance: An update. *Sports Med* 15(1):14-23.

90th Percentile ADC	Conclusions
Adults: 5.2 mg/kg Children: <2 mg/kg	The authors report slight declines in ADC when comparing the MRCA surveys of 1975 and 1989, but slight increases when comparing the USDA NFCS surveys of 1977 and 1987.
Adults: 3.2–5.2 mg/kg	Men and nonpregnant women in the same age groups consumed similar amounts of caffeine.
	The authors conclude that the percentage of American adults who consume caffeine is increasing when comparing the 1977 GRAS surveys and 1998 CSFII (82% and 87%).

papers cannot be validly and reliably compared when trying to quantify a change in average caffeine consumption in recent years because the methodology is poorly defined. Finally, no paper includes caffeine obtained through dietary supplements.

[a]National Academy of Sciences.

[b]U.S. Department of Agriculture.

Doubt, T. J., and S. S. Hsieh. 1991. Additive effects of caffeine and cold water during submaximal leg exercise. *Med Sci Sports Exerc* 23(4):435-442.

Energy drinks: Behind the buzz. 2007. *Consum Rep* 72(9):6.

Frary, C. D., R. K. Johnson, and M. Q. Wang. 2005. Food sources and intakes of caffeine in the diets of persons in the United States. *J Am Diet Assoc* 105(1):110-113.

Graham, D. M. 1978. Caffeine—It's identity, dietary sources, intake and biological effects. *Nutr Rev* 36(4):97-102.

Graham, T. E., J. W. Rush, and M. H. van Soeren. 1994. Caffeine and exercise: Metabolism and performance. *Can J Appl Physiol* 19(2):111-138.

IOM (Institute of Medicine). 2001. *Caffeine for the sustainment of mental task performance: Formulations for military operations.* Washington, DC: National Academy Press.

Killgore, D. S., E. L. Lipizzi, G. H. Kamimori, and T. J. Balkin. 2007. Caffeine effects on risky decision making after 75 hours of sleep deprivation. *Aviat Space Environ Med* 78(10):957-962.

Knight, C. A., I. Knight, D. C. Mitchell, and J. E. Zepp. 2004. Beverage caffeine intake in U.S. consumers and subpopulations of interest: Estimates from the Share of Intake Panel Survey. *Food Chem Toxicol* 42(12):1923-1930.

McLellan, T. M., G. H. Kamimori, D. M. Voss, T. Charmaine, and S. J. R. Smith. 2007. Caffeine effects on physical and cognitive performance during sustained operations. *Aviat Space Environ Med* 78(9):871-877.

Nawrot P., S. Jordan, J. Eastwood, J. Rotstein, A. Hugenholtz, and M. Feeley. 2003. Effects of caffeine on human health. *Food Addit Contam* 20(1):1-30.

Nehlig, A. 1999. Are we dependent upon coffee and caffeine? A review on human and animal data. *Neurosci Biobehav Rev* 23(4):563-576.

Neuhäuser-Berthold, M., S. Beine, S. C. Verwied, and P. M. Lührmann. 1997. Coffee consumption and total body water homeostasis as measured by fluid balance and bioelectrical impedance analysis. *Ann Nutr Metab* 41(1):29-36.

Nielsen, S. J., and B. M. Popkin. 2004. Changes in beverage intake between 1977 and 2001. *Am J Prev Med* 27(3):205-210.

Pao, E. M., K. Fleming, P. M. Guenther, and S. J. Mickel. 1982. Foods commonly eaten by individuals: Amount per day and per eating occasion. USDA Home Economics Research Report No. 44.

Pardo, L. R., G. Y. Alvarez, T. D. Barral, and A. M. Farré. 2007. Caffeine: A nutrient, a drug, or a drug of abuse. *Adicciones* 19(2):225-238.

Porkka-Heiskanen, T. 1999. Adenosine in sleep and wakefulness. *Ann Med* 31(2):125-129.

Price, N. J., J. M. Mullington, S. Kapoor, S. Samuel, M. P. Szuba, and D. F. Dinges. 2000. Plasma norepinephrine during 66 hr of sustained low-dose caffeine intake and 88 hr of sleep deprivation. *Sleep* 23(Suppl 1):A119.

Reid, T. R., and B. Sacha. 2005. Caffeine. *National Geographic* 207(1):2-33.

Roache, J. D., and R. R. Griffiths. 1987. Interactions of diazepam and caffeine: Behavioral and subjective dose effects in humans. *Pharmacol Biochem Behav* 26(4):801-812.

Rogers, N. L., and D. F. Dinges. 2005. Caffeine: Implications for alertness in athletes. *Clin Sports Med* 24(2):e1-e13.

Rogers, N. L., N. J. Price, M. P. Szuba, H. P. Van Dongen, and D. F. Dinges. 2001. Effect of sustained caffeine on core body temperature during 88 hours of sustained wakefulness. *Sleep* 24(Abstract Suppl):A172-A173.

Spriet, L. L. 1995. Caffeine and performace. *Int J Sport Nutr* 5(Suppl):S84-S99.

Tarnopolsky, M. A. 1994. Caffeine and endurance performance. *Sports Med* 18(2):109-125.

Vallerand, A. L., I. Jacobs, M. F. Kavanagh. 1989. Mechanism of enhanced cold tolerance by an ephedrine-caffeine mixture in humans. *J Appl Physiol* 67(1):438-444.

Van Dongen, H. P., N. J. Price, J. M. Mullington, M. P. Szuba, S. C. Kapoor, and D. F. Dinges. 2001. Caffeine eliminates psychomotor vigilance deficits from sleep inertia. *Sleep* 24(7):813-819.

CHROMIUM

Background

Chromium,[2] an essential trace mineral, is important for the metabolism of carbohydrate, fat, and protein. Chromium enhances the action of insulin and is associated with improved glucose tolerance and lipid-lipoprotein profiles. In 2001, the Food and Nutrition Board of the Institute of Medicine (IOM) determined the Recommended Dietary Allowance for chromium to be 35 μg for adult males and 25 μg for adult females. Relatively high concentrations of chromium are found in processed meats, ready-to-eat bran cereals, whole-grain products, green beans, and broccoli, and relatively low concentrations in foods high in simple sugars (Lukaski, 1999). Estimates of nutrient intakes indicate that the diets of most Americans provide sufficient amounts of chromium (ODS, 2005; Vincent, 2003a).

[2]The monographs were developed in order to evaluate the review process outlined in Chapter 5. The monographs present scientific reviews of safety and efficacy, but do not attempt to provide a final assessment of safety or efficacy.

Absorption of dietary chromium in the intestines ranges from 0.5 percent to 2.0 percent. This variation is related to intake of the mineral: As dietary intake of chromium increases, absorption of the mineral decreases. Moreover, both dietary and nondietary factors can moderate chromium absorption. For example, foods containing ascorbic acid promote chromium absorption, while foods containing phytates, which bind to chromium, inhibit transport of the mineral across the intestinal tract (Lukaski, 1999). Chromium absorption is also reduced by medicines that alter stomach acidity, such as antacids, corticosteroids, and proton pump inhibitors, and by other medicines including beta-blockers, insulin, nonsteroidal anti-inflammatory drugs, and prostaglandin inhibitors (ODS, 2005).

Although chromium deficiency is rare, patients maintained on intravenous solutions that do not contain the mineral can suffer from impaired control of blood glucose levels, elevated triglyceride and cholesterol levels, and peripheral neuropathy. Treatment with chromium rapidly reversed these symptoms (Lukaski, 1999; ODS, 2005; Stoecker, 2001; Vincent, 2003a). Marginal intake of chromium coupled with physiological stressors such as physical trauma and acute exercise that might occur in a military setting increases the possibility of chromium deficiency (Lukaski, 1999).

Chromium in the form of chromium picolinate, which is the salt of chromium with three molecules of the intermediary metabolite picolinic acid, has been widely promoted as a dietary supplement for stimulating weight loss, increasing lean body mass, promoting longevity, and enhancing fitness (Evans, 1989; IOM, 2000; Pittler et al., 2003). Chromium picolinate is found both as a single-ingredient dietary supplement and as a component of multivitamin and multimineral products including pills, energy drinks, energy bars, and chewing gums (Andersson et al., 2007). Although chromium picolinate is the most widely used form of the mineral, chromium nicotinate, chromium chloride, and chromium histidine are also found in dietary supplements. The various forms of the mineral differ in absorbability; data indicating that the picolinate form was absorbed more readily than the nicotinate or chloride form contributed to the popularity of the picolinate form of the mineral in dietary supplements (DiSilvestro and Dy, 2007). However, more recent research demonstrating that chromium histidine is absorbed almost twice as well as chromium picolinate could lead to an increase in the use of supplements containing this form of the mineral (Anderson et al., 2004).

Putative Benefits

Initial support for a beneficial role of chromium picolinate supplements in the management of body composition came from a 1989 study. College-age athletes participating in a strength-training program who were given 200 mg of chromium picolinate for 6 weeks lost more weight and gained more lean body mass than athletes not taking the supplement (Evans, 1989). This report was followed by a spectacular rise in the sales of chromium picolinate, making it one of the most widely used nutrient supplements for weight loss and/or muscle development (Sharpe et al., 2006; Vincent, 2003b). The study by Evans, however, presents methodological problems; for instance, there was no control over prior training, and differences found in anthropomorphic measurements appeared to be functionally not significant (Lefavi et al., 1992).

Although chromium picolinate continues to be vigorously marketed and used, the supplement's ability to alter body composition is questionable (Hallmark et al., 1996; Lukaski et al., 2007; Nissen and Sharp, 2003; Pittler et al., 2003; Stallings and Vincent, 2006; Vincent, 2003a,b). A 2003 meta-analysis of 10 double-blind, randomized control trials concluded that individuals taking 200 to 400 μg of chromium picolinate on a daily basis for 6 to 14 weeks lost approximately 1.1 kg more (i.e., 0.08–0.2 kg/week) during the intervention and increased lean body mass to a slightly greater degree than those taking a placebo (Pittler et al., 2003). More detailed examination revealed that data from only two of the trials accounted for most of the observed differences in body composition between individuals taking chromium picolinate and those taking a placebo. These findings suggest that the effects of chromium picolinate on weight loss and body composition are small and of marginal clinical significance (Pittler et al., 2003). More recent studies have confirmed this suggestion (Lukaski et al., 2007). Taken together, the results of studies evaluating the effects of chromium picolinate on body weight and composition indicate that the supplement is not a useful adjunct to either weight reduction or body building programs.

Safety Concerns

No frequent, consistent adverse events have been reported in studies assessing the use of chromium picolinate for periods of up to 3 months. However, a few isolated reports of detrimental effects of taking chromium picolinate, including weight loss, changes in cognitive behavior, allergic skin disorders, renal failure, and liver dysfunction have appeared in the literature (Jeejeebhoy, 1999; Lamson and Plaza, 2002; Lukaski, 1999; Vincent, 2003b; Wani et al., 2006). Additional studies addressing the genotoxic and cytotoxic effects of trivalent chromium complexes have led to the conclusion that these toxic effects of chromium are not a concern for individuals taking supplements containing the mineral (Andersson et al., 2007; Hininger et al., 2007; Lamson and Plaza, 2002). Taking the preceding findings together, there is insufficient evidence to indicate concern about the safety of chromium-containing supplements as presently used, and therefore, a Tolerable Upper Intake Level has not been established by the IOM (IOM, 2005; Lukaski, 1999; ODS, 2005).

Considerations Specific to the Military

Studies on the effects of chromium picolinate on body weight and composition have not been conducted in military settings. However, research involving individuals engaged in strength-training programs similar to those that might be used in a military setting (e.g., weight lifters, varsity wrestlers) indicates that the benefits of chromium picolinate for decreasing body weight while increasing lean body mass are limited at best.

Relevant data and conclusions on efficacy and safety reviews and publications identified for chromium are shown in Table 4-2 on pages 156–159.

References

Anderson, R. A., M. M. Polansky, and N. A. Bryden. 2004. Stability and absorption of chromium and absorption of chromium and absorption of chromium histidinate complexes by humans. *Biol Trace Elem Res* 101(3):211-218.

Andersson, M. A., K. V. P. Grawe, O. M. Karlsson, L. A. Abramsson-Zetterberg, and B. E. Hellman. 2007. Evaluation of the potential genotoxicity of chromium picolinate in mammalian cells *in vivo* and *in vitro*. *Food Chem Toxicol* 45(7):1097-1106.

Campbell, W. W., L. J. Joseph, S. L. Davey, D. Cyr-Campbell, R. A. Anderson, and W. J. Evans. 1999. Effects of resistance training and chromium picolinate on body composition and skeletal muscle in older men. *J Appl Physiol* 86(1):29-39.

Diaz, M. L., B. A. Watkins, Y. Li, R. A. Anderson, and W. W. Campbell. 2008. Chromium picolinate and conjugated linoleic acid do not synergistically influence diet- and exercise-induced changes in body composition and health indexes in overweight women. *J Nutr Biochem* 19(1):61-68.

DiSilvestro, R. A., and E. Dy. 2007. Comparison of acute absorption of commercially available chromium supplements. *J Trace Elem Med Biol* 21(2):120-124.

Evans, G. W. 1989. The effect of chromium picolinate on insulin controlled parameters in humans. *Int J Biosoc Med Res* 11(2):163-180.

Hallmark, M. A., T. H. Reynolds, C. A. DeSouza, C. O. Dotson, R. A. Anderson, and M. A. Rogers. 1996. Effects of chromium and resistive training on muscle strength and body composition. *Med Sci Sports Exerc* 28(1):139-144.

Hininger, I., R. Benaraba, M. Osman, H. Faure, A. M. Roussel, and R. A. Anderson. 2007. Safety of trivalent chromium complexes: No evidence for DNA damage in human HACaT keratinocytes. *Free Radic Biol Med* 42(12):1759-1765.

IOM (Institute of Medicine). 2000. *Dietary reference intakes for vitamin A, vitamin K, arsenic, boron, chromium, copper, iodine, iron, manganese, molybdenum, nickel, silicon, vanadium, and zinc.* Washington, DC: National Academy Press.

IOM. 2005. *Nutrient composition of rations for short-term, high-intensity combat operations.* Washington, DC: The National Academies Press.

Jeejeebhoy, K. N. 1999. The role of chromium in nutrition and therapeutics and as a potential toxin. *Nutr Rev* 57(11):329-335.

Lamson, D. W., and S. M. Plaza. 2002. The safety and efficacy of high-dose chromium. *Altern Med Rev* 7(3):218-235.

Lefavi, R., R. A. Anderson, R. E. Keith, G. D. Wilson, J. L. McMillan, and M. H. Stone. 1992. Efficacy of chromium supplementation in athletes: Emphasis on anabolism. *Int J Sport Nutr* 2(2):111-122.

Livolsi, J. M., G. M. Adams, and P. L. Laguna. 2001. The effect of chromium picolinate on muscular strength and body composition in women athletes. *J Strength Cond Res* 15(2):161-166.

Lukaski, H. C. 1999. Chromium as a supplement. *Annu Rev Nutr* 19:279-302.

Lukaski, H. C., W. A. Siders, and J. G. Penland. 2007. Chromium picolinate supplementation in women: Effects on body weight, composition, and iron status. *Nutrition* 23(3): 187-195.

Martin, J., Z. Q. Wang, X. H. Zhang, D. Watchel, J. Volaufova, D. E. Matthews, and W. T. Cefalu. 2006. Chromium picolinate supplementation attenuates body weight gain and increases insulin sensitivity in subjects with type 2 diabetes. *Diabetes Care* 29(8):1826-1832.

Nissen, S. L., and R. L. Sharp. 2003. Effect of dietary supplements on lean mass and strength gains with resistance exercise: A meta-analysis. *J Appl Physiol* 94(2):651-659.

ODS (Office of Dietary Supplements). 2005. *Dietary supplement fact sheet: Chromium.* http://ods.od.nih.gov/factsheets/chromium.asp (accessed September 5, 2007).

Pittler, M. H., C. Stevinson, and E. Ernst. 2003. Chromium picolinate for reducing body weight: Meta-analysis of randomized trials. *Int J Obes Relat Metab Disord* 27(4): 522-529.

Sharpe, P. A., M. L. Granner, J. M. Conway, B. E. Ainsworth, and M. Dobre. 2006. Availability of weight-loss supplements: Results of an audit of retail outlets in a southeastern city. *J Am Diet Assoc* 106(12):2045-2051.

Stallings, D., and J. B. Vincent. 2006. Chromium: A case study in how not to perform nutritional research. *Curr Topics Nutraceut Res* 4(2):89-112.

Stoecker, B. J. 2001. Chromium. In *Present knowledge in nutrition*, 8th ed., edited by B. A. Bowman and R. M. Russell. Washington, DC: ILSI Press. Pp. 366-372.

Trumbo, P. R., and K. C. Ellwood. 2006. Chromium picolinate intake and risk of type 2 diabetes: An evidence-based review by the United States Food and Drug Administration. *Nutr Rev* 64(8):357-363.

Vincent, J. B. 2003a. Recent advances in the biochemistry of chromium (III). *J Trace Elem Exp Med* 16(4):227-236.

Vincent, J. B. 2003b. The potential value and toxicity of chromium picolinate as a nutritional supplement, weight loss agent and muscle development agent. *Sports Med* 33(3):213-230.

Wani, S., C. Weskamp, J. Marple, and L. Spry. 2006. Acute tubular necrosis associated with chromium picolinate-containing dietary supplement. *Ann Pharmacother* 40(3): 563-566.

CREATINE

Background

Creatine[3] is a natural component of the body that is synthesized principally in the liver and composed of the essential amino acids methionine, arginine, and glycine. The daily turnover of creatine is about 2 g/day (Shao and Hathcock, 2006), with about half coming from the diet and half from

[3]The monographs were developed in order to evaluate the review process outlined in Chapter 5. The monographs present scientific reviews of safety and efficacy, but do not attempt to provide a final assessment of safety or efficacy.

endogenous synthesis with catabolism through nonenzymatic production of creatinine. The principal dietary sources are protein foods such as meat, fish, and poultry, since most creatine (approximately 95 percent) is found in skeletal muscle. Creatine's primary role in human metabolism is as an intracellular storage form of high-energy phosphate bonds that can serve as a source of energy without the requirement for oxidative metabolism when the minute storage amount of adenosine-5′-triphosphate is consumed during brief periods of high energy consumption, as during high-intensity muscular activity. Thus, as might be expected, short-term creatine administration primarily benefits anaerobic performance, while longer-term use increases the development of strength and fosters lean tissue accretion with resistance exercise (Volek et al., 2006); there is evidence suggesting that this increase is primarily caused by an anticatabolic effect in skeletal muscle (Parise et al., 2001).

Creatine supplementation is thought to increase the size of the creatine phosphate pool in muscle, and a pattern of nonresponsiveness in a significant minority of subjects may be attributable to an already optimal pool of creatine phosphate (Calfee and Fadale, 2006). Although creatine was initially provided with up to a week of loading with 20–30 g/day followed by 5 g/day, the current mode of use is to provide the smaller dose daily in relation to the beginning or end of exercise (Bemben and Lamont, 2005; Shao and Hathcock, 2006).

Putative Benefits

Nearly 100 randomized trials of creatine supplementation have been conducted in the past decade, generally with beneficial results on short, repeated bouts of high-intensity exercise (Bemben and Lamont, 2005). Despite considerable variability in results, there is an average greater gain of 2–5 pounds of muscle mass and 5–15 percent of muscle power and strength with creatine compared to placebo (Bemben and Lamont, 2005; Shao and Hathcock, 2006). Although studies have been conducted mostly in men, similar results for improvement of performance in high-intensity activity or exercise or increased strength and improved body composition (lean body mass gains) with resistance training have been found in women (Volek et al., 2006). As might be anticipated from the mode of action, there is little or no evidence for improvement in endurance or aerobic performance (Bemben and Lamont, 2005).

A recent review of the literature confirms the lack of effect for submaximal aerobic training in young men and women (Reardon et al., 2006), for tennis-specific training (Pluim et al., 2006), multiple sprint running performance (Glaister et al., 2006), and sprint skating in hockey players (Cornish et al., 2006). Thus, creatine can be a relatively safe and effective ergogenic aid, but its value for any specific activity does need to be examined. For the military, an additional cogent application is suggested by the recent preliminary report that creatine supplementation showed a positive effect on cognitive and psychomotor performance and mood state following 24 hours of sleep deprivation (McMorris et al., 2006). This is in agreement with the fact that creatine is found in the brain, and creatine monohydrate supplementation increases brain creatine content (Dechent et al., 1999). A study by Warber et al. (2002) confirmed the ability of creatine to increase muscle strength and lean tissue but showed no benefit for the military obstacle course.

There is also substantial evidence from animal studies that creatine intake may be useful in protecting against traumatic brain injury, perhaps through improvement of mitochondrial bioenergetics (Scheff and Dhillon, 2004; Sullivan et al., 2000).

Safety Concerns

The Tolerable Upper Intake Level (UL) for creatine was not derived from a recent risk assessment based on cumulative studies in animals and humans. Rather, a newer assessment method, the Observed Safe Level, was utilized. It suggests that the evidence for safety is strong for chronic intakes of 5 g/day (Shao and Hathcock, 2006). Although there was some concern about gastrointestinal side effects (Calfee and Fadale, 2006), these were either mild or not found in randomized trials (Shao and Hathcock, 2006). There is also concern about two noted cases of renal function compromise (Calfee and Fadale, 2006; Shao and Hathcock, 2006), one of whom had underlying renal disease, and a third case of reversible renal failure in a healthy 24-year-old taking creatine as well as multiple other supplements used for bodybuilding (Thorsteinsdottir et al., 2006).

Interactions with Other Dietary Supplements or Medications

Research on the pharmacokinetics of creatine is limited, but effects of caffeine and carbohydrate intake on creatine transporters have been noted (Persky et al., 2003). The limited data and studies available do suggest important interactions with caffeine that are relevant particularly because caffeine, widely used in the military, is so often employed as an ergogenic aid. One study reported an ergogenic effect of the combination (Doherty et al., 2002); another reported opposing effects on muscle relaxation time that were nullified when creatine and caffeine were combined (Hespel et al., 2002). Several studies in human subjects have demonstrated improvements in glucose tolerance with creatine taken alone (Derave et al., 2003; Gualano et al., 2007) or combined with protein supplementation (Op't Eijnde et al.,

2006), a popular combination for users of creatine. Although statin drugs interact with numerous other drugs, low levels of toxicity were found with use in combination with other drugs (Law and Rudnicka, 2006). The absence of reported interactions of creatine with the common statin drugs presumably implies a very low level of concern; most likely the absence of reported interactions is because populations that take statins are different from those who consume creatine. There is also a paucity of data on the interaction of creatine with analgesics and nonsteroidal anti-inflammatory drugs, an instance in which the two patient populations should overlap in a significant manner. However, there is one interesting report of a significant positive interaction—the combination of creatine with cyclooxygenase-2 inhibitors produced additive neuroprotective effects and extended survival by 30 percent—in an animal model of amyotrophic lateral sclerosis (Klivenyi et al., 2004). Finally, although vitamin supplementation is probably common among those who take creatine supplements, data about significant interactions are sparse. There is one report that creatine lowers homocysteine concentration (Korzun, 2004), which might be of some interest, given the effect of vitamins B_{12}, pyridoxine, and folic acid on homocysteine.

Considerations Specific to the Military

Although studies are not definitive, some trials with creatine in subjects involved in high-intensity activities and sports with a high likelihood of injury have shown very little evidence for concern (Greenwood et al., 2003; Hoffman et al., 2006; Santos et al., 2004). Performance is often enhanced or injury lessened. This suggests that there is, if anything, improvement in conditions where injury is common (e.g., sports), and no evidence for bleeding complications.

There are no data on creatine intake and tolerance of cold. The available studies suggest either no impact or improvement in tolerance of thermal stress (Kilduff et al., 2004; Mendel et al., 2005; Volek et al., 2001; Weiss and Powers, 2006). There are no data available on the effect of creatine use at high altitudes.

Given the large amount of creatine usually provided and its intracellular location, there have been concerns about dehydration or local fluid retention and even risk of heatstroke (Bailes et al., 2002). However, in clinical trials and experience in sports usage, there is little evidence for cramping, diarrhea, or dehydration (Graham and Hatton, 1999; Greenwood et al., 2003; Santos et al., 2004; Smith and Dahm, 2000). There was an increase noted in all fluid volumes in one study of creatine use (Weiss and Powers, 2006). A trial of 175 subjects showed few adverse effects, although edematous limbs presumed secondary to fluid retention were seen more commonly in those taking creatine than those in the placebo group (Groeneveld et al.,

2005). However, a single randomized study of musculotendinous injury, which might be considered a consequence of overhydrated tissues, did not demonstrate this effect (Watsford et al., 2003). Although fluid retention may be related to the intracellular location of creatine, this does not seem to present a major concern in terms of effects on body weight.

Diarrhea was generally not a problem associated with creatine use (Graham and Hatton, 1999; Greenwood et al., 2003; Santos et al., 2004; Smith and Dahm, 2000). In the trial of 175 subjects, severe diarrhea, responsive to discontinuation of creatine, was seen in two subjects (Groeneveld et al., 2005). No data are available on infectious disease and creatine intake.

There has been concern about renal dysfunction as well as two reported cases of renal failure and three deaths in American wrestlers, but minimal impact of creatine intake on renal function was seen in short- and intermediate-term trials (Pline and Smith, 2005; Pritchard and Kalra, 1998; Watsford et al., 2003). Thus, renal function compromise may represent an idiosyncratic reaction, perhaps related to dose or related by association only. It does, however, remain a concern.

Relevant data and conclusions on efficacy and safety reviews and publications identified for creatine are shown in Table 4-3 on pages 160–181.

References

Bailes, J. E., R. C. Cantu, and A. L. Day. 2002. The neurosurgeon in sport: Awareness of the risks of heatstroke and dietary supplements. *Neurosurgery* 51(2):283-286.

Bemben, M., and H. Lamont. 2005. Creatine supplementation and exercise performance: Recent findings. *Sports Med* 35(2):107-125.

Calfee, R., and P. Fadale. 2006. Popular ergogenic drugs and supplements in young athletes. *Pediatrics* 117(3):e577-e589.

Cornish, S., P. Chilibeck, and D. Burke. 2006. The effect of creatine monohydrate supplementation on sprint skating in ice-hockey players. *J Sports Med Phys Fitness* 46:90-98.

Dechent, P., P. Pouwels, B. Wilken, F. Hanefeld, and J. Frahm. 1999. Increase of total creatine in human brain after oral supplementation of creatine-monohydrate. *Am J Physiol Regul Integr Comp Physiol* 277(3):R698-R704.

Derave, W., B. O. Eijnde, P. Verbessem, M. Ramaekers, M. Van Leemputte, E. A. Richter, and P. Hespel. 2003. Combined creatine and protein supplementation in conjunction with resistance training promotes muscle GLUT-4 content and glucose tolerance in humans. *J Appl Physiol* 94(5):1910-1916.

Doherty, M., P. M. Smith, R. C. Davison, and M. G. Hughes. 2002. Caffeine is ergogenic after supplementation of oral creatine monohydrate. *Med Sci Sports Exerc* 34(11): 1785-1792.

Glaister, M., R. Lockey, C. Abraham, A. Staerck, J. Goodwin, and G. McInnnes. 2006. Creatine supplementation and multiple sprint running performance. *J Strength Cond Res* 20(2):273-277.

Graham, A. S., and R. C. Hatton. 1999. Creatine: A review of efficacy and safety. *J Am Pharm Assoc (Wash)* 39(6):803-810.

Greenwood, M., R. B. Kreider, C. Melton, C. Rasmussen, S. Lancaster, E. Cantler, and P. Milnor. 2003. Creatine supplementation during college football training does not increase the incidence of cramping or injury. *Mol Cell Biochem* 244(1-2):83-88.

Groeneveld, G. J., C. Beijer, J. H. Veldink, S. Kalmijn, J. H. Wokke, and L. H. van den Berg. 2005. Few adverse effects of long-term creatine supplementation in a placebo-controlled trial. *Int J Sports Med* 26(4):307-313.

Gualano, B., R. B. Novaes, G. G. Artioli, T. O. Freire, D. F. Coelho, F. B. Scagliusi, P. S. Rogeri, H. Roschel, C. Ugrinowitsch, and A. H. Lancha, Jr. 2008. Effects of creatine supplementation on glucose tolerance and insulin sensitivity in sedentary healthy males undergoing aerobic training. *Amino Acids* 34(2):245-250.

Hespel, P., B. Op't Eijnde, and M. Van Leemputte. 2002. Opposite actions of caffeine and creatine on muscle relaxation time in humans. *J Appl Physiol* 92(2):513-518.

Hoffman, J., N. Ratamess, J. Kang, G. Mangine, A. Faigenbaum, and J. Stout. 2006. Effect of creatine and beta-alanine supplementation on performance and endocrine responses in strength/power athletes. *Int J Sport Nutr Exerc Metab* 16(4):430-446.

Kilduff, L. P., E. Georgiades, N. James, R. H. Minnion, M. Mitchell, D. Kingsmore, M. Hadjicharlambous, and Y. P. Pitsiladis. 2004. The effects of creatine supplementation on cardiovascular, metabolic, and thermoregulatory responses during exercise in the heat in endurance-trained humans. *Int J Sport Nutr Exerc Metab* 14(4):443-460.

Klivenyi, P., M. Kiaei, G. Gardian, N. Y. Calingasan, and M. F. Beal. 2004. Additive neuroprotective effects of creatine and cyclooxygenase 2 inhibitors in a transgenic mouse model of amyotrophic lateral sclerosis. *J Neurochem* 88(3):576-582.

Korzun, W. J. 2004. Oral creatine supplements lower plasma homocysteine concentrations in humans. *Clin Lab Sci* 17(2):102-106.

Law, M., and A. R. Rudnicka. 2006. Statin safety: A systematic review. *Am J Cardiol* 97(8): S52-S60.

McMorris, T., R. Harris, J. Swain, J. Corbett, K. Collard, R. Dyson, L. Dye, C. Hodgson, and N. Draper. 2006. Effect of creatine supplementation and sleep deprivation, with mild exercise, on cognitive and psychomotor performance, mood state, and plasma concentrations of catecholamines and cortisol. *Psychopharmacology (Berl)* 185(1):93-103.

Mendel, R. W., M. Blegen, C. Cheatham, J. Antonio, and T. Ziegenfuss. 2005. Effects of creatine on thermoregulatory responses while exercising in the heat. *Nutrition* 21(3): 301-307.

Op't Eijnde, B., H. Jijakli, P. Hespel, and W. J. Malaisse. 2006. Creatine supplementation increases soleus muscle creatine content and lowers the insulinogenic index in an animal model of inherited type 2 diabetes. *Int J Mol Med* 17(6):1077-1084.

Parise, G., S. Mihic, D. MacLennan, K. E. Yarasheski, and M. A. Tarnopolsky. 2001. Effects of acute creatine monohydrate supplementation on leucine kinetics and mixed-muscle protein synthesis. *J Appl Physiol* 91(3):1041-1047.

Persky, A. M., G. A. Brazeau, and G. Hochhaus. 2003. Pharmacokinetics of the dietary supplement creatine. *Clin Pharmacokinet* 42(6):557-574.

Pline, K. A., and C. L. Smith. 2005. The effect of creatine intake on renal function. *Ann Pharmacother* 39(6):1093-1096.

Pluim, B., A. Ferrauti, F. Broekhof, M. Deutekom, A. Gotzmann, H. Kuipers, and K. Weber. 2006. The effects of creatine supplementation on selected factors of tennis specific training. *Br J Sports Med* 40(6):507-511.

Pritchard, N. R., and P. A. Kalra. 1998. Renal dysfunction accompanying oral creatine supplements. *Lancet* 351(9111):1252-1253.

Reardon, T., P. Ruell, S. Fiatarone, C. Thompson, and K. Rooney. 2006. Creatine supplementation does not enhance submaximal aerobic training adaptations in healthy young men and women. *Eur J Appl Physiol* 98(3):234-241.

Santos, R. V., R. A. Bassit, E. C. Caperuto, and L. F. Costa Rosa. 2004. The effect of creatine supplementation upon inflammatory and muscle soreness markers after a 30 km race. *Life Sci* 75(16):1917-1924.

Scheff, S. W., and H. S. Dhillon. 2004. Creatine-enhanced diet alters levels of lactate and free fatty acids after experimental brain injury. *Neurochem Res* 29(2):469-479.

Shao, A., and J. Hathcock. 2006. Risk assessment for creatine monohydrate. *Regul Toxicol Pharmacol* 45(3):242-251.

Smith, J., and D. L. Dahm. 2000. Creatine use among a select population of high school athletes. *Mayo Clin Proc* 75(12):1257-1263.

Sullivan, P. G., J. D. Geiger, M. P. Mattson, and S. W. Scheff. 2000. Dietary supplement creatine protects against traumatic brain injury. *Ann Neurol* 48(5):723-729.

Thorsteinsdottir, B., J. Grande, and V. Garovic. 2006. Acute renal failure in a young weight lifter taking multiple food supplements, including creatine monohydrate. *J Ren Nutr* 16(4):341-345.

Volek, J. S., S. A. Mazzetti, W. B. Farquhar, B. R. Barnes, A. L. Gomez, and W. J. Kraemer. 2001. Physiological responses to short-term exercise in the heat after creatine loading. *Med Sci Sports Exerc* 33(7):1101-1108.

Volek, J., C. Forsythe, and W. Kraemer. 2006. Nutritional aspects of women strength athletes. *Br J Sports Med* 40(9):742-748.

Warber, J., W. Thorian, J. Patton, C. Champagne, P. Mitotti, and H. Lieberman. 2002. The effect of creatine monohydrate supplementation on obstacle course and multiple bench press performance. *J Strength Cond Res* 16:500-509.

Watsford, M. L., A. J. Murphy, W. L. Spinks, and A. D. Walshe. 2003. Creatine supplementation and its effect on musculotendinous stiffness and performance. *J Strength Cond Res* 17(1):26-33.

Weiss, B. A., and M. E. Powers. 2006. Creatine supplementation does not impair the thermoregulatory response during a bout of exercise in the heat. *J Sports Med Phys Fitness* 46(4):555-563.

DEHYDROEPIANDROSTERONE (DHEA)

Background

Dehydroepiandrosterone[4] (DHEA), a steroid compound considered a prohormone, is secreted by the adrenal glands and produced in the brain. It can be converted to a variety of steroid hormones, including estrogen and testosterone. Most of the circulating DHEA in the body is in the sulfated form, DHEA-S. Blood concentrations peak in early adulthood and decline with age; at 70+ years old, they are approximately at 10–20 percent of peak levels (Allolio and Arlt, 2002). Some epidemiological studies demonstrate a correlation between lower blood DHEA and increased mortality in men (Allolio and Arlt, 2002). This fact, as well as the loss of lean body mass and muscle function with age, has prompted some to explore the use of DHEA as a supplement for aging individuals. There is some evi-

[4]The monographs were developed in order to evaluate the review process outlined in Chapter 5. The monographs present scientific reviews of safety and efficacy, but do not attempt to provide a final assessment of safety or efficacy.

dence linking DHEA to cognitive function including mood and sexuality (Allolio and Arlt, 2002). DHEA may exert its actions via conversion to estrogens or androgens or via direct action as a neurosteroid on receptors in the brain (Allolio and Arlt, 2002). Blood DHEA is reduced in some clinical conditions, including anorexia nervosa, cancer, lupus, HIV, kidney disease, and diabetes. Some drugs are known to reduce blood DHEA (e.g., dexamethasone, insulin, carbamazepine, phenytoin) while others (e.g., benfluorex, diltiazem) increase concentration of this prohormone (Kroboth et al., 1999; Salek et al., 2002). Although many other prohormones came under tighter regulation by the U.S. Food and Drug Administration in 2004 (the Anabolic Steroid Control Act), DHEA was exempt from this act and thus can still be sold as a dietary supplement (Handelsman, 2005).

Putative Benefits

Because the primary indication for use has been to restore reduced blood DHEA concentration to values typical of young adults, most studies have been performed on older individuals (60+ years of age). Most of these studies show that ingestion of DHEA can increase the blood DHEA concentration of elderly individuals to that of young adults (Morales et al., 1998; Percheron et al., 2003). There is a gender difference in DHEA's effect on other steroid hormones in that women usually also have an increase in testosterone while men have an increase in estrogen (Allolio and Arlt, 2002). Although one of the earlier clinical trials reported a reduction in body fat, increase in lean body mass, and increase in muscle strength in men taking 100 mg/d DHEA for 6 months, this study had a small subject number (9 men and 10 women, ages 50–65 years) and no placebo group (Morales et al., 1998). Most subsequent studies using larger groups of subjects for up to 2 years report similar effects on blood hormone concentration but no effects on body composition or muscle function (e.g., Baulieu et al., 2000; Nair et al., 2006). One exception is a study reporting improved insulin sensitivity and reduced visceral and subcutaneous fat in subjects over 65 years of age subsequent to ingestion of 50 mg/d DHEA for 6 months (Villareal and Holloszy, 2004). Another study reported a modest but significant increase in bone mineral density in 87 elderly men (>60 years old), but as this change was much less than that reported for other therapeutic interventions, the authors concluded that this was of limited value (Nair et al., 2006). The few studies performed on younger individuals involved in resistance training did not report a benefit on lean tissue or strength gain (Bahrke and Yesalis, 2004; Brown et al., 2006). A Cochrane review of several randomized, placebo-controlled trials that investigated the effects of DHEA on individuals over 50 years of age concluded that DHEA did not improve cognitive function in older individuals (Evans et al., 2007).

Although there is limited data, a few studies suggest potential benefit on mood and sexuality, especially in older women (Allolio and Arlt, 2002; Baulieu et al., 2000). In conclusion, while DHEA may be of medical value for people with certain clinical problems, including adrenal insufficiency, or for those under chronic glucocorticoid treatment, the largest, longest, and best-designed studies do not identify benefits of DHEA on body composition, muscle function, or cognitive function.

Safety Concerns

Negative effects of DHEA ingestion were primarily observed in women (and were likely secondary to an increase in endogenously synthesized testosterone) and included acne, hirsutism, and reduction in serum high-density lipoprotein (HDL) cholesterol (Allolio and Arlt, 2002). Because of the effects of DHEA on steroid hormones, there has been concern about its potential effects on development of hormone-sensitive cancers such as breast and prostate. One study observed no effect on prostate size or serum prostate-specific antigen (PSA) in men who consumed 75 mg/d of DHEA for 2 years (Nair et al., 2006). However, this may not be long enough to detect an effect on neoplasia. Epidemiological and case-control studies of pre- and postmenopausal women who later developed breast cancer have identified an increase in breast cancer risk for those with the highest blood DHEA levels (Kaaks et al., 2005a,b; Missmer et al., 2004; Raven and Hinson, 2007). This suggests, but does not prove, an association between DHEA supplementation and risk of breast cancer. Caution is appropriate, at least in women already at higher risk of breast cancer, and for long-term users.

Studies measuring typical health-related blood panels, including liver function, do not report a change attributable to DHEA taken in typical doses (50–100 mg/d) (Morales et al., 1998; Nair et al., 2006). However, because rodent studies have identified hepatic carcinogenic properties of DHEA (Mayer and Forstner, 2004) in rats fed 0.45–1 percent of their diet as DHEA for 52–100 weeks, safety cannot be assured.

Although there is modest evidence for enhancement of neoplasia—mostly from large epidemiological studies in women, with some evidence for hepatic cancer in animal models—performance of additional research (i.e., clinical trials) is not warranted because of DHEA's potential health risk combined with little evidence of benefit.

Considerations Specific to the Military

There are no reports of studies evaluating DHEA in conditions that would be specific to the military. However, there is no reason to suspect that effects would be different in different environmental or working conditions. In addition, study subjects were generally older than active duty military personnel. Most studies with participants who were demographically similar to the military population did not reveal benefits, so the research conducted does not support the value of DHEA as a performance enhancer for military personnel.

Relevant data and conclusions on efficacy and safety reviews and publications identified for DHEA are shown in Table 4-4 on pages 182–191.

References

Allolio, B., and W. Arlt. 2002. DHEA treatment: Myth or reality? *Trends Endo Metab* 13(7):288-294.

Bahrke, M. S., and C. E. Yesalis. 2004. Abuse of anabolic androgenic steroids and related substances in sport and exercise. *Curr Opin Pharmacol* 4:614-620.

Baulieu, E. E., G. Thomas, S. Legrain, N. Lahlou, M. Roger, B. Debuire, V. Faucounau, L. Girard, M. P. Hervy, F. Latour, M. C. Leaud, A. Mokrane, H. Pitti-Ferrandi, C. Trivalle, O. de Acharriere, S. Nouveau, B. Rakoto-Arison, J. C. Souberbielle, J. Raison, Y. Le Bouc, A. Raynaud, X. Girerd, and F. Forette. 2000. Dehydroepiandrosterone (DHEA), DHEA sulfate, and aging: Contribution of the DHEAge study to a sociobiomedical issue. *Proc Natl Acad Sci* 97(8):4279-4284.

Brown, G. A., M. Vukovich, and D. S. King. 2006. Testosterone prohormone supplements. *Med Sci Sports Exerc* 38(8):1451-1461.

Evans, G. J., R. Malouf, F. Huppert, and J. K. van Niekerk. 2007. Dehydroepiandrosterone (DHEA) supplementation for cognitive function in healthy elderly people (review). *Cochrane Database Syst Rev* 4:CD006221.

Handelsman, D. J. 2005. Editorial: Andro and the prosteroids: Bolting the stable door. *J Clin Endocrinol Metab* 90(2):1249-1251.

Kaaks, R., F. Berrino, T. Key, S. Rinaldi, L. Dossus, C. Biessy, G. Secreto, P. Amiano, S. Bingham, H. Boeing, H. B. Bueno de Mesquita, J. Chang-Claude, F. Clavel-Chapelon, A. Fournier, C. H. van Gils, C. A. Gonzalez, A. B. Gurrea, E. Critselis, K. T. Khaw, V. Krogh, P. H. Lahmann, G. Nagel, A. Olsen, N. C. Onland-Moret, K. Overvad, D. Palli, S. Panico, P. Peeters, J. R. Quirós, A. Roddam, A. Thiebaut, A. Tjønneland, M. D. Chirlaque, A. Trichopoulou, D. Trichopoulos, R. Tumino, P. Vineis, T. Norat, P. Ferrari, N. Slimani, and E. Riboli. 2005a. Serum sex steroids in premenopausal women and breast cancer risk within the European Prospective Investigation into Cancer and Nutrition (EPIC). *J Natl Cancer Inst* 97(10):755-765.

Kaaks, R., S. Rinaldi, T. J. Key, F. Berrino, P. H. M. Peeters, C. Biessy, L. Dossus, A. Lukanova, S. Bingham, K.-T. Khaw, N. E. Allen, H. B. Bueno de Mesquita, C. H. van Gils, D. Grobbee, H. Boeing, P. H. Lahmann, G. Nagel, J. Chang-Claude, F. Clavel-Chapelon, A. Fournier, A. Thiébaut, C. A. González, J. R. Quirós, M.-J. Tormo, E. Ardanaz, P. Amiano, V. Krogh, V. Palli, S. Panico, R. Tumino, P. Vineis, A. Trichopoulou, V. Kalapothaki, D. Trichopoulos, P. Ferrari, T. Norat, R. Saracci, and E. Riboli. 2005b. Postmenopausal serum androgens, oestrogens and breast cancer risk: The European Prospective Investigation into Cancer and Nutrition. *Endocr Relat Cancer* 12(4):1071-1082.

Kroboth, P. D., F. S. Salek, A. L. Pittenger, T. J. Fabian, and R. F. Frye. 1999. DHEA and DHEA-S: A review. *J Clin Pharmacol* 39(4):327-348.

Mayer, D., and K. Forstner. 2004. Impact of dehydroepiandrosterone on hapatocarcinogenesis in the rat (review). *Int J Oncol* 25:1021-1030.

Missmer, S. A., A. H. Eliassen, R. L. Barbieri, and S. E. Hankinson. 2004. Endogenous estrogen, androgen, and progesterone concentrations and breast cancer risk among postmenopausal women. *J Natl Cancer Inst* 96(24):1856-1865.

Morales, A. J., R. H. Haubricht, J. Y. Hwang, H. Asakura, and S. S. Yen. 1998. The effect of six months with a 100 mg daily dose of dehydroepiandrosterone (DHEA) on circulating sex steroids, body composition and muscle strength in age-advanced men and woman. *Clin Endo* 49(4):421-432.

Muller, M., A. W. van den Beld, Y. T. van der Schouw, D. E. Grobbee, and S. W. J. Lamberts. 2006. Effects of dehydroepiandrosterone and atamestane supplementation on frailty in elderly men. *J Clin Endocrinol Metab* 91(10):3988-3991.

Nair, K. S., R. A. Rizza, P. O'Brien, K. Dhatariya, K. R. Short, A. Nehra, J. L. Vittone, G. G. Klee, A. Basu, R. Basu, C. Cobelli, G. Toffolo, C. Dalla Man, D. J. Tindall, L. J. III, G. E. Smith, S. Khosla, and M. D. Jensen. 2006. DHEA in elderly women and DHEA or testosterone in elderly men. *New Eng J Med* 355(16):1647-1659.

Percheron, G., J. Hogrel, S. Denot-Ledunois, G. Fayet, F. Forette, E. Baulieu, M. Fardeau, and J. Marini. 2003. Effect of 1-year oral administration of dehydroepiandrosterone to 60- to 80-year-old individuals on muscle function and cross-sectional area. *Arch Intern Med* 163(6):720-727.

Raven, P. W., and J. P. Hinson. 2007. Dehydroepiandrosterone (DHEA) and the menopause: An update. *Menopause Int* 13(2):75-78.

Salek, F. S., K. L. Bigos, and P. D. Broboth. 2002. The influence of hormones and pharmaceutical agents on DHEA and DHEA-S concentrations: A review of clinical studies. *J Clin Pharmacol* 42(3):247-266.

Villareal, D. T., and J. O. Holloszy. 2004. Effect of DHEA on abdominal fat and insulin action in elderly women and men: A randomized controlled trial. *JAMA* 292(18):2243-2248.

EPHEDRA

Background

The genus *Ephedra*[5] is composed of 40 different species all belonging to the family Ephedraceae (Andraws et al., 2005; Mahady et al., 1999). The correct scientific name for the most commonly used form of *Ephedra* is *Ephedra sinica* Stapf; however, other ephedrine-containing species of the same genus are also used. While there are no botanical synonyms used for this plant, there are numerous vernacular (common) names used worldwide for *Ephedra* (for a listing, see Mahady et al., 1999).

Ephedra sinica is a small, green, almost leafless shrub native to many parts of the world. *Ephedra* species are found in China, India, Mongolia, and Afghanistan, as well as regions of the Mediterranean and North and Central America (Mahady et al., 1999). *Ephedra* herb has a pinelike odor and an astringent taste, often having a numbing action on the tongue (Blumenthal and King, 1995). The traditional Chinese name by which it is

[5]The monographs were developed in order to evaluate the review process outlined in Chapter 5. The monographs present scientific reviews of safety and efficacy, but do not attempt to provide a final assessment of safety or efficacy.

commonly known, *ma huang*, is thought to refer to the astringent action (*ma*) and the yellow color (*huang*) of the twigs (Tyler et al., 1988).

In traditional Chinese medicine, *Ephedra*-containing preparations have been used for 5,000 years for the treatment of colds, influenzas, fever, headache, bronchial asthma, nasal congestion, coughs, and wheezing (Blumenthal and King, 1995; Mahady et al., 2001). In Western medicine, some of the alkaloids in *Ephedra*, such as ephedrine and pseudoephedrine, are employed as drug therapy for the treatment of bronchial asthma, nasal congestion, acute bronchospasm, and idiopathic orthostatic hypertension (Mahady et al., 2001). In the United States, the Food and Drug Administration (FDA) has approved several alkaloids in *Ephedra* as ingredients in over-the-counter nasal decongestants and bronchodilator drugs. Pseudoephedrine is approved as an oral decongestant for the symptomatic treatment of the common cold, hay fever, allergic rhinitis, upper respiratory allergies, and sinusitis. Ephedrine has been approved as topical therapy only for the treatment of nasal congestion and asthma (Blumenthal and King, 1995). The plant and its alkaloids are also used for modern purposes that include weight loss and enhancement of athletic performance; however, the usefulness of *Ephedra* for these indications remains to be proven.

Standardized extracts and other commercial products of *Ephedra* are prepared from the dried stem or aerial part of *Ephedra sinica* Stapf and other ephedrine-containing species of the same genus. The chemical constituents of *Ephedra* include (–)-ephedrine in concentrations of 40–90 percent of the total alkaloid fraction, accompanied by (+)-pseudoephedrine. Other compounds in the alkaloid complex include trace amounts of (–)-norephedrine, (+)-norpseudoephedrine, (–)-methylephedrine and (+)-methylpseudoephedrine. Although the total alkaloid content can exceed 2 percent depending on the species, not all *Ephedra* species contain ephedrine or alkaloids (Mahady et al., 1999).

The daily dose of *Ephedra*-containing products varies depending on the concentration of ephedrine in the preparation: for crude plant material, 1–6 g daily, generally given as a decoction; for liquid extract (1:1 in 45 percent alcohol), 1–3 mL daily; for tincture (1:4 in 45 percent alcohol), 6–8 mL daily (Mahady et al., 1999).

Putative Benefits

Ephedrine acts as a stimulant in the central nervous system (ODS, 2007). Of the *Ephedra* alkaloids, ephedrine is the most potent thermogenic agent. It may function as an anorectic by acting on the satiety center in the hypothalamus. A review of all of the clinical trials for *Ephedra* is beyond the scope of this work, and only clinical trials or case reports involving weight loss and athletic performance were assessed.

Limited data from a meta-analysis of the clinical trials for *Ephedra*-containing supplements showed an increase in weight loss of 0.6–0.8 kg per month as compared with placebo. *Ephedra* taken in combination with caffeine resulted in a weight loss of 1.0 kg/month when compared with placebo, observed for only a 6-month period (Keisler and Hosey, 2005). No long-term data exist.

The majority of the studies published in the literature show no effect on athletic performance (Keisler and Hosey, 2005). Clinical trials have assessed the effects of ephedrine hydrochloride (HCl) (the synthetic drug form of ephedrine) and other *Ephedra* alkaloids such as pseudoephedrine in combination with caffeine. In various exercise modalities, ephedrine and related alkaloids have not been shown to result in any significant performance improvements (Magkos and Kavouras, 2004).

The committee identified and reviewed various studies in which the effects of use of *Ephedra*–caffeine combinations on either performance (Bell et al., 2001; Jacobs et al., 2003), weight loss (Boozer et al., 2002; Coffey et al., 2004; Hackman et al., 2006), or adverse events (Haller et al., 2005; Kalman et al., 2002; Vukovich et al., 2005) were investigated (see Table 4-5 on pages 192–229). Caffeine–ephedrine mixtures have been reported to provide a greater ergogenic benefit than either drug alone. However, the published scientific data are too heterogeneous to allow conclusions to be drawn. An increase in athletic performance is a uniform finding observed during submaximal steady-state aerobic exercise, short- and long-distance running, and maximal and supramaximal anaerobic cycling, as well as weight lifting. The ingestion of ephedrine in combination with caffeine increases blood glucose and lactate concentrations during exercise, whereas similar qualitative effects on lipid fuels (free fatty acids and glycerol) are less pronounced. In parallel, epinephrine and dopamine concentrations are significantly increased, while the effects on norepinephrine are not significant. No physiologically significant effects on pulmonary gas exchange were observed during short-term intense exercise following the ingestion of caffeine, ephedrine, or a combination of the two. However, tests during longer and/or more demanding efforts have shown some sporadic enhancements. An increase in heart rate, exceeding that caused by exercise alone, is a relatively consistent concomitant effect of the caffeine-ephedrine mixture. Finally, evidence to date strongly suggests that the combination of caffeine and synthetic ephedrine HCl may be effective in decreasing the rating of perceived exertion; this appears to be independent of the type of activity being performed (Magkos and Kavouras, 2004).

Safety Concerns

Haller and Benowitz (2000) reviewed 140 case reports of adverse events associated with the use of dietary supplements that were reported to the FDA from 1997 to 1999. Of these reports, 43 cases (31 percent) were considered definitely or probably associated with the use of *Ephedra* alkaloids (for simplicity, products containing ephedrine alkaloids will be referred to as "ephedra"), and another 44 cases (31 percent) possibly related. Of events related to ephedra, 47 percent involved cardiovascular symptoms and 18 percent were central nervous system events. Hypertension was the adverse effect most frequently reported (17 reports), followed by palpitations, tachycardia, or both (13 reports); stroke (10 reports); and seizures (7 reports). There were 10 events resulting in death, and 13 resulted in permanent disability. Sixty-three percent of ephedra users were under the age of 45 years (Haller and Benowitz, 2000). Use of ephedra-containing supplements is associated with both ischemic and hemorrhagic stroke, cardiac arrhythmias including ventricular tachycardia, coronary vasospasm, acute myocardial infarction, tachycardia-induced cardiomyopathy, and sudden death (Dhar et al., 2005). Increased coronary vasoconstriction, tachycardia, and hypertension reported associated with use of ephedra may be due to induction of myocardial ischemia and infarction. Hemorrhagic stroke is likely secondary to hypertension or cerebral vasculitis (Dhar et al., 2005). Other adverse events such as hearing loss (Schweinfurth and Pribitkin, 2003), psychosis (Jacobs and Hirsch, 2000), rhabdomyolysis (Moawad et al., 2006; Stahl et al., 2006), seizures (Haller et al., 2005), and visual disturbances (Moawad et al., 2006; Simsek et al., 2006) have also been reported.

Products containing *Ephedra* and ephedra alkaloids are contraindicated in patients with coronory thrombosis, diabetes, glaucoma, coronary heart disease, hypertension, thyroid disease, impaired circulation to the cerebrum, pheochromocytoma, or enlargement of the prostate (Mahady et al., 1999).

In 2004, because of concerns over cardiovascular effects including increased blood pressure and irregular heart rhythm, the FDA banned the sale of dietary supplements containing ephedra. The final FDA rule, published February 6, 2004, became effective on April 12, 2004, and has remained unchanged in spite of attempts by industry to have this ruling overturned (Rados, 2004).

Interactions with Other Dietary Supplements or Medications

Ephedrine (ephedrine sulfate) is both an α- and a β-adrenergic agonist, and also acts as an indirect sympathomimetic drug by enhancing the release of norepinephrine from sympathetic neurons. Indirect sympathomimetic agents given in combination with monoamine oxidase inhibitors may induce severe hypertension, hyperpyrexia, seizures, arrhythmias, and possibly death (Hansten and Horn, 2000).

Ephedra in combination with cardiac glycosides or halothane (anesthesia) may cause heart rhythm disturbances; with guanethidine, it may enhance the sympathomimetic effect; with ergot alkaloid derivatives or oxytocin, it may increase the risk of high blood pressure (Mahady et al., 1999).

Considerations Specific to the Military

Owing to the strong impetus in the military to maintain prescribed weight and enhance physical performance, past studies reported that the use of ephedra-containing products was high (Brasfield, 2004; Deuster et al., 2003). Although the use of ephedra is currently banned in the United States, the availability of botanicals that are chemically similar to ephedra and might mimic its effects raises safety concerns. The likelihood of adverse events resulting from the misuse of over-the-counter medications containing ephedra might be small, but continues to be of concern.

While the effects of ephedra on alertness, physical activity, and caloric intake may be beneficial, the ingestion of products containing ephedra alkaloids is more likely to have negative effects on hydration, thermal regulation, gastrointestinal tract function, kidney stone development, liver function, mood, and recovery from injury, and be dangerous to cardiovascular health.

Relevant data and conclusions on efficacy and safety reviews and publications identified for ephedra are shown in Table 4-5 on pages 192–229.

References

Abourashed, E. A., A. T. El-Alfy, I. A. Khan, and L. Walker. 2003. Ephedra in perspective: A current review. *Phytother Res* 17(7):703-712.

Andraws, R., P. Chawla, and D. L. Brown. 2005. Cardiovascular effects of ephedra alkaloids: A comprehensive review. *Prog Cardiovasc Dis* 47(4):217-225.

Bell, D. G., I. Jacobs, and K. Ellerington. 2001. Effect of caffeine and ephedrine ingestion on anaerobic exercise performance. *Med Sci Sports Exerc* 33(8):1399-1403.

Bell, D. G., T. M. McLellan, and C. M. Sabiston. 2002. Effect of ingesting caffeine and ephedrine on 10-km run performance. *Med Sci Sports Exerc* 34(2):344-349.

Bent, S., T. N. Tiedt, M. C. Odden, and M. G. Shlipak. 2003. The relative safety of ephedra compared with other herbal products. *Ann Intern Med* 138(6):468-471.

Blumenthal, M., and P. King. 1995. A review of the botany, chemistry, medicinal uses, safety concerns and legal status of *Ephedra* and its alkaloids. *Herbalgram* 34:22-57.

Boerth, J. M., and C. F. Caley. 2003. Possible case of mania associated with ma-huang. *Pharmacotherapy* 23(3):380-383.

Boozer, C. N., P. A. Daly, P. Homel, J. L. Solomon, D. Blanchard, J. A. Nasser, R. Strauss, and T. Meredith. 2002. Herbal ephedra/caffeine for weight loss: A 6-month randomized safety and efficacy trial. *Int J Obes Relat Metab Disord* 26(5):593-604.

Brasfield, K. 2004. Dietary supplement intake in the active duty enlisted population. *US Army Med Dep J* (Oct-Dec):44-56.

Charatan, F. 2003. Ephedra supplement may have contributed to sportsman's death. *Br Med J* 326(7387):464.

Chen, C., J. Biller, S. J. Willing, and A. M. Lopez. 2004. Ischemic stroke after using over the counter products containing ephedra. *J Neurol Sci* 217(1):55-60.

Chen-Scarabelli, C., S. E. Hughes, G. Landon, P. Rowley, Z. Allebban, N. Lawson, L. Saravolatz, J. Gardin, D. Latchman, and T. M. Scarabelli. 2005. A case of fatal ephedra intake associated with lipofuscin accumulation, caspase activation and cleavage of myofibrillary proteins. *Eur J Heart Fail* 7(5):927-930.

Coffey, C. S., D. Steiner, B. A. Baker, and D. B. Allison. 2004. A randomized double-blind placebo-controlled clinical trial of a product containing ephedrine, caffeine, and other ingredients from herbal sources for treatment of overweight and obesity in the absence of lifestyle treatment. *Int J Obes Relat Metab Disord* 28(11):1411-1419.

Deuster, P. A., A. Sridhar, W. J. Becker, R. Coll, K. K. O'Brien, and G. Bathalon. 2003. Health assessment of U.S. Army Rangers. *Mil Med* 168(1):57-62.

Dhar, R., C. W. Stout, M. S. Link, M. K. Homoud, J. Weinstock, and N. A. Estes III. 2005. Cardiovascular toxicities of performance-enhancing substances in sports. *Mayo Clin Proc* 80(10):1307-1315.

Goldberg, L. D., D. Elliot, and K. Kuehl. 2002. Effect of caffeine and ephedrine ingestion on anaerobic exercise performance (Letter). *Med Sci Sports Exerc* 34(1):181-182.

Hackman, R. M., P. J. Havel, H. J. Schwartz, J. C. Rutledge, M. R. Watnik, E. M. Noceti, S. J. Stohs, J. S. Stern, and C. L. Keen. 2006. Multinutrient supplement containing ephedra and caffeine causes weight loss and improves metabolic risk factors in obese women: A randomized controlled trial. *Int J Obes* (Lond) 30(10):1545-1556.

Haller, C., and N. L. Benowitz. 2000. Adverse cardiovascular and central nervous system events associated with dietary supplements containing ephedra alkaloids. *N Engl J Med* 343(25):1833-1838.

Haller, C., K. H. Meier, and K. R. Olson. 2005. Seizures reported in association with use of dietary supplements. *Clin Toxicol* 1:23-30.

Hansten, P. D., and J. R. Horn. 2000. *The top 100 drug interactions: A guide to patient management.* Edmonds, WA: H & H Publications.

Jacobs, I., H. Pasternak, and D. G. Bell. 2003. Effects of ephedrine, caffeine, and their combination on muscular endurance. *Med Sci Sports Exerc* 35(6):987-994.

Jacobs, K. M., and K. A. Hirsch. 2000. Psychiatric complications of Ma-huang. *Psychosomatics* 41:58-62.

Jordan, J., J. R. Shannon, A. Diedrich, B. Black, D. Robertson, and I. Biaggioni. 2004. Water potentiates the pressor effect of ephedra alkaloids. *Circulation* 109(15):1823-1825.

Kalman, D., T. Incledon, I. Gaunaurd, H. Schwartz, and D. Krieger. 2002. An acute clinical trial evaluating the cardiovascular effects of an herbal ephedra-caffeine weight loss product in healthy overweight adults. *Int J Obes Relat Metab Disord* 26(10):1363-1366.

Keisler, B. D., and R. G. Hosey. 2005. Ergogenic aids: An update on ephedra. *Curr Sports Med Rep* 4(4):231-235.

Libman, R. B., B. L. Menna, and S. Gulati. 2005. Case report: Consequences of ephedra use in an athlete. *Lancet* 366(Suppl 1):S22.

LoVecchio, F., B. Sawyers, and P. A. Eckholdt. 2005. Transient ischemic attack associated with Metabolife 356 use. *Am J Emerg Med* 23(2):199-200.

Magkos, F., and S. A. Kavouras. 2004. Caffeine and ephedrine: Physiological, metabolic and performance-enhancing effects. *Sports Med* 34(13):871-889.

Maglione, M., K. Miotto, M. Iguchi, L. Hilton, and P. Shekelle. 2005. Psychiatric symptoms associated with ephedra use. *Expert Opin Drug Saf* 4(5):879-884.

Mahady, G. B., H. H. S. Fong, and N. R. Farnsworth. 1999. Herba Ephedrae. *WHO monographs on selected medicinal plants.* Vol. I. Geneva, Switzerland: World Health Organization.

Mahady, G. B., H. H. S. Fong, and N. R. Farnsworth. 2001. *Botanical dietary supplements: Quality, safety and efficacy.* Lisse, The Netherlands: Swets and Zeilinger.

Miller, S. C. 2004. Safety concerns regarding ephedrine-type alkaloid-containing dietary supplements. *Mil Med* 169(2):87-93.

Moawad, F. J., J. D. Hartzell, T. J. Biega, and C. J. Lettieri. 2006. Transient blindness due to posterior reversible encephalopathy syndrome following ephedra overdose. *South Med J* 99(5):511-514.

Morgenstern, L. B., C. M. Viscoli, W. N. Kernan, L. M. Brass, J. P. Broderick, E. Feldmann, J. L. Wilterdink, T. Brott, and R. I. Horwitz. 2003. Use of ephedra-containing products and risk for hemorrhagic stroke. *Neurology* 60(1):132-135.

Naik, S. D., and R. S. Freudenberger. 2004. Ephedra-associated cardiomyopathy. *Ann Pharmacother* 38(3):400-403.

ODS (Office of Dietary Supplements). 2003. *Ephedra and ephedrine alkaloids for weight loss and athletic performance.* http://ods.od.nih.gov/factsheets/ephedraandephedrine.asp (accessed April 17, 2008).

Peters, C. M., J. O. O'Neill, J. B. Young, and C. Bott-Silverman. 2005. Is there an association between ephedra and heart failure? A case series. *J Card Fail* 11(1):9-11.

Rados, C. 2004. Ephedra ban: No shortage of reasons. *FDA Consum* 38(2):6-7.

Rakovec, P., M. Kozak, and M. Sebestjen. 2006. Ventricular tachycardia induced by abuse of ephedrine in a young healthy woman. *Wien Klin Wochenschr* 118(17-18):558-561.

Schweinfurth, J., and E. Pribitkin. 2003. Sudden hearing loss associated with ephedra use. *Am J Health Syst Pharm* 60(4):375-377.

Shekelle, P. G., M. L. Hardy, S. C. Morton, M. Maglione, W. A. Mojica, M. J. Suttorp, S. L. Rhodes, L. Jungvig, and J. Gagne. 2003. Efficacy and safety of ephedra and ephedrine for weight loss and athletic performance: A meta-analysis. *JAMA* 289(12):1537-1545.

Simsek, S., A. Khazen, and P. J. Lansink. 2006. Visual impairment and ephedra. *Eur J Intern Med* 17(2):147.

Stahl, C. E., C. V. Borlongan, M. Szerlip, and H. Szerlip. 2006. No pain, no gain—Exercise-induced rhabdomyolysis associated with the performance enhancer herbal supplement ephedra. *Med Sci Monit* 12(9):CS81-CS84.

Tyler, V. E., L. R. Brady, and J. E. Robbers. 1988. *Pharmacognosy*, 9th ed. Philadelphia, PA: Lea and Febiger.

Verduin, M. L., and L. A. Labbate. 2002. Psychosis and delirium following Metabolife use. *Psychopharmacol Bull* 36(3):42-45.

Vukovich, M. D., R. Schoorman, C. Heilman, P. Jacob III, and N. L. Benowitz. 2005. Caffeine-herbal ephedra combination increases resting energy expenditure, heart rate and blood pressure. *Clin Exp Pharmacol Physiol* 32(1-2):47-53.

Walton, R., and G. H. Manos. 2003. Psychosis related to ephedra-containing herbal supplement use. *South Med J* 96(7):718-720.

GARLIC

Background

Garlic[6] is a perennial, erect, bulbous herb, with the bulb giving rise to a number of narrow, keeled, grasslike leaves above the ground (Mahady et al., 1999). Botanical researchers believe that garlic originated in central Asia (Koch and Lawson, 1996; Mahady et al., 1999), but its botanical name, *Allium sativum,* may have been derived from the Celtic word *áll*, meaning warm or pungent (Mahady et al., 2001; Srivastava et al., 1995). Botanical synonyms that may appear in the scientific literature include *Porvium sativum* Rehb. (Mahady et al., 1999). Due to its widespread use throughout the world, there are numerous vernacular (common) names for garlic (for a listing, see Mahady et al., 1999). Currently, garlic is commercially cultivated in Argentina, China, Egypt, France, Hungary, India, Italy, Japan, Mexico, Spain, the United States, and the Czech Republic and Slovakia (Koch and Lawson, 1996; Scientific Technical & Research Commission, 1985).

Garlic is one of the earliest documented examples of a food plant that was also used for the prevention and treatment of disease (Mahady et al., 1999; Srivastava et al., 1995). The medical history of garlic dates back approximately 4,000 years, when its medicinal uses were described in Chinese, Indian, and Sumerian literature (Mahady et al., 2001; Srivastava et al., 1995). In 1550 BCE, the importance of garlic in Egyptian medical practice was illustrated in the *Codex Ebers*, a famous Egyptian papyrus recording over 800 medical formulas. Garlic is contained in 22 of them, for treatment of various ailments including body weakness, headaches, and throat tumors (Srivastava et al., 1995). Cloves of garlic were often found among the ruins of the tombs of Egyptian pharaohs, including Tutankhamen (Mahady et al., 2001). During the first century CE, the Roman naturalist Pliny the Elder advocated garlic for the treatment of epilepsy, hoarseness, hemorrhoids, and tuberculosis. The Greek physician Dioscorides recommended garlic to clean the arteries, and Hippocrates (460–370 BCE) prescribed garlic for a wide variety of ailments including infections (Mahady et al., 2001). The therapeutic properties of garlic are also mentioned in the Bible and the Talmud. In medieval Europe, garlic was purported to confer immunity from the bubonic plague, and individual resistance to the plague was often attributed to its consumption (Mahady et al., 2001; Srivastava et al., 1995).

Standardized extracts and other commercial products of garlic are prepared from the fresh or dried bulbs of *Allium sativum* L. (Liliaceae)

[6]The monographs were developed in order to evaluate the review process outlined in Chapter 5. The monographs present scientific reviews of safety and efficacy, but do not attempt to provide a final assessment of safety or efficacy.

(*European pharmacopoeia*, 1996; Mahady et al., 1999; Sendl, 1995). The important chemical constituents of garlic bulbs are organosulfur compounds (Mahady et al., 1999). Approximately 82 percent of the total sulfur content of a garlic bulb is composed of the cysteine sulfoxides (e.g., alliin) and the nonvolatile γ-glutamylcysteine peptides. The thiosulfinates (e.g., allicin), ajoenes (e.g., *E*-ajoene, *Z*-ajoene), vinyldithiins (e.g., 2-vinyl-(4H)-1,3-dithiin, 3-vinyl-(4H)-1,2-dithiin), and sulfides (e.g., diallyl disulfide, diallyl trisulfide), however, are not naturally occurring compounds. These compounds are degradation products that are produced from the naturally occurring cysteine sulfoxide, alliin. When a garlic bulb is crushed, minced, or otherwise processed, the compartmentalized alliin comes in contact with the enzyme alliinase from the adjacent vacuoles, resulting in hydrolysis and immediate condensation of the reactive intermediate (allylsulfenic acid) to form allicin. Allicin is an unstable compound, and will undergo additional reactions to form other derivatives, depending on environmental or processing conditions (Mahady et al., 1999; Reuter and Sendl, 1994; Sendl, 1995). Analysis of various commercial garlic products shows the variation in sulfur chemical profiles that are reflective of the processing procedure. For example, processed bulb or dried garlic bulb powder products contain mainly alliin and allicin, while the volatile oil contains almost entirely diallyl sulfide, diallyl disulfide, diallyl trisulfide, and diallyl tetrasulfide. Oil macerates, on the other hand, contain mainly 2-vinyl-[4H]-1,3-dithiin; 3-vinyl-[4H]-1,3-dithiin; *cis*-ajoene; and *trans*-ajoene (Lawson, 1991; Sendl, 1995; Ziegler and Sticher, 1989).

Putative Benefits

Modern therapeutic applications for products containing garlic include its use as an adjunct to dietetic management of hyperlipidemia and the prevention of atherosclerotic (age-associated) vascular changes (Mahady et al., 1999). However, results from recent clinical trials that included a low-cholesterol diet for 2 to 4 weeks prior to garlic treatments failed to show any benefits of garlic supplementation when used in conjunction with a cholesterol-lowering diet (Mahady et al., 2001; Pittler and Ernst, 2007). Other reviews of the scientific literature assessing the effectiveness of garlic in reductions in serum cholesterol, low-density lipoproteins, oxidation, platelet aggregation, and hypertension show that 44 percent of clinical trials demonstrated a reduction in total cholesterol, with the most profound effect observed in garlic's ability to reduce platelet aggregation. Mixed results have been obtained in the area of blood pressure and oxidative-stress reduction (Ackermann et al., 2001; Rahman and Lowe, 2006).

Garlic has been reported to reduce the growth of various antibiotic-resistant microorganisms and reduce the minimum inhibitory concentrations of specific antibiotics in vitro (Cai et al., 2007; Cutler and Wilson, 2004; Tsao and Yin, 2001). Pure compounds from garlic, such as ajoene and allicin, have both antibacterial and antifungal activities in vitro, in vivo, and in human studies; however, these results need to be repeated in controlled clinical trials. One 12-week double-blind clinical trial involving 146 subjects treated daily with garlic or placebo showed a reduction in the symptoms of the common cold and a reduction in the duration of illness in those receiving garlic compared to those receiving placebo (Pittler and Ernst, 2007).

Other medical uses claimed for garlic include treatment of asthma, bronchitis, dyspepsia, fever, lower urinary tract infections, ringworm, and rheumatism; however, there are no clinical data to support these claims (Mahady et al., 1999).

Safety Concerns

Garlic has been reported to reduce the activity of the cytochrome P450 enzyme isomer CYP2E1, thus affecting liver function and health (Hu et al., 2005). Consumption of large doses of garlic-containing dietary supplements may increase the risk of postoperative bleeding (Mahady et al., 1999). Use of supplements containing garlic is contraindicated in patients with a known allergy to garlic, and there is often a cross-sensitivity to onions and tulips (Mahady et al., 1999).

Interactions with Other Dietary Supplements or Medications

The level of safety for garlic is reflected by its worldwide use as a seasoning in food. However, in therapeutic doses, garlic may cause postoperative bleeding, especially when used in combination with anticoagulants such as warfarin. Two case reports suggest that the combination of warfarin and garlic products may increase clotting time and potentially cause postoperative bleeding (Mahady et al., 1999). Therefore, daily use of garlic-containing dietary supplements with concurrent administration of anticoagulants and antiplatelet drugs is not recommended.

The possible interaction of garlic with chlorpropamide resulting in hypoglycemia has been reported. Daily administration of garlic-containing supplements has been reported to reduce the plasma concentrations of protease inhibitors, reducing their efficacy and increasing the potential for serious gastrointestinal adverse events.

Considerations Specific to the Military

The use of supplements containing garlic would likely have no impact on high-intensity physical activity, caloric restriction, hydration, mood, alertness, or ability to function at high altitude or in extreme temperatures. However, garlic supplementation has been reported to cause gastric upset including heartburn, nausea, vomiting, and diarrhea (Mahady et al., 1999). Because of the increased risk of bleeding, especially when taken concurrently with anticoagulants, the use of garlic as a dietary supplement might expose military subpopulations to unnecessary risks when they are in combat situations. Garlic-containing supplements should be discontinued 2 weeks prior to any surgical procedures or combat deployment.

Relevant data and conclusions on efficacy and safety reviews and publications identified for garlic are shown in Table 4-6 on pages 230–237.

References

Ackermann, R. T., C. D. Mulrow, G. Ramirez, C. D. Gardner, L. Morbidoni, and V. A. Lawrence. 2001. Garlic shows promise for improving some cardiovascular risk factors. *Arch Intern Med* 161(6):813-824.

Ankri, S., and D. Mirelman. 1999. Antimicrobial properties of allicin from garlic. *Microbes Infect* 1(2):125-129.

Cai, Y., R. Wang, F. Pei, and B. B. Liang. 2007. Antibacterial activity of allicin alone and in combination with beta-lactams against *Staphylococcus* spp. and *Pseudomonas aeruginosa. J Antibiot (Tokyo)* 60(5):335-338.

Cutler, R. R., and P. Wilson. 2004. Antibacterial activity of a new, stable, aqueous extract of allicin against methicillin-resistant *Staphylococcus aureus. Br J Biomed Sci* 61(2):71-74.

European pharmacopoeia. 1996. 3rd ed. Strasbourg: Council of Europe.

Hu, Z., X. X. Yang, P. C. L. Ho, S. Y. Chan, P. W. S. Heng, E. Chan, W. Duan, H. L. Koh, and S. F. Zhou. 2005. Herb-drug interactions. *Drugs* 65(9):1239-1282.

Koch, H. P., and L. D. Lawson. 1996. *Garlic, the science and therapeutic application of* Allium sativum *L. and related species*, 2nd ed. Baltimore: Williams & Wilkins.

Lawson, L. 1991. HPLC analysis of allicin and other thiosulfinates in garlic clove homogenates. *Planta Medica* 57:263-270.

Ledezma, E., and R. Apitz-Castro. 2006. Ajoene the main active compound of garlic (*Allium sativum*): A new antifungal agent. *Rev Iberoam Micol* 23(2):75-80.

Mahady, G. B., H. H. S. Fong, and N. F. Farnsworth. 1999. Bulbus *Allii sativi. WHO monographs on selected medicinal plants.* Vol. 1. Geneva, Switzerland: World Health Organization.

Mahady, G. B., H. H. S. Fong, and N. F. Farnsworth. 2001. *Botanical dietary supplements: Quality, safety and efficacy.* Lisse, the Netherlands: Swets & Zeilinger.

Martin, K. W., and E. Ernst. 2003. Herbal medicines for treatment of bacterial infections: A review of controlled clinical trials. *J Antimicrob Chemother* 51(2):241-246.

Milner, J. 2006. Preclinical perspectives on garlic and cancer. *J Nutr* 136(3):827S-831S.

Pittler, M. H., and E. Ernst. 2007. Clinical effectiveness of garlic (*Allium sativum*). *Mol Nutr Food Res* 51:1382-1385.

Rahman, K., and G. M. Lowe. 2006. Garlic and cardiovascular disease: A critical review. *J Nutr* 136(3):736S-740S.

Reuter, H. D., and A. Sendl. 1994. *Allium sativum* and *Allium ursinum*: Chemistry, pharmacology, and medicinal applications. In *Economic and medicinal plants research*, Vol. 6, edited by H. Wagner and N. R. Farnsworth. London: Academic Press. Pp. 55-113.

Scientific Technical and Research Commission. 1985. *African pharmacopoeia*, 1st ed., Vol. 1. Lagos, Nigeria: Organization of African Unity.

Sendl, A. 1995. *Allium sativum* and *Allium ursinum*: Part 1. Chemistry, analysis, history, botany. *Phytomedicine* 4:323-339.

Sengupta, A., S. Ghosh, and S. Bhattacharjee. 2004. Allium vegetables in cancer prevention. *Asian Pac J Cancer Prev* 5(3):237-245.

Srivastava, K. C., A. Bordia, and S. K. Verma. 1995. Garlic (*Allium sativum*) for disease prevention. *South African Journal of Science* 91:68-77.

Tsao, S., and M. Yin. 2001. In vitro activity of garlic oil and four diallyl sulphides against antibiotic-resistant *Pseudomonas aeruginosa* and *Klebsiella pneumoniae*. *J Antimicrob Chemother* 47(5):665-670.

Ziegler, S. J., and O. Sticher. 1989. HPLC of S-alk(en)yl-L-cysteine derivatives in garlic including quantitative determination of (+)-S-allyl-L-cysteine sulfoxide (alliin). *Planta Medica* 55:372-378.

GINKGO BILOBA

Background

Ginkgo biloba[7] is a tall, deciduous tree, known to be extremely resistant to insects, bacterial and viral infections, and air pollution (Mahady, 2001, 2002; Major, 1967; Van Beek et al., 1998). The tree is native to China, and the earliest documentation describes the tree as originating in a region south of the Yangtze River (Huh and Staba, 1992). Many specimens of *Ginkgo biloba* are thought to be over 1,000 years old. *Ginkgo biloba* was not introduced into Europe and North America until the middle and latter part of the 18th century; it is currently grown as an ornamental shade tree in Europe, Japan, Australia, Southeast Asia, and the United States (Huh and Staba, 1992; Mahady, 2002). It is commercially cultivated in China, France, Korea, and the United States (Mahady, 2002).

Medical therapy with ginkgo dates back approximately 5,000 years to the origins of traditional Chinese medicine, when ginkgo was described in ancient Chinese medical texts such as *Chen Noung Pen T'sao*, *Shi Wu Ben Cao*, and *Ri Yong Ben Cao* (Mahady, 2001, 2002). In China, the seeds (nuts) of the ginkgo tree are considered a tonic, and the medicinal uses of ginkgo seeds were reported in the *Pen Ts'ao Kang Mu* (Great Herbal of 1596) written by Li Shih-Chen (Van Beek et al., 1998). *Ginkgo* seeds were used for the treatment of alcohol abuse, asthma, bladder inflammation, coughs, and leukorrhoea; in the modern Chinese pharmacopoeia, prepara-

[7]The monographs were developed in order to evaluate the review process outlined in Chapter 5. The monographs present scientific reviews of safety and efficacy, but do not attempt to provide a final assessment of safety or efficacy.

tions of the leaves of *Ginkgo biloba* are the official treatment of heart and lung diseases (Mahady, 2002; Van Beek et al., 1998). In 1965, the German physician and pharmacist Dr. Willmar Schwabe introduced a standardized *Ginkgo biloba* leaf extract into Western medical practice (Mahady, 2001).

Only a few ginkgo extracts have ever been tested in randomized controlled clinical trials. The most widely investigated ginkgo standardized leaf extract, EGb 761, is manufactured by Dr. Willmar Schwabe BmbH & Company in Karlsruhe, Germany. EGb 761 contains 22–27 percent flavonoid glycosides; 5–7 percent terpene lactones, of which approximately 2.8–3.4 percent consists of ginkgolides A, B, and C and 2.6–3.2 percent bilobalide; and <5 ppm of ginkgolic acids (Mahady et al., 1999; Van Beek et al., 1998). Today, EGb 761 is used worldwide for the treatment of memory-related disorders and peripheral arterial occlusive diseases and shows some promise for the treatment and prevention of cardiovascular disease and stroke (Mahady, 2001, 2002).

Putative Benefits

Results from meta-analysis and reviews of the clinical trials indicate that standardized leaf extracts of *Ginkgo biloba* may reduce the symptoms of age-associated memory impairment and dementia, including Alzheimer's disease, and may be of some benefit for the treatment of intermittent claudication (Birks et al., 2002; Mahady, 2001, 2002; Mahady et al., 1999). However, many of the early trials used poor methodology and small sample size, and publication bias could not be excluded. The evidence that ginkgo has predictable and clinically significant benefit for people with dementia or cognitive impairment is inconsistent; the studies would require adequately designed randomized control trials (Birks and Grimley Evans, 2007). The usefulness of ginkgo for the treatment of tinnitus (i.e., ringing in the ears) is limited and thus far unconvincing (Hilton and Stuart, 2004).

Its effectiveness in improving cognitive function in healthy subjects has not been well investigated and is also controversial. Ten randomized, placebo-controlled studies involving approximately 1,077 healthy volunteers have measured the effects of various doses of specific *Ginkgo biloba* extracts on attention, cognition, executive function, reaction times, and quality of life (Burns et al., 2006; Cieza et al., 2003; Elsabagh et al., 2005; Kennedy et al., 2000; Mattes and Pawlik, 2004; Mix and Crews, 2002; Solomon et al., 2002; Stough et al., 2001; Subhan and Hindmarch, 1984; Warot et al., 1991). The dose of ginkgo extract used ranged from 120 mg/d to 720 mg/d and the length of treatment from a single dose to 4 months. In the most recent study by Burns et al. (2006), no statistically significant difference was found between the group receiving a low dose of ginkgo (120 to 180 mg/d) and that receiving placebo for any of the cognition tests performed in either young (18–43 years old) or older (55–79 years old) healthy volunteers. In the acute dosing studies, administration of a single dose of ginkgo extract (120 to 600 mg/d) improved performance on sustained attention tasks and pattern recognition memory task, while administration of chronic doses to healthy individuals showed no effect (Elsabagh et al., 2005; Kennedy et al., 2000; Subhan and Hindmarch, 1984; Warot et al., 1991). These studies presented limitations such as small subject numbers, lack of dose–response, and lack of standardized tests.

Two larger randomized, placebo-controlled studies assessed the effects of ginkgo in healthy adults over 60 years of age (Mix and Crews, 2002; Solomon et al., 2002). Mix and Crews used a standardized *Ginkgo biloba* extract at a higher dose, 180 mg/d versus 120 mg/d used in the Solomon et al. (2002) study. Salomon et al. (2002) analyzed a modified intent-to-treat population and indicated that there were no significant differences between treatment groups on any outcome measure after chronic administration of ginkgo to healthy subjects. In this study, ginkgo did not enhance performance on standard neuropsychological tests of learning, memory, attention, and concentration or naming and verbal fluency (Solomon et al., 2002). Conversely, the results of the study by Mix and Crews (2002) demonstrated that healthy older participants who received 180 mg of the extract EGb 761 daily for 6 weeks exhibited significant improvement on standard recognition test tasks involving 30 minutes of free recall and recognition ($P < .01$) of noncontextual, auditory–verbal material, as compared with the placebo controls. By treatment end, the follow-up self-report questionnaire showed that significantly more older adults in the ginkgo group rated their overall abilities to remember as "improved" as compared with the placebo controls. The results of this study, from both objective, standardized, neuropsychological tests and a subjective, follow-up self-report questionnaire, suggest that extract EGb 761 is effective in enhancing certain neuropsychological or memory processes of cognitively intact adults 60 years of age and older (Mix and Crews, 2002). Thus, the results of these two studies are conflicting. These two studies measured different outcomes, supporting the need for further studies with larger populations and standardized methodologies and products.

In summary, for younger healthy subjects, high acute dosing of ginkgo may enhance mental performance for short periods of time, while chronic dosing does not appear to be effective. In older healthy subjects with no cognitive deficits, the data about beneficial effects on mental performance are still conflicting, with one study showing benefits with the chronic use of a higher dose of ginkgo (180 mg/d) and one study showing that a lower dose (120 mg/d) was not effective.

The Chinese Pharmacopoeia includes an official monograph on use of *Ginkgo biloba* for the treatment of cardiovascular disease (Mahady, 2002).

In pilot studies, ginkgo is reported to reduce nanoplaque formation in high-risk cardiovascular patients (Rodriguez et al., 2007) and is used in the treatment of acute ischemic stroke (Liu, 2006; Zeng et al., 2005); however, the data are poor, and large-scale randomized controlled clinical trials are needed before any therapeutic recommendations can be made.

Ginkgo has been reported to have a protective effect on liver function in various animal models due to its strong antioxidant and anti-inflammatory effects (Harputluoglu et al., 2006; Naik and Panda, 2007; Yuan et al., 2007; Zhou et al., 2007). *Ginkgo biloba* extracts inhibit the activities of cytochrome P450 (CYP) enzymes CYP1A2, CYP2D6, CYP2E1, or CYP3A4 in elderly subjects (Gurley et al., 2005).

Ginkgo extracts have been shown to reduce nephrotoxicity due to hypoxia, cisplatin, adriamycin, and diabetic-induced neuropathy in animal models (Abd-Ellah and Mariee, 2007; Gulec et al., 2006; Welt et al., 2007). In one small Chinese clinical study, ginkgo extract was reported to improve the renal function of patients with nephritic syndrome (Zhong et al., 2007).

Safety Concerns

A recent review of the clinical data has concluded that use of *Ginkgo biloba* appears to be safe, with no excess side effects compared with placebo (Birks and Grimley Evans, 2007). However, 15 published case reports described a temporal association between the use of ginkgo and bleeding events (Bent et al., 2005). Most cases involved serious medical conditions, including eight episodes of intracranial bleeding. However, 13 of the case reports identified other risk factors for the increased bleeding, and only six reports clearly stated that when subjects stopped using ginkgo, bleeding did not recur. In three reports, bleeding times were increased when patients were taking ginkgo. The review concluded that a structured assessment of published case reports suggests a possible causal association between the use of ginkgo and bleeding events (Bent et al., 2005). Given these data, it is recommended that products containing *Ginkgo biloba* not be taken with other prescription medications that may also cause bleeding, such as anticoagulants.

Interactions with Other Dietary Supplements or Medications

Ginkgo biloba extract has been reported to interact with trazodone, warfarin, acetylsalicyclic acid, ibuprofen, ticlopidine, tolbutamide, and chlorpropamide (see Table 4-7 on pages 238–259). In addition, *Ginkgo biloba* extract (120 mg/d) decreased plasma insulin by 26 percent in hyperinsulinemic patients with type 2 diabetes mellitus who were taking antihyperglycemic drugs. Ginkgo may increase the hepatic clearance of insulin and antihyperglycemic drugs.

Ginkgo biloba extracts inhibit cytochrome P450 (CYP) enzymes CYP1A2, CYP2D6, CYP2E1, or CYP3A4 activities in elderly subjects (Gurley et al., 2005). Because many medications, including antiarrhythmics, antibiotics, calcium channel blockers, corticosteroids, immunosuppressants, HMG-CoA reductase inhibitors, anxiolytics, and some neuropsychiatric medications are metabolized in the liver by the cytochrome P450 enzyme complex, *Ginkgo biloba* has the potential to negatively affect drug metabolism and produce an adverse reaction.

Considerations Specific to the Military

High acute dosing of ginkgo may enhance mental performance for short periods of time, while chronic dosing does not appear to be effective. Ginkgo extracts have the potential to relieve symptoms of altitude sickness that might result with high-altitude military activities. The clinical trial methodologies from published studies are poor, however, and data are conflicting. The largest clinical study showed no effect on altitude sickness (Gertsch et al., 2004).

The ingestion of ginkgo-containing products has been reported to cause bleeding, particularly when used in combination with aspirin or warfarin. Postoperative bleeding has also been reported. Although a recent review of the clinical data has concluded that *Ginkgo biloba* appears to be safe in use with no excess side effects compared with placebo (Birks and Grimley Evans, 2007), chronic daily use of *Ginkgo biloba* extracts, in therapeutic doses, may have the potential to cause serious bleeding events postsurgery and in combat situations.

Ginkgo extracts have been reported to cause gastrointestinal tract disturbances such as nausea, vomiting, and diarrhea. Upon initiation of ginkgo therapy, transient headaches have also been reported. These headaches are associated with increased blood circulation to the brain and usually resolve over a week of daily administration of the product. Allergic skin reactions have been reported (Mahady et al., 1999).

There is no apparent reason to believe that the physiological effects of *Ginkgo biloba* will be altered by physical activity, diets with caloric restriction, or inadequate hydration. There is also no scientific evidence that *Ginkgo biloba* would improve other outcomes that are vital to military performance, such as alertness, immune function, or mood.

Relevant data and conclusions on efficacy and safety reviews and publications identified for ginkgo are shown in Table 4-7 on pages 238–259.

References

Abd-Ellah, M. F., and A. D. Mariee. 2007. *Ginkgo biloba* leaf extract (EGb 761) diminishes adriamycin-induced hyperlipidaemic nephrotoxicity in rats: Association with nitric oxide production. *Biotechnol Appl Biochem* 46(Pt 1):35-40.

Bent, S., H. Goldberg, A. Padula, and A. L. Avins. 2005. Spontaneous bleeding associated with *Ginkgo biloba*: A case report and systematic review of the literature. *J Gen Intern Med* 20(7):657-661.

Betz, J., and R. Costello. 2006. Studies on natural products. *Arch Intern Med* 166(3): 370-371.

Birks, J., and J. Grimley Evans. 2007. *Ginkgo biloba* for cognitive impairment and dementia. *Cochrane Database Syst Rev* (2):CD003120.

Birks, J., E. V. Grimley, and M. Van Dongen. 2002. *Ginkgo biloba* for cognitive impairment and dementia. *Cochrane Database Syst Rev* 2(4):CD003120.

Burns, N. R., J. Bryan, and T. Nettelbeck. 2006. *Ginkgo biloba*: No robust effect on cognitive abilities or mood in healthy young or older adults. *Hum Psychopharmacol* 21(1): 27-37.

Carlson, J. J., J. W. Farquhar, E. DiNucci, L. Ausserer, J. Zehnder, D. Miller, K. Berra, L. Hagerty, and W. L. Haskell. 2007. Safety and efficacy of a *Ginkgo biloba*-containing dietary supplement on cognitive function, quality of life, and platelet function in healthy, cognitively intact older adults. *J Am Diet Assoc* 107(3):422-432.

Chow, T., V. Browne, H. L. Heileson, D. Wallace, J. Anholm, and S. M. Green. 2005. *Ginkgo biloba* and acetazolamide prophylaxis for acute mountain sickness: A randomized, placebo-controlled trial. *Arch Intern Med* 165(3):296-301.

Cieza, A., P. Maier, and E. Poppel. 2003. Effects of *Ginkgo biloba* on mental functioning in healthy volunteers. *Arch Med Res* 34(5):373-381.

Elsabagh, S., D. E. Hartley, O. Ali, E. M. Williamson, and S. E. File. 2005. Differential cognitive effects of *Ginkgo biloba* after acute and chronic treatment in healthy young volunteers. *Psychopharmacology* (Berl) 179(2):437-446.

Gertsch, J. H., T. B. Seto, J. Mor, and J. Onopa. 2002. *Ginkgo biloba* for the prevention of severe acute mountain sickness (AMS) starting one day before rapid ascent. *High Alt Med Biol* 3(1):29-37.

Gertsch, J. H., B. Basnyat, E. W. Johnson, J. Onopa, and P. S. Holck. 2004. Randomised, double blind, placebo controlled comparison of *Ginkgo biloba* and acetazolamide for prevention of acute mountain sickness among Himalayan trekkers: The prevention of high altitude illness trial (PHAIT). *Br Med J* 328(7443):797-802.

Gulec, M., M. Iraz, H. R. Yilmaz, H. Ozyurt, and I. Temel. 2006. The effects of *Ginkgo biloba* extract on tissue adenosine deaminase, xanthine oxidase, myeloperoxidase, malondialdehyde, and nitric oxide in cisplatin-induced nephrotoxicity. *Toxicol Ind Health* 22(3):125-130.

Gurley, B. J., S. F. Gardner, M. A. Hubbard, D. K. Williams, W. B. Gentry, Y. Cui, and C. Y. Ang. 2005. Clinical assessment of effects of botanical supplementation on cytochrome P450 phenotypes in the elderly: St. John's wort, garlic oil, *Panax ginseng* and *Ginkgo biloba*. *Drugs Aging* 22(6):525-539.

Harputluoglu, M. M., U. Demirel, H. Ciralik, I. Temel, S. Firat, C. Ara, M. Aladag, M. Karincaoglu, and F. Hilmioglu. 2006. Protective effects of *Ginkgo biloba* on thioacetamide-induced fulminant hepatic failure in rats. *Hum Exp Toxicol* 25(12):705-713.

Hilton, M., and E. Stuart. 2004. *Ginkgo biloba* for tinnitus. *Cochrane Database Syst Rev* (2):CD003852.

Hu, Z. P., X. X. Yang, P. C. Lui, S. Y. Chan, P. W. Heng, E. Chan, W. Duan, H. L. Koh, and S. F. Zhou. 2005. Herb-drug interactions: A literature review. *Drugs* 65(9):1239-1282.

Huh, H., and E. J. Staba. 1992. The botany and chemistry of *Ginkgo biloba* L. *J Herbs, Spices Med Plants* 1:91-124.

Kennedy, D. O., A. B. Scholey, and K. A. Wesnes. 2000. The dose-dependent cognitive effects of acute administration of *Ginkgo biloba* to healthy young volunteers. *Psychopharmacology* (Berl) 151(4):416-423.

Liu, J. 2006. The use of *Ginkgo biloba* extract in acute ischemic stroke. *Explore (NY)* 2(3):262-263.

Mahady, G. B. 2001. *Ginkgo biloba*: A review of quality, safety and efficacy. *Nutr Clin Care* 4(3):140-147.

Mahady, G. B. 2002. *Ginkgo biloba* for the prevention and treatment of cardiovascular disease: A review of the literature. *J Cardiovasc Nurs* 16(4):21-32.

Mahady, G. B., H. H. S. Fong, and N. R. Farnsworth. 1999. Folium Ginkgo. *WHO Monographs on selected medicinal plants.* Vol 1. Geneva, Switzerland: World Health Organization.

Major, R. T. 1967. The Ginkgo, the most ancient living tree. *Science* 157(3794):1270-1273.

Mattes, R. D., and M. K. Pawlik. 2004. Effects of *Ginkgo biloba* on alertness and chemosensory function in healthy adults. *Hum Psychopharmacol* 19(2):81-90.

Mix, J. A., and W. D. Crews, Jr. 2002. A double-blind, placebo-controlled, randomized trial of *Ginkgo biloba* extract EGb 761 in a sample of cognitively intact older adults: Neuropsychological findings. *Hum Psychopharmacol* 17(6):267-277.

Naik, S. R., and V. S. Panda. 2007. Antioxidant and hepatoprotective effects of *Ginkgo biloba* phytosomes in carbon tetrachloride-induced liver injury in rodents. *Liver Int* 27(3):393-399.

Rodriguez, M., L. Ringstad, P. Schafer, S. Just, H. W. Hofer, M. Malmsten, and G. Siegel. 2007. Reduction of atherosclerotic nanoplaque formation and size by *Ginkgo biloba* (EGb 761) in cardiovascular high-risk patients. *Atherosclerosis* 192(2):438-444.

Roncin, J. P., F. Schwartz, and P. D'Arbigny. 1996. EGb 761 in control of acute mountain sickness and vascular reactivity to cold exposure. *Aviat Space Environ Med* 67(5):445-452.

Solomon, P. R., F. Adams, A. Silver, J. Zimmer, and R. DeVeaux. 2002. Ginkgo for memory enhancement: A randomized controlled trial. *JAMA* 288(7):835-840.

Stough, C., J. Clarke, J. Lloyd, and P. J. Nathan. 2001. Neuropsychological changes after 30-day *Ginkgo biloba* administration in healthy participants. *Int J Neuropsychopharmacol* 4(2):131-134.

Subhan, Z., and I. Hindmarch. 1984. The psychopharmacological effects of *Ginkgo biloba* extract in normal healthy volunteers. *Int J Clin Pharmacol Res* 4(2):89-93.

Van Beek, T. A., E. Bombardelli, P. Morazzoni, and F. Peterlongo. 1998. *Ginkgo biloba* L. *Fitoterapia* 69(3):195-244.

Warot, D., L. Lacomblez, P. Danjou, E. Weiller, C. Payan, and A. J. Puech. 1991. Comparative effects of *Ginkgo biloba* extracts on psychomotor performances and memory in healthy subjects. *Therapie* 46(1):33-36.

Welt, K., J. Weiss, R. Martin, T. Hermsdorf, S. Drews, and G. Fitzl. 2007. *Ginkgo biloba* extract protects rat kidney from diabetic and hypoxic damage. *Phytomedicine* 14(2-3):196-203.

Wolf, H. R. 2006. Does *Ginkgo biloba* special extract EGb 761 provide additional effects on coagulation and bleeding when added to acetylsalicylic acid 500 mg daily? *Drugs R D* 7(3):163-172.

Yuan, G., Z. Gong, J. Li, and X. Li. 2007. *Ginkgo biloba* extract protects against alcohol-induced liver injury in rats. *Phytother Res* 21(3):234-238.

Zeng, X., M. Liu, Y. Yang, Y. Li, and K. Asplund. 2005. Ginkgo biloba for acute ischaemic stroke. *Cochrane Database Syst Rev* (4):CD003691.

Zhong, Z. M., L. Yu, Z. Y. Weng, Z. H. Hao, L. Zhang, Y. X. Zhang, and W. Q. Dong. 2007. Therapeutic effect of *Ginkgo biloba* leaf extract on hypercholestrolemia in children with nephrotic syndrome. *Nan Fang Yi Ke Da Xue Xue Bao* 27(5):682-684.

Zhou, J. B., X. K. Yang, Q. F. Ye, Y. Z. Ming, and Z. J. Xia. 2007. Effect of extract of *Ginkgo biloba* leaves on the precondition of liver graft in rat liver transplantation. *Zhong Nan Da Xue Xue Bao Yi Xue Ban* 32(1):54-58.

GINSENG

Background

Some of the most popular and well-known dietary supplements come from a group of plants known generically as ginseng.[8] The primary commercial species (scientific name, *Panax ginseng* C.A. Meyer), is commonly referred to as Korean or Asian ginseng. The plant is indigenous to the mountainous regions of Korea, Japan, China (Manchuria), and Russia (eastern Siberia) (Hu, 1976; Mahady et al., 1999). However, most commercial ginseng is now cultivated, as wild *Panax ginseng* is a protected species in both Russia and China (Carlson, 1986). Commercial products are prepared from cultivated ginseng imported from China and Korea (Hu, 1976; Mahady et al., 1999).

In China, the root or rhizome (underground stem) and other parts of the plant have been used medicinally (Hu, 1976). However, the root is certainly the most prominent part and sales of root-derived products dominate the commercial market. The plant is a slow-growing perennial herb, and the roots are usually not harvested until the fifth or sixth year of growth, when the ginsenosides (the active constituents) are at their highest concentration (Hu, 1976; Mahady et al., 2001). After harvesting, *Panax ginseng* roots are prepared for commercial use by one of two methods to prevent rotting and microbial contamination. Ginseng root prepared by drying and bleaching the roots using sulfur dioxide is called "white ginseng." The root is also sometimes peeled to remove the outer coating (skin). "Red ginseng" is prepared by steaming the root for 3 hours and then air-drying it. The steamed root turns a caramel color and is resistant to invasion by fungi and pests (Hu, 1976; Mahady et al., 2001; Shibata et al., 1985).

The main active chemical constituents of *Panax ginseng* include the triterpene saponins, known as the ginsenosides (Mahady et al., 1999). More than 30 are based on the dammarane structure, with one, ginsenoside Ro, being an oleanolic acid derivative (Cui, 1995; Mahady et al., 1999; Shibata et al., 1985). The ginsenosides are derivatives of either protopanaxadiol or protopanaxatriol. The most important constituents are the ginsenosides Rb_{-1}, Rb_{-2}, Rc, Rd, Rf, Rg_{-1}, and Rg_{-2} (Mahady et al., 1999, 2001).

[8]The monographs were developed in order to evaluate the review process outlined in Chapter 5. The monographs present scientific reviews of safety and efficacy, but do not attempt to provide a final assessment of safety or efficacy.

Putative Benefits

While the genus name *Panax* derives from the Greek word *panacea*, meaning "cure-all," its application according to traditional Chinese medicine is actually very specific (Hu, 1976; Mahady et al., 2001; Sonnenborn and Proppert, 1991). *Panax ginseng* is used to treat older patients with chronic illnesses, especially given during periods of convalescence, to restore the person to a normal state of good health (Hu, 1976; Mahady et al., 2001).

Up until 1937, *Panax ginseng* was an official compendial drug in the United States, listed in the *The Dispensatory of the United States of America*. The U.S. Food and Drug Administration currently regards ginseng as a food and ginseng-containing products as dietary supplements (Mahady et al., 2001). According to the World Health Organization's (WHO's) *WHO Monographs on Selected Medicinal Plants*, *Panax ginseng* is used as a tonic or immune stimulant for enhancement of mental and physical capacity during fatigue, chronic illness, and convalescence (Mahady et al., 1999).

The hypothesis that *Panax ginseng* might be used as an ergogenic agent in healthy subjects is a more modern idea; in 2001 and 2003, two small controlled clinical trials investigated the ergogenic effects of standardized *Panax ginseng* extract G115 in healthy subjects (Engels et al., 2001, 2003). Both studies failed to find ergogenic benefits in the recovery from short, supramaximal exercise or in the Wingate Anaerobic test (an all-out-effort, 30-second leg cycle test). These studies confirm the lack of ergogenic effects for *Panax ginseng* in healthy subjects seen in previous studies (Lieberman, 2001). Thus, to date, there are no compelling data that suggest that *Panax ginseng* has any positive effects on physical performance in healthy individuals.

One randomized placebo-controlled clinical trial assessed the effects of *Panax ginseng* extract G115 at a dose of 200 to 400 mg/day on mood and other psychological parameters in 83 young healthy subjects (Cardinal and Engels, 2001). After 8 weeks of treatment, no improvements were observed in any measured parameter, indicating that ginseng has no beneficial effects on mood or memory in young healthy subjects (Cardinal and Engels, 2001). Two smaller clinical studies assessed the cognitive effects of *Panax ginseng* extract G115 at a dose of 200 mg or 400 mg in 30 or 27 healthy young adults respectively (Reay et al., 2005, 2006). The 2006 study showed that both *Panax ginseng* or glucose enhanced the performance of a mental arithmetic task and ameliorated the increase in subjective feelings of mental fatigue experienced by participants during the later stages of the sustained, cognitively demanding task performance. No evidence of synergistic effects was observed when glucose and *Panax ginseng* G115 were administered together (Reay et al., 2006). The 2005 trial showed that improvements in behavioral effects were associated with the oral administration of 200 mg of *Panax ginseng* G115 extract, and included significant improvements ($P < .05$) in the Serial Sevens subtraction task performance and a significant reduction in the subjective mental fatigue test throughout all of the post-dose completions of the 10-minute battery (with the exception of one time point in each case) (Reay et al., 2005). The study concluded that *Panax ginseng* may improve performance and subjective feelings of mental fatigue during sustained mental activity and that these effects may be related to the acute glucoregulatory properties of the extract (Reay et al., 2005). Some of the problems with these investigations include the small sample sizes, lack of dose–response, poor methodology, and the short delay between intake and testing, all making the studies difficult to interpret.

The effects of a combination of *Panax ginseng* extract G115 and *Ginkgo biloba* extracts look more promising in terms of improving mood and memory in healthy subjects. In four randomized placebo-controlled trials, the combination of ginkgo plus *Panax ginseng* was investigated in one large (n=256) and three small (n=20) clinical studies (Kennedy et al., 2001, 2002; Scholey and Kennedy, 2002; Wesnes et al., 2000). Results from the smaller studies suggest an enhancement in quality of memory and improvements in secondary memory and accuracy as well as improvements in mood in healthy subjects (Kennedy et al., 2001, 2002; Scholey and Kennedy, 2002). However, the quality of these studies is low due to the small number of subjects and poor methods. In the larger study, treatment of healthy volunteers with a combination of ginseng and ginkgo significantly improved the Index of Memory Quality (Wesnes et al., 2000). Improvements averaging 7.5 percent were seen in a number of aspects of memory, including working and long-term memory. These memory enhancements were observed throughout the 12-week dosing period as well as after a 2-week washout (Wesnes et al., 2000). *Panax ginseng* extracts, particularly the water-soluble polysaccharides from these extracts, are reported in animals to have immune-stimulating effects against infections (Lee and Han, 2006; Quan et al., 2007; Song et al., 2003) and radiation damage (Han et al., 2005; Kim et al., 2007). Five clinical trials assessed the effects of ginseng on immune function (reviewed in Kaneko and Nakanishi, 2004; Mahady et al., 2001). The studies in general used poor methods and had few subjects, but showed an increase in immune function via an increase in natural killer cell activity, T-cell ratios, phagocytosis by macrophages, and antibody titers when administered in addition to an anti-influenza polyvalent vaccination (Kaneko and Nakanishi, 2004; Mahady et al., 2001).

Safety Concerns

With few exceptions, *Panax ginseng* appears to be safe if administered in recommended therapeutic doses (Mahady et al., 1999).

In a 2-year uncontrolled study involving 133 patients who were taking large doses of ginseng (up to 15 g/d compared to a normal dose of 2 g/d), 14 patients presented with symptoms of hypertension, nervousness, irritability, diarrhea, skin eruptions, and insomnia, which were collectively called ginseng abuse syndrome (GAS) (Coon and Ernst, 2002; Mahady et al., 2001). Critical analysis of this report has shown that there were no controls, nor was there analysis to determine the type of ginseng being ingested or the constituents of the preparation taken. Additionally, the authors of this improperly designed study did not take into account the concomitant ingestion of prescription drugs and/or alcohol by the subjects.

In a follow-up study, when the ginseng dose was decreased to 1.7 g/d, the symptoms of GAS were rare, indicating that excessive and uncontrolled intake of ginseng products should be avoided. One case of ginseng-associated cerebral arteritis has been reported in a patient consuming a high dose of a rice-wine extract of ginseng root (approximately 6 g in one dose). Two cases of mydriasis and disturbance in accommodation as well as dizziness have been reported after ingestion of large doses (3–9 g) of an unspecified type of ginseng preparation (Coon and Ernst, 2002; Mahady et al., 2001).

Mahady et al. (2001) indicated that ginseng supplementation has also been reported to cause estrogenic-like adverse effects in both pre- and postmenopausal women, including seven cases of mastalgia and one case of vaginal bleeding in a postmenopausal woman. These effects have not been confirmed. Ginseng supplementation was associated with the development of Stevens-Johnson syndrome (SJS) in one patient, but the type of the ginseng was not identified, and the patient had been taking both acetylsalicylic acid and unspecified antibiotics 6 days prior to the development of SJS (Mahady et al., 2001).

In one human study, administration of *Panax ginseng* to elderly subjects was followed by a statistically significant inhibition of cytochrome 2D6; however, the magnitude of the effect (approximately 7 percent) was not clinically relevant (Gurley et al., 2005).

Interactions with Other Dietary Supplements or Medications

Panax ginseng reduces the blood concentrations of alcohol and warfarin, induces mania when used concomitantly with phenelzine (a monoamine oxidase inhbitor), and may increase the efficacy of influenza vaccination (Hu et al., 2005). While co-administration of ginseng with warfarin did not appear to alter the international normalized ratio (INR) or platelet aggregation in one clinical trial (Jiang et al., 2004), alterations were observed in another study (Yuan et al., 2004). Considering the potential seriousness of this interaction, co-administration of warfarin with products containing *Panax ginseng* is not recommended.

With few exceptions, *Panax ginseng* appears to be safe if administered in recommended therapeutic doses (Mahady et al., 1999).

Considerations Specific to the Military

Although there is no evidence to believe that *Panax ginseng* would have different effects under the extreme conditions of military operations (e.g., high physical activity, caloric restriction, or high altitude), there are no data available from which to draw conclusions.

According to Coon and Ernst (2002), the most commonly experienced adverse events are headache, sleep disorders, and gastrointestinal disorders. Although the consumption of *Panax ginseng* might not cause dehydration per se, some adverse gastrointestinal effects (e.g., vomiting, diarrhea) might result in dehydration.

Panax ginseng has been shown to have vasodilating effects in animal models and in one human study. Administration of *Panax ginseng* to volunteers subjected to cold stress increased tolerability in the ice water tolerance test (Kaneko and Nakanishi, 2004). This effect was thought to be due to dilation of the blood vessels, increased blood flow under cold stress, decreased pain from ischemia, and protection from local tissue damage.

Relevant data and conclusions on efficacy and safety reviews and publications identified for ginseng are shown in Table 4-8 on pages 260–269.

References

Cardinal, B. J., and H. J. Engels. 2001. Ginseng does not enhance psychological well-being in healthy, young adults: Results of a double-blind, placebo-controlled, randomized clinical trial. *J Am Diet Assoc* 101(6):655-660.

Carlson, A. W. 1986. Ginseng: America's botanical drug connection to the Orient. *Econ Bot* 40(2):233-249.

Cheng, T. O. 2005. Ginseng and other herbal medicines that interact with warfarin. *Int J Cardiol* 104(2):227.

Coon, J. T., and E. Ernst. 2002. *Panax ginseng*: A systematic review of adverse effects and drug interactions. *Drug Saf* 25(5):323-344.

Cui, J. F. 1995. Identification and quantification of ginsenosides in various commercial ginseng preparations. *Eur J Pharm Sci* 3(2):77-85.

Engels, H. J., I. Kolokouri, T. J. Cieslak II, and J. C. Wirth. 2001. Effects of ginseng supplementation on supramaximal exercise performance and short-term recovery. *J Strength Cond Res* 15(3):290-295.

Engels, H. J., M. M. Fahlman, and J. C. Wirth. 2003. Effects of ginseng on secretory IgA, performance, and recovery from interval exercise. *Med Sci Sports Exerc* 35(4):690-696.

Gurley, B. J., S. F. Gardner, M. A. Hubbard, D. K. Williams, W. B. Gentry, Y. Cui, and C. Y. Ang. 2005. Clinical assessment of effects of botanical supplementation on cytochrome P450 phenotypes in the elderly: St. John's wort, garlic oil, *Panax ginseng* and *Ginkgo biloba*. *Drugs Aging* 22(6):525-539.

Han, S. K., J. Y. Song, Y. S. Yun, and S. Y. Yi. 2005. Ginsan improved Th1 immune response inhibited by gamma radiation. *Arch Pharm Res* 28(3):343-350.

Hu, S. Y. 1976. The genus *Panax* (ginseng) in Chinese medicine. *Econ Bot* 30(1):11-28.

Hu, Z., X. Yang, P. C. Ho, S. Y. Chan, P. W. Heng, E. Chan, W. Duan, H. L. Koh, and S. Zhou. 2005. Herb-drug interactions: A literature review. *Drugs* 65(9):1239-1282.

Jiang, X., K. M. Williams, W. S. Liauw, A. J. Ammit, B. D. Roufogalis, C. C. Duke, R. O. Day, and A. J. McLachlan. 2004. Effect of St. John's wort and ginseng on the pharmacokinetics and pharmacodynamics of warfarin in healthy subjects. *Br J Clin Pharmacol* 57(5):592-599.

Kaneko, H., and K. Nakanishi. 2004. Proof of the mysterious efficacy of ginseng: Basic and clinical trials: Clinical effects of medical ginseng, korean red ginseng: Specifically, its anti-stress action for prevention of disease. *J Pharmacol Sci* 95(2):158-162.

Kennedy, D. O., A. B. Scholey, and K. A. Wesnes. 2001. Differential, dose dependent changes in cognitive performance following acute administration of a *Ginkgo biloba/Panax ginseng* combination to healthy young volunteers. *Nutr Neurosci* 4(5):399-412.

Kennedy, D. O., A. B. Scholey, and K. A. Wesnes. 2002. Modulation of cognition and mood following administration of single doses of *Ginkgo biloba*, ginseng, and a ginkgo/ginseng combination to healthy young adults. *Physiol Behav* 75(5):739-751.

Kim, H. J., M. H. Kim, Y. Y. Byon, J. W. Park, Y. Jee, and H. G. Joo. 2007. Radioprotective effects of an acidic polysaccharide of *Panax ginseng* on bone marrow cells. *J Vet Sci* 8(1):39-44.

Lee, J. H., and Y. Han. 2006. Ginsenoside Rg1 helps mice resist to disseminated candidiasis by Th1 type differentiation of CD4+ T cell. *Int Immunopharmacol* 6(9):1424-1430.

Lieberman, H. R. 2001. The effects of ginseng, ephedrine, and caffeine on cognitive performance, mood and energy. *Nutr Rev* 59(4):91-102.

Mahady, G. B., H. H. S. Fong, and N. R. Farnsworth. 1999. *WHO monographs of selected medicinal plants*. Vol. 1. Geneva, Switzerland: World Health Organization.

Mahady, G. B., H. H. S. Fong, and N. R. Farnsworth. 2001. *Botanical dietary supplements: Quality, safety and efficacy*. Lisse, the Netherlands: Swets and Zeilinger.

Quan, F. S., R. W. Compans, Y. K. Cho, and S. M. Kang. 2007. Ginseng and salviae herbs play a role as immune activators and modulate immune responses during influenza virus infection. *Vaccine* 25(2):272-282.

Reay, J. L., D. O. Kennedy, and A. B. Scholey. 2005. Single doses of *Panax ginseng* (G115) reduce blood glucose levels and improve cognitive performance during sustained mental activity. *J Psychopharmacol* 19(4):357-365.

Reay, J. L., D. O. Kennedy, and A. B. Scholey. 2006. Effects of *Panax ginseng*, consumed with and without glucose, on blood glucose levels and cognitive performance during sustained "mentally demanding" tasks. *J Psychopharmacol* 20(6):771-781.

Rosado, M. F. 2003. Thrombosis of a prosthetic aortic valve disclosing a hazardous interaction between warfarin and a commercial ginseng product. *Cardiology* 99(2):111.

Scholey, A. B., and D. O. Kennedy. 2002. Acute, dose-dependent cognitive effects of *Ginkgo biloba, Panax ginseng* and their combination in healthy young volunteers: Differential interactions with cognitive demand. *Hum Psychopharmacol* 17(1):35-44.

Shibata, S., O. Tanaka, J. Shoji, and H. Saito. 1985. Chemistry and pharmacology of panax. In *Economic and medicinal plants research*. Vol. 1, edited by H. Wagner and N. R. Farnsworth. London-San Diego-New York: Academic Press. Pp. 217-284.

Song, Z., C. Moser, H. Wu, V. Faber, A. Kharazmi, and N. Hoiby. 2003. Cytokine modulating effect of ginseng treatment in a mouse model of *Pseudomonas aeruginosa* lung infection. *J Cyst Fibros* 2(3):112-119.

Sonnenborn, U., and Proppert, Y. 1991. Ginseng (*Panax ginseng* C. A. Meyer). *Brit J Phytotherapy* 2:3-14.

Wesnes, K. A., T. Ward, A. McGinty, and O. Petrini. 2000. The memory enhancing effects of a *Ginkgo biloba/Panax ginseng* combination in healthy middle-aged volunteers. *Psychopharm* (Berl) 152(4):353-361.

Yuan, C. S., G. Wei, L. Dey, T. Karrison, L. Nahlik, S. Maleckar, K. Kasza, M. Ang-Lee, and J. Moss. 2004. Brief communication: American ginseng reduces warfarin's effect in healthy patients: A randomized, controlled trial. *Ann Intern Med* 141(1):23-27.

β-HYDROXY-β-METHYLBUTYRATE (HMB)

Background

β-Hydroxy-β-methylbutyrate[9] (HMB) is a metabolic derivative of the amino acid leucine. The first step of catabolism of leucine is transamination to α-ketoisocaproate, followed by production of HMB via KIC-kioxygenase. Under normal conditions, approximately 5 percent of leucine is converted to HMB (Baxter et al., 2005). There have been over 20 human clinical trials investigating the effects of HMB on body composition, muscle function, and safety factors concerning HMB intake (Alon et al., 2002; Bohn et al., 2002; Nissen and Sharp, 2003; Nissen et al., 2000; Palisin and Stacy, 2005; Slater and Jenkins, 2000; van Someren et al., 2005).

The mechanism of action appears to be primarily via reduction in muscle protein catabolism. Specifically, HMB has been shown in vitro to attenuate the protein degradation induced by proteolysis-inducing factor (PIF) through the ubiquitin-proteasome proteolytic pathway by inhibition of protein kinase C and resulting stabilization of the IκB/NFκB complex (Smith et al., 2004). This is compatible with the finding that HMB is most effective in individuals undergoing substantial muscle catabolism (e.g., elderly people, AIDS and cancer patients, untrained individuals beginning a resistance exercise program). HMB's role as precursor for cholesterol synthesis in muscle cells has been suggested as a mechanism for an effect of HMB of decreasing muscle damage following strenuous exercise (Baxter et al., 2005).

Putative Benefits

Altogether, the literature supports the value of HMB to increase fat-free mass gain in untrained subjects undergoing resistance training (Alon et al., 2002; Bohn et al., 2002; Nissen and Sharp, 2003; Palisin and Stacy, 2005; Slater and Jenkins, 2000) and in elderly or clinically catabolic subjects (e.g., patients with cancer or AIDS) without resistance training (Alon et al., 2002; Palisin and Stacy, 2005). One meta-analysis of nine studies determined that the net increase in lean mass gain in untrained men consuming 3 g/d of

[9]The monographs were developed in order to evaluate the review process outlined in Chapter 5. The monographs present scientific reviews of safety and efficacy, but do not attempt to provide a final assessment of safety or efficacy.

HMB during resistance training was 0.28 percent per week greater than in those consuming a placebo (Nissen and Sharp, 2003). Some studies support an increase in muscle function (e.g., strength) as well as mass (Slater and Jenkins, 2000). One meta-analysis calculated a net increase in strength gain of 1.40 percent per week for subjects consuming HMB compared to placebo (Nissen and Sharp, 2003). The value of HMB for well-trained athletes is less often observed than for individuals initiating a resistance training program (Palisin and Stacy, 2005). Several studies reported reduction in markers of muscle damage and/or soreness following *strenuous* exercise associated with the use of HMB (Bohn et al., 2002; van Someren et al., 2005). However, the majority of studies do not support a unique value of this supplement for reduction of markers (e.g., serum creatine kinase) or functional impairment (e.g., strength, soreness, range of motion) associated with skeletal muscle injury following *resistance* exercise (Bloomer, 2007).

Almost all human clinical trials that supported a benefit of HMB used a dose of 3 g/d for 4 to 24 weeks. None of the studies involving shorter periods of supplementation (e.g., 6 to 10 days) reported any benefits (Palisin and Stacy, 2005). Most studies used between 28 and 35 subjects, with 9 to 18 subjects per group. Some of the studies used HMB in combination with arginine and lysine in elderly or clinically catabolic subjects (Palisin and Stacy, 2005). Those studies reported anabolic effects of the combination supplement compared to placebo, but as the isoenergetic placebo was not isonitrogenous, it is not possible to attribute the benefits to HMB per se.

Safety Concerns for HMB

Toxicological studies in rats show no negative effects for HMB given at up to 5 percent of the diet for 91 days (Baxter et al., 2005). Many of the human studies of HMB ingestion measured health-related blood factors, psychological function, and frequency of adverse events. There was virtually no indication of negative side effects of the supplement, with several suggestions of improvement in some measures of blood cholesterol and blood pressure, especially in those who began with elevated levels. However, the long-term effects of chronic ingestion are not known, as most of the studies were performed for relatively brief periods (up to 12 weeks). A minority of studies used doses greater than 3 g/d (i.e., 6 g/d). There were no clear benefits or side effects associated with this higher dose compared to 3 g/d. No interactions with food components or drugs were noted, and none would be expected based on the theoretical metabolism of the compound.

There is no evidence to support a safety concern for this supplement taken in doses of 3 g/d for up to 24 weeks.

Considerations Specific to the Military

HMB may help to slightly increase lean tissue gains for new military recruits undergoing vigorous resistance training but is less likely to be of value for well-trained individuals, and its high cost relative to other potentially anabolic supplements (e.g., creatine) may reduce the practicality of HMB use. Although negative effects on liver or kidney function have not been reported in any study, individuals with compromised function of either of these organs are advised not to use these supplements.

Relevant data and conclusions on efficacy and safety reviews and publications identified for HMB are shown in Table 4-9 on pages 270–277.

References

Alon, T., D. Bagchi, and H. G. Preuss. 2002. Supplementing with beta-hydroxy-beta-methylbutyrate (HMB) to build and maintain muscle mass: A review. *Res Comm Mol Path Pharma* 111(1-4):139-152.

Baxter, J. H., J. L. Carlos, J. Thurmond, R. N. Rehani, J. Bultman, and D. Frost. 2005. Dietary toxicity of calcium β-hydroxy-β-methyl butyrate (CaHMB). *Food Chem Toxic* 43(12):1731-1741.

Bloomer, R. J. 2007. The role of nutritional supplements in the prevention and treatment of resistance exercise-induced skeletal muscle injury. *Sports Med* 37(6):519-532.

Bohn, A. M., S. Betts, and T. L. Schwenk. 2002. Creatine and other nonsteroidal strength-enhancing aids. *Curr Sports Med Rep* 1(4):239-245.

Crowe, M. J., D. M. O'Connor, and J. E. Lukins. 2003. The effects of beta-hydroxy-beta-methylbutyrate (HMB) and HMB/creatine supplementation on indices of health in highly trained athletes. *Int J Sport Nutr Exerc Metab* 13(2):184-197.

Flakoll, P., R. Sharp, S. Baier, D. Levenhagen, C. Carr, and S. Nissen. 2004. Effect of beta-hydroxy-beta-methylbutyrate, arginine, and lysine supplementation on strength, functionality, body composition, and protein metabolism in elderly women. *Nutrition* 20(5):445-451.

Hoffman, J. R., J. Cooper, M. Wendell, J. Im, and J. Kang. 2004. Effects of beta-hydroxy-beta-methylbutyrate on power performance and indices of muscle damage and stress during high-intensity training. *J Strength Cond Res* 18(4):747-752.

May, P. E., A. Barber, J. T. D'Olimpio, A. Hourihane, and N. N. Abumrad. 2002. Reversal of cancer-related wasting using oral supplementation with a combination of beta-hydroxy-beta-methylbutyrate, arginine, and glutamine. *Am J Surg* 183(4):471-479.

Nissen, S., and R. L. Sharp. 2003. Effect of dietary supplements on lean mass and strength gains with resistance exercise: A meta-analysis. *J Appl Physiol* 94(2):651-659.

Nissen, S., R. L. Sharp, L. Panton, M. Vukovich, S. Trappe, and J. C. Fuller. 2000. β-Hydroxy-β-Methylbutyrate (HMB) supplementation in humans is safe and may decrease cardiovascular risk factors. *J Nutr* 130(8):1937-1945.

Palisin, T., and J. J. Stacy. 2005. β-Hydroxy-β-Methylbutyrate and its use in athletics. *Curr Sports Med Rep* 4(4):220-223.

Ransone, J., K. Neighbors, R. Lefavi, and J. Chromiak. 2003. The effect of beta-hydroxy beta-methylbutyrate on muscular strength and body composition in collegiate football players. *J Strength Cond Res* 17(1):34-39.

Rathmacher, J. A., S. Nissen, L. Panton, R. H. Clark, P. E. May, A. E. Barber, J. D'Olimpio, and N. N. Abumrad. 2004. Supplementation with a combination of beta-hydroxy-beta-methylbutyrate (HMB), arginine, and glutamine is safe and could improve hematological parameters. *J Parenter Enteral Nutr* 28(2):65-75.

Slater, G. J., and D. Jenkins. 2000. β-Hydroxy-β-Methylbutyrate (HMB) supplementation and the promotion of muscle growth and strength. *Sports Med* 30(2):105-116.

Smith, H. J., S. M. Wyke, and M. J. Trisdale. 2004. Mechanism of the attenuation of proteolysis-inducing factor stimulated protein degradation in muscle by β-Hydroxy-β-Methylbutyrate. *Cancer Res* 64(23):8731-8735.

van Someren, K. A., A. J. Edwards, and G. Howatson. 2005. Supplementation with β-Hydroxy-β-Methylbutyrate (HMB) and α-ketoisocaproic acid (KIC) reduces signs and symptoms of exercise-induced muscle damage in man. *Int J Sport Nutr Exerc Metab* 15(4):413-424.

MELATONIN

Background

Melatonin[10] is a light-sensitive hormone synthesized from tryptophan (i.e., it is a metabolite of 5-hydroxytryptamine). It is secreted by the pineal gland, and is a mediator in circadian processes. Because the pineal gland is neurobiologically part of the endogenous circadian system in humans and many other complex animals, the secretory profile of melatonin is circadian (i.e., about a day in length). Plasma levels of melatonin peak during the period of darkness (nighttime) in all mammal species (Arendt and Skene, 2005). A 10- to 50-fold increase in blood melatonin concentration occurs 1 to 2 hours after dusk (Lewy et al., 1992), suggesting that endogenous melatonin has a role in facilitating sleep (e.g., it lowers core body temperature by increasing heat loss prior to sleep). Similarly, exogenous melatonin has acute sleepiness-inducing and temperature-lowering effects during "biological daytime." The half-life of endogenous melatonin in the bloodstream is less than 1 hour, making hangover effects in the morning relatively rare (Morin et al., 2007).

Due to widespread belief that endogenous melatonin has a key role in the "natural" promotion or regulation of sleep, exogenous melatonin has become one of the most frequently requested over-the-counter sleep aids (Wagner et al., 1998). Among 31,044 people who completed the 2002 Alternative Health/Complementary and Alternative Medicine supplement to the National Health Interview Survey, 5.2 percent reported using melatonin. Of those users, 27.5 percent reported insomnia as a reason for taking the supplement (Bliwise and Ansari, 2007). Women were five times

[10]The monographs were developed in order to evaluate the review process outlined in Chapter 5. The monographs present scientific reviews of safety and efficacy, but do not attempt to provide a final assessment of safety or efficacy.

as likely to report melatonin use as men, and 13.9 percent of them described taking melatonin for anxiety and/or depression.

Putative Benefits

Laboratory studies of melatonin in treating sleep disorders have shown mixed results in various measures of sleep quality. Melatonin is typically administered orally, with dosages ranging from 0.3 to 5 mg in both regular and time-release capsules. In one placebo-controlled study of patients with primary insomnia, melatonin treatment reduced sleep onset latency by an average of 4.0 minutes, increased sleep efficiency by 2.2 percent, and increased total sleep duration by 12.8 minutes (Brzezinski et al., 2005). Another meta-analysis found that melatonin decreased sleep-onset latency by an average of 7.2 minutes in insomniacs and by an average of 38.8 minutes in patients with delayed sleep phase syndrome (Buscemi et al., 2005). However, there was no significant difference between melatonin and placebo. Most reviews of the effects of exogenous melatonin on insomnia conclude that the consensus is that the majority of studies find no benefits of melatonin for insomnia, and/or that the studies are inadequate, and that larger, long-term studies are needed to determine efficacy (Buscemi et al., 2005; Turek and Gillette, 2004). In contrast to the absence of evidence that exogenous melatonin administration can improve physiological signs and subjective symptoms of insomnia, an extensive scientific literature shows that exogenous melatonin can be an effective chronobiotic (Arendt and Skene, 2005). That is, when its ingestion is timed appropriately (i.e., most effective around dusk and dawn), it will shift the phase of the human circadian clock (i.e., recalibrate sleep, core body temperature, and endogenous production of melatonin and cortisol) to earlier or later times.

Thus, the literature reveals that ingestion of melatonin 1 hour before the desired sleep time can be effective for insomnia associated with jet lag (Morin et al., 2007). Exogenous melatonin has also been tested in several different ways to facilitate adjustment to night-shift work. Although exogenous melatonin has been shown to have some benefit in adjustment to jet lag when used prior to the desired sleep time, there is considerably less scientific evidence for its efficacy in promoting adjustment to night-shift work, perhaps because circadian synchronizers such as bright light also promote phase adjustment to jet lag, while they promote no adjustment to night-shift work. The authors of the leading scientific review on the effects of exogenous melatonin concluded that due to the large number of poorly controlled studies, use of melatonin for adaptation to night-shift work is unproven but promising (Arendt and Skene, 2005).

Safety Concerns

Although available as an over-the-counter product in the United States, melatonin is classified as a drug in Canada and is available only by prescription in the United Kingdom. One recent review concluded that there is no long-term safety data on the use of exogenous melatonin or on the optimal dose and formulation for any application (Arendt and Skene, 2005). Another review concluded that melatonin is generally regarded as safe in recommended doses for short-term use, and is likely safe when taken orally for up to 2 years at a maximum dose of 5 mg/d (Morin et al., 2007). A placebo-controlled study showed that the occurrence of adverse events was similar for melatonin and placebo. The most commonly reported adverse effects were headaches, dizziness, nausea, and drowsiness (Buscemi et al., 2006).

Exogenous melatonin is a vasodilator—it lowers core body temperature, and it can affect skin blood flow, which suggests it is not advisable in cold environments, where it may accelerate heat loss (Weekley, 1993).

While one study reported a case of exogenous melatonin being linked to psychosis, other case reports suggest it helps prevent psychotic symptoms from severe reactions to jet lag (Katz et al., 2001).

Interactions with Other Dietary Supplements or Medications

To the extent that melatonin is sedating, it has the potential for unwanted synergy with other sedating agents. Therefore, in people engaged in safety-sensitive activities that require alertness and quick responses, this supplement should not be taken in conjunction with other sedating or hypnotic substances. Of the 109 medications most frequently prescribed for military personnel, 13 have sedating side effects (e.g., hypnotics, anxiolytics, antidepressants, opioids).

Considerations Specific to the Military

Although there is evidence that exogenous melatonin has chronobiotic effects—helping to phase shift circadian rhythms in jet lag and night-shift work—the timing of intake in relation to the effect (i.e., phase response curve) is essential. The decrease in core body temperature seen as a common effect of melatonin poses a risk to military personnel in cold environments, and drowsiness can adversely effect both physical and mental performance. However, melatonin could counteract disruptions in sleep and the thermoregulatory and central nervous systems, which would be of benefit for active duty military personnel. Therefore, consideration should be given to the tasks performed and circumstances; for instance, its use might be limited to the needed adjustment to jet lag and/or night-shift work and in a thermal environment that is above freezing.

Relevant data and conclusions on efficacy and safety reviews and publications identified for melatonin are shown in Table 4-10 on pages 278–281.

References

Arendt, J., and D. J. Skene. 2005. Melatonin as a chronobiotic. *Sleep Med Rev* 9(1):25-39.

Bliwise, D. L., and F. P. Ansari. 2007. Insomnia associated with valerian and melatonin usage in the 2002 National Health Interview Survey. *Sleep* 30(7):881-884.

Brzezinski, A., M. G. Vangel, R. J. Wurtman, G. Norrie, I. Zhdanova, A. Ben-Shushan, and I. Ford. 2005. Effects of exogenous melatonin on sleep: A meta-analysis. *Sleep Med Rev* 9(1):41-50.

Buscemi, N., B. Vandermeer, N. Hooton, R. Pandya, L. Tjosvold, L. Hartling, G. Baker, T. P. Klassen, and S. Vohra. 2005. The efficacy and safety of exogenous melatonin for primary sleep disorders—A meta-analysis. *J Gen Intern Med* 20(12):1151-1158.

Buscemi, N., B. Vandermeer, N. Hooton, R. Pandya, L. Tjosvold, L. Hartling, S. Vohra, T. P. Klassen, and G. Baker. 2006. Efficacy and safety of exogenous melatonin for secondary sleep disorders and sleep disorders accompanying sleep-restriction: Meta-analysis. *BMJ* 332(7538):385-393.

Katz, G., R. Durst, and H. Y. Knobler. 2001. Exogeneous melatonin, jet lag, and psychosis: Preliminary case results. *J Clin Psychopharmacol* 21(3):349-351.

Lewy, A. J., S. Ahmed, J. M. Jackson, and R. L. Sack. 1992. Melatonin shifts human circadian rhythms according to a phase–response curve. *Chronobiol Int* 9(5):380-392.

Morin, A. K., C. I. Jarvis, and A. M. Lynch. 2007. Therapeutic options for sleep-maintenance and sleep-onset insomnia. *Pharmacotherapy* 27(1):89-110.

Turek, F. W., and M. U. Gillette. 2004. Melatonin, sleep and circadian rhythms: Rationale for development of specific melatonin agonists. *Sleep Med* 5(6):523-532.

Wagner, J., M. L. Wagner, and W. A. Hening. 1998. Beyond benzodiazepines: Alternative pharmacologic agents for the treatment of insomnia. *Ann Pharmacother* 32(6):680-686.

Weekley, L. B. 1993. Effects of melatonin on pulmonary and coronary vessels are exerted through perivascular nerves. *Clin Auton Res* 3(1):45-47.

QUERCETIN

Background

There are more than 5,000 different flavonoid compounds in plants that can be subdivided into six major subclasses. One subclass is the flavonols, which include quercetin,[11] myricetin, and kaempferol. Flavonols are three-ring compounds chemically characterized as flavan-3,4-diols. These compounds are especially prevalent in onions, kale, broccoli, apples, and

[11]The monographs were developed in order to evaluate the review process outlined in Chapter 5. The monographs present scientific reviews of safety and efficacy, but do not attempt to provide a final assessment of safety or efficacy.

berries (Ross and Kasum, 2002). Quercetin is the most frequently studied of all flavonoids (Formica and Regelson, 1995).

The absorption and bioavailability of quercetin has been extensively studied. Recent reviews point to evidence that quercetin is readily absorbed from foods or supplements, although there is some variability depending on the specific food matrix in which it is consumed and whether the molecule has a glycoside linkage (Erdman et al., 2007; Ross and Kasum, 2002). The maximal blood concentration of quercetin is reached within a few hours of ingestion with reported half-lives of between 11 and 28 hours. Results from several studies suggest that repeated consumption of foods containing quercetin will maintain blood concentrations of this flavonol (Ross and Kasum, 2002). In persons consuming their habitual diets, blood concentrations ranging between about 15 and 24 μg/L (50–80 nmole/L) were noted compared to about 42 μg/L (140 nmole/L) after a diet high in vegetables, fruits, and berries, respectively (Erlund, 2004). Long-term feeding of quercetin to rats leads to accumulation in many tissues including lungs, testes, kidney, heart, liver, thymus, and muscle (de Boer et al., 2005).

Putative Benefits

A variety of in vitro trials have provided support for antioxidant activity of quercetin and other flavonoids. It is quite difficult, however, to demonstrate that specific food components in isolation such as flavonoids have biologically important antioxidant effects in vivo. These flavonols have also been reported to have utility as antibiotic, antiallergenic, antidiarrheal, antiulcer, and anti-inflammatory agents. Other studies of these compounds have shown inhibition of cellular proliferation in a variety of cancer cell models, although some studies have used concentrations of the flavonoids that are 100 times or higher than achieved by eating diets high in flavonoid-containing foods.

Epidemiological evaluations of diets high in flavonoids provide some support of the theory that flavonoid intake is related to reduction in risk factors of cardiovascular disease. Most recently, an ILSI-North America (International Life Sciences Institute-North America) workshop group concluded that "[d]ata presented support the concept that certain flavonoids in the diet can be associated with significant health benefits, including heart health" (Erdman et al., 2007). For example, Lotito and Frei (2006) demonstrated that quercetin and some other flavonols were able to inhibit endothelial adhesion molecule expression in human aortic endothelial cells. There is also a great deal of interest in the role of flavonoids in the reduction of inflammation and inflammatory states that are thought to be related to a variety of diseases such as cardiovascular disease.

The effects of quercetin on immunological responses have been studied in several testing systems. For example, Formica and Regelson (1995) stated that flavonoids appear to inhibit enzyme pathways involved in lymphocyte activation via their ability to scavenge free radicals.

In a double-blind, randomized, crossover study, MacRae and Mefferd (2006) investigated whether 6 weeks of supplementation with an antioxidant would enhance the performance of elite male cyclists in 30-km time trials. The supplement contained a variety of nutrient and nonnutrient antioxidants, and included a total of 600 mg of quercetin. The results showed that the supplement improved the time trial performance and enhanced power output. These findings could not be attributed to quercetin, however, as there was no quercetin-only supplement. Nieman et al. (2007) tested whether 1,000 mg/d of quercetin would have an effect on upper respiratory tract infections (URTI) and exercise-induced changes in immune function in trained male cyclists (n=40). Participants were randomized to receive quercetin or placebo supplements twice daily under double-blind conditions for 3 weeks prior to, during, and 2 weeks following a 3-day period in which subjects cycled at high output for 3 hours per day. The results of this trial showed no effects on natural killer cell activity, PHA-stimulated lymphocyte proliferation, polymorphonuclear oxidative burst activity, or salivary immunoglobulin A (IgA) output. However, the incidence of URTI during the 2-week postexercise period differed significantly between groups ($P = .004$), with quercetin resulting in only one versus nine episodes of URTI in the placebo group. Interestingly, plasma quercetin was increased from 113 µg/L in the placebo group to 1,158 µg/L in supplemented groups. The authors concluded that even in the absence of demonstrated effects of the supplement on multiple measures of immune function, quercetin may have a direct antiviral mechanism.

Davis et al. (2007) evaluated the effects of 7 days of an oral gavage of quercetin (either 12.5 or 25 mg/kg body weight) on tissue mitochondrial enzymes and performance on a treadmill in previously sedentary mice. Both dose levels of quercetin were associated with significant increases in mitochondrial content in skeletal muscle and brain cells as well as increased endurance capacity in the mice.

Safety Concerns

The safety of quercetin was extensively reviewed by Okamoto (2005). He notes that although the National Toxicology Program had reported some studies showing carcinogenic effects in rats, most in vivo studies indicated that quercetin is not carcinogenic. Moreover, in 1999, the International Agency for Research on Cancer concluded that quercetin is not classifiable as to its carcinogenicity to humans (IARC, 1999). One phase I clinical trial of the effects of quercetin on the inhibition of tyrosine kinase activity has been completed, and antitumor activity was shown (Ferry et al., 1996).

Numerous published in vitro trials have reported the effects of querctin on a variety of cell culture types and a wide range of outcomes. Many have focused on cell proliferation in cancer cell lines. There is a clear, though not consistent, effect of dose level on whether quercetin inhibits cancer cell growth or causes cellular damage. For example, van der Woude et al. (2005) showed a biphasic effect of quercetin in several breast cancer cell lines in which, at a low dose level (10–20 μmol/L), quercetin increases cell proliferation, while at higher doses (40–80 μmol/L), there is decreased proliferation. In contrast, Watjen et al. (2005) showed in a rat hepatoma cell line that lower concentrations of quercetin (as low as 10–25 μmol/L) and other flavonoids protected against DNA strand breaks and induced apoptosis, but at higher concentrations (between 50–250 μmol/L) caused DNA damage. Thus, dose level may play a critical role in whether quercetin supplementation has helpful or adverse outcomes.

To put the concentrations used in typical cell culture studies into perspective, it was estimated that blood concentrations of quercetin ranging between about 50 nmol/L and about 140 nmol/L are reached for persons consuming their habitual diets and diets high in vegetables, fruits, and berries, respectively (Erlund, 2004). Nieman et al. (2007) reported achieving levels of 1,158 μg/L, or about 3.8 μmol/L, in test subjects receiving 1,000 mg of quercetin daily for several weeks. These blood levels are substantially below those of most in vitro trials. It is not known whether concentrations of quercetin higher than plasma levels might be achieved in other tissues after consuming quercetin. However, it appears that the majority of in vitro studies have involved quercetin levels that are not achieved even with high-dose dietary supplements. The applicability of the findings of these high-dose in vitro studies to human health and safety is questionable.

Overall, Okamoto (2005) concluded that it is unlikely that administration of quercetin at a typical dosage could cause any adverse effect. There do not appear to be any safety concerns about quercetin supplements at doses of 1,000 mg daily or less. However, most dietary supplements currently on the market contain mixtures of compounds, not just quercetin in isolation. There are no clear interactions of quercetin with other dietary supplements or medications.

Considerations Specific to the Military

There are no clear indications that quercetin supplements have adverse effects upon issues of military concern (e.g., high-intensity physical activity, injury/bleeding, temperature extremes, high altitude, dehydration, diarrhea, infectious disease, risk of kidney stones, weight considerations).

Relevant data and conclusions on efficacy and safety reviews and publications identified for quercetin are shown in Table 4-11 on pages 282–283.

References

Davis, J. M., E. A. Murphy, M. D. Carmichael, J. B. Davis, J. D. Gangemi, and E. P. Mayer. 2007. Effect of quercetin feedings on tissue mitochondrial enzymes and performance in mice. *Am Coll Sports Med* Abstract.

de Boer, V. C. J., A. A. Dihal, H. van der Woude, I. C. W. Arts, S. Wolffram, G. M. Alink, I. M. C. M. Rietjens, J. Kiejer, and P. C. H. Hollman. 2005. Tissue distribution of quercetin in rats and pigs. *J Nutr* 135(7):1718-1725.

Erdman, J. W., Jr., D. Balentine, L. Arab, G. Beecher, J. T. Dwyer, J. Folts, J. Harnly, P. Hollman, C. L. Keen, G. Mazza, M. Messina, A. Scalbert, J. Vita, G. Williamson, and J. Burrowes. 2007. Flavonoids and heart health: Proceedings of the ILSI North America flavonoids workshop, May 31–June 1, 2005. Washington, DC. *J Nutr* 137(3):718S-737S.

Erlund, I. 2004. Review of the flavonoids quercetin, hesperetin, and naringenin. Dietary sources, bioactivities, bioavailability, and epidemiology. *Nutr Res* 24(10):851-874.

Ferry, D. R., A. Smith, J. Malkhandi, D. W. Fyfe, P. G. de Takats, D. Anderson, J. Baker, and D. J. Kerr. 1996. Phase I clinical trial of the flavonoid quercetin: Pharmacokinetics and evidence for *in vivo* tyrosine kinase inhibition. *Clin Cancer Res* 2(4):659-668.

Formica, J. V., and W. Regelson. 1995. Review of the biology of quercetin and related bioflavonoids. *Food Chem Toxicol* 33(12):1061-1080.

IARC (International Agency for Research on Cancer). 1999. IARC monographs on the evaluation of carcinogenic risks to humans. *IARC* 73:497-515.

Lotito, S. B., and B. Frei. 2006. Dietary flavonoids attenuate tumor necrosis factor α-induced adhesion molecule expression in human aortic endothelial cells. *J Biol Chem* 281(48): 37102-37110.

MacRae, H. S. H., and K. M. Mefferd. 2006. Dietary antioxidant supplementation combined with quercetin improves cycling time trial performance. *Int J Sport Nutr Exerc Metab* 16(4):405-419.

Nieman, D. C., D. A. Henson, S. J. Gross, D. P. Jenkins, J. M. Davis, E. A. Murphy, M. D. Carmichael, C. L. Dumke, A. C. Utter, S. R. Mcanulty, L. S. Mcanulty, and E. P. Mayer. 2007. Quercetin reduces illness but not immune perturbations after intensive exercise. *Med Sci Sports Exerc* 39(9):1561-1569.

Okamoto, T. 2005. Safety of quercetin for clinical application (review). *Int J Molec Med* 16(2):275-278.

Ross, J. A., and C. M. Kasum. 2002. Dietary flavonoids: Bioavailability, metabolic effects and safety. *Annu Rev Nutr* 22:19-34.

van der Woude, H., G. M. Alink, and I. M. C. M. Rietjens. 2005. The definition of hormesis and its implications for *in vitro* to *in vivo* extrapolation and risk assessment. *Crit Rev Toxicol* 35(6):603-607.

Watjen, W., G. Michels, B. Steffan, P. Niering, Y. Chovolou, A. Kampkooter, Q-H. Tran-Thi, P. Proksch, and R. Kahl. 2005. Low concentrations of flavonoids are protective in rat H411E cells whereas high concentrations cause DNA damage and apoptosis. *J Nutr* 135(3):525-531.

SPORTS BARS

Background

Sports bars[12] are a vehicle for provision of calories, macronutrients, and micronutrients for active individuals. Although more concentrated and thus a lighter-weight form of energy than sports drinks, they do not contribute to hydration. This category cannot be easily summarized—there is a very broad range of sports bars commercially available. Most bars contain substantial amounts of carbohydrate and protein, moderate to low amounts of fat, and a total of 100–300 kcal/bar. Most companies fortify these products with vitamins or minerals, and some add herbs or other compounds purported to improve health or performance (e.g., creatine, antioxidants). Sports bars can serve as a snack contributing to the overall carbohydrate and protein needs of service members, especially those with higher energy demands. For example, the Military Dietary Reference Intake for protein is 91 g/d for an 80-kg male. For sustained operations, the carbohydrate and protein needs for an 80-kg male have been estimated at 450 g/d and 100–120 g/d, respectively (IOM, 2005). A more detailed review of the value of protein and carbohydrate for military personnel is presented in the previous IOM report, *Nutrient Composition of Rations for Short-Term, High-Intensity Combat Operations* (2005).

Energy supplements in the form of gels are another vehicle for ingestion of carbohydrate during activity. The energy in these products (approximately 100 kcal) typically comes only from carbohydrate, but they may be fortified with electrolytes or other micronutrients. They are intended to serve as a concentrated source of carbohydrate (one or two packages per hour is the suggested rate of ingestion) during prolonged periods of exertion.

Putative Benefits

Very few published studies have examined the effect of sports bars on physical performance. One study observed that consumption of a bar containing a mix of macronutrients (7 g fat, 14 g protein, 19 g carbohydrate) increased use of fat during exercise of 330 minutes in duration, but reduced ability to complete a high-intensity time trial following the submaximal exercise bout compared to ingestion of an equal amount of energy as carbohydrate (glucose polymer) alone (Rauch et al., 1999). Thus, if carbohydrate and fluids are the limiting factor for physical performance, consumption of

[12]The monographs were developed in order to evaluate the review process outlined in Chapter 5. The monographs present scientific reviews of safety and efficacy, but do not attempt to provide a final assessment of safety or efficacy.

a sports drink would likely be a better choice during exercise than a sports bar. However, sports bars may be especially valuable after exercise when a concentrated source of energy and carbohydrate is beneficial, and adequate fluids are available and ingested. These products can also serve to boost energy (and nutrient) intake between meals in individuals with high energy demand.

Safety Concerns

Sports bars, like sports gels, need to be ingested with copious amounts of water since they do not provide sufficient fluid to prevent dehydration. Research shows that ingestion of gels with a small amount of water impaired endurance exercise performance in a hot environment relative to ingestion of the same amount of carbohydrate in a sports drink (Ebert et al., 2007). Some individuals may experience gastrointestinal distress when using gels during exercise (Burke et al., 2005).

A minor safety concern is the potential for excess energy intake from the additional calories provided to those whose activity level or environment does not require additional energy. Many bars are highly fortified, so there is potential for overconsumption of micronutrients, including the potential to exceed the upper limit for some minerals. It is valuable to train personnel to read the labels of the bars so users are aware of the unique composition, energy, and nutrient value of the product and how it fits into their daily diet. The safety of added ingredients other than macronutrients and required micronutrients cannot be summarized but needs to be assessed individually.

Considerations Specific to the Military

Sports bars are a convenient vehicle to carry fuel for active individuals. These bars typically have long shelf lives and so can be transported and stored without refrigeration until needed. This may be important for various military environments and circumstances. If consumed during exercise, they should be consumed with sufficient water to maintain hydration.

Relevant data and conclusions on efficacy and safety reviews and publications identified for sports bars are shown in Table 4-12 on pages 284–285.

References

Burke, L. M., C. Wood, D. B. Pyne, D. R. Telford, and P. U. Saunders. 2005. Effect of carbohydrate intake on half-marathon performance of well-trained runners. *Int J Sport Nutr Exerc Metab* 15(6):573-589.

Ebert, T. R., D. T. Martin, N. Bullock, I. Mujika, M. J. Quod, L. A. Farthing, L. M. Burke, and R. T. Withers. 2007. Influence of hydration status on thermoregulation and cycling hill climbing. *Med Sci Sports Exerc* 39(2):323-329.

IOM (Institute of Medicine). 2005. *Nutrient composition of rations for short-term, high-intensity combat operations.* Washington, DC: The National Academies Press.

Rauch, H. G., J. A. Hawley, M. Woodey, T. D. Noakes, and S. C. Dennis. 1999. Effects of ingesting a sports bar versus glucose polymer on substrate utilisation and ultra-endurance performance. *Int J Sports Med* 20(4):252-257.

SPORTS DRINKS

Background

Sports drinks[13] were developed to supply carbohydrate as a fuel and maintain hydration or enhance rehydration in response to the stresses of exercise. Most sports drinks contain 6–8 percent carbohydrate (as combinations of various forms including glucose, fructose, sucrose, high-fructose corn syrup, multidextrans) and electrolytes (10–25 mmol/L sodium and 3–5 mmol/L potassium) (Maughan and Murray, 2001). They are typically used prior to exercise to ensure fluid balance and to top off carbohydrate stores; during exercise to maintain hydration and provide carbohydrate fuel; and after exercise to replace body fluids, electrolytes, and carbohydrate. Some newer sports drinks have protein added, with the claim that this will enhance hydration and muscle protein balance.

Some newer beverages marketed to active individuals also include additional compounds such as vitamins, minerals, herbs, and stimulants. These products contributed to a recent broad market for "energy drinks" or "functional beverages." Some of these products are claimed to improve mood, athletic performance, or health. These products blur the line between foods and supplements. Some manufacturers may attempt to sell functional beverages as supplements because of the differences in regulation between supplements and foods. Very little research has been done to validate the effects of these beverages on health or performance.

Putative Benefits

Much research has been performed using traditional sports drinks with virtually no evidence of harm. On the contrary, there is much research that demonstrates evidence of benefit of carbohydrate ingestion for prolonged, moderately intense endurance exercise (especially in a hot environment).

[13]The monographs were developed in order to evaluate the review process outlined in Chapter 5. The monographs present scientific reviews of safety and efficacy, but do not attempt to provide a final assessment of safety or efficacy.

Most studies demonstrate that consumption of sports drinks (at up to 1 g/min carbohydrate) can improve endurance performance of exercise at 70 percent of aerobic capacity for 60 min or more (Jeukendrup, 2004; Maughan and Murray, 2001). Some studies support a benefit for exercise bouts of approximately an hour, but this finding is not consistent. More recent studies that performed simulating sport activities such as soccer or basketball report improved performance and/or perception of effort (Winnick et al., 2005).

The fluids and electrolytes provided by sports drinks can maintain plasma volume during exercise better than plain water and more rapidly rehydrate the body following dehydration. The electrolytes in these drinks help maintain the drive to drink such that more total fluid volume is typically ingested than if water alone is provided.

There is some evidence that consumption of carbohydrate during exercise reduces the immune suppression that can occur with strenuous exercise (Nieman, 2007).

As reviewed by Gibala (2007), addition of protein to a carbohydrate beverage ingested during endurance exercise improves protein balance but does not consistently affect performance. Additional well-designed research is necessary to confirm the effects of protein on health and performance during exercise. Several studies suggest that sports beverages containing protein may improve muscle protein balance after strenuous exercise (Gibala, 2007), which also requires additional validation. Enhancement of muscle protein balance by protein ingestion following resistance exercise has been repeatedly observed, but most hydration-type sports beverages that do contain protein would not provide the amount observed to have a substantial effect. Protein-carbohydrate products marketed specifically for recovery following resistance exercise typically have the recommended 6 g or more of protein per serving that may improve acute muscle balance. Very limited research suggests that consumption of these products or foods containing carbohydrate and protein shortly after every resistance workout will enhance lean tissue gains (Koopman et al., 2007).

Safety Concerns

There is little reason to be concerned about harm from the various "traditional" sports drinks containing electrolytes and 6–8 percent carbohydrate, other than provision of extra calories to those whose physical activities and environment do not warrant the additional hydration and energy. Substantial overconsumption of any hypotonic fluid, including sports drinks, could cause hyponatremia (blood sodium <135 mmol/L), a very rare but potentially fatal condition caused by retention of fluids in vascular space in spite of efflux of blood sodium (Gardner, 2002; Montain et al., 2001). Data from the military estimated this risk to be very low, at 0.10 per 1,000 soldier-years (Craig, 1999). The risk may be higher for those whose sweat is very salty and for those drinking extreme amounts of fluid. Evaluation of cases of hyponatremia among military personnel showed that all had consumed more than 5 L (usually 10–20 L) of water during a period of a few hours (Gardner, 2002). The incidence of hyponatremia is higher in female marathon runners than in male marathon runners, but the reported incidence in the military is similar to the gender distribution of the Army (15 percent female and 85 percent male) (Montain et al., 2001). Weight gain during prolonged exercise suggests evidence of possible hyponatremia. The risk of hyponatremia can be reduced by consuming an appropriate amount (not to exceed 150 percent of losses during exercise, typically not greater than 1.5 L/h) of sodium-containing fluid. The value of ingestion of an electrolyte-containing beverage compared to water for superior maintenance of blood sodium during exertion has been shown in experimental studies (Barr et al., 1991) and with theoretical models (Montain et al., 2006).

Considerations Specific to the Military

Sports drinks are most likely to be of benefit for military personnel working in hot, humid environments where sweat loss is substantial. In addition, those personnel who are doing considerable amounts of exercise (>1 h/d) as part of their duties may perform better, feel better, and become less dehydrated if they consume a sports drink at regular intervals. The amount consumed should attempt to match the loss of body weight (i.e., sweat loss) and/or provide aproximately 1 g/min carbohydrate.

Relevant data and conclusions on efficacy and safety reviews and publications identified for sports drinks are shown in Table 4-13 on pages 286–287.

References

Barr, S. I., D. L. Costill, and W. Fink. 1991. Fluid replacement during prolonged exercise: Effects of water, saline, or no fluid. *Med Sci Sports Exerc* 23:811-817.

Craig, S. C. 1999. Hyponatremia associated with heat stress and excessive water consumption: The impact of education and a new Army fluid replacement policy. *MSMR* 5:1-9.

Gardner, J. W. 2002. Death by water intoxication. *Military Med* 5:432-434.

Gibala, M. 2007. Protein metabolism and endurance exercise. *Sports Med* 37(4-5):337-340.

Jeukendrup, A. 2004. Carbohydrate intake during exercise and performance. *Nutrition* 20(7-8):669-677.

Koopman, R., W. H. Saris, A. J. Wagenmakers, and L. J. van Loon. 2007. Nutritional interventions to promote post-exercise muscle protein synthesis. *Sports Med* 37(10):895-906.

Maughan, R., and R. Murray. 2001. *Sports drinks: Basic science and practical aspects.* Boca Raton, FL: CRC Press.

Montain, S. J., M. N. Sawka, and C. B. Wenger. 2001. Hyponatremia associated with exercise: Risk factors and pathogenesis. *Exerc Sports Sci Rev* 29(3):113-117.

Montain, S. J., S. N. Cheuvront, and M. N. Sawka. 2006. Exercise associated hyponatremia: Quantitative analysis to understand the etiology. *Brit J Sports Med* 40:98-105.

Nieman, D. C. 2007. Marathon training and immune function. *Sports Med* 37(4-5): 412-415.

Winnick, J. J., J. M. Davis, R. S. Welsh, M. D. Carmichael, E. A. Murphy, and J. A. Blackmon. 2005. Carbohydrate feedings during team sport exercise preserve physical and CNS function. *Med Sci Sports Exerc* 37(2):306-315.

TYROSINE

Background

Tyrosine,[14] a large neutral amino acid found in most protein-containing foods, is the metabolic precursor for the catecholamine neurotransmitters dopamine, epinephrine, and norepinephrine. These neurotransmitters play a significant role in mediating neural functions such as attention, arousal, and mood. Under normal conditions, the brain receives sufficient quantities of tyrosine from the diet to provide adequate amounts of these neurotransmitters. However, in stressful situations in which there are increases in the activity of catecholaminergic neurons and subsequent depletion of these neurotransmitters, tyrosine supplementation may prove useful.

Both norepinephrine and dopamine play an important role in the performance of cognitive tasks involving psychomotor skills, decision making, vigilance, and memory. Decrements in these tasks are often observed in stressful situations resulting from conditions such as extremes in environmental temperature, sleep deprivation, and high altitudes. It has been hypothesized that these stress-induced decrements in cognitive performance are the result of increased activity within catecholaminergic neurons, and the consequent reduction of norepinephrine and dopamine within the central nervous system. It has been further suggested that increasing the synthesis of these neurotransmitters could ameliorate stress-induced deficits in mental functioning.

Putative Benefits

One way to increase levels of dopamine, epinephrine, and norepinephrine is to provide more of their metabolic precursor, tyrosine. Indeed, research using young military and nonmilitary personnel of normal weight

[14]The monographs were developed in order to evaluate the review process outlined in Chapter 5. The monographs present scientific reviews of safety and efficacy, but do not attempt to provide a final assessment of safety or efficacy.

has shown that tyrosine supplements can reverse a portion of the deficits in cognitive performance observed in cold environments (Ahlers et al., 1994; Mahoney et al., 2007; O'Brien et al., 2007; Shurtleff et al., 1994), at high altitudes (Bandertet and Lieberman, 1989), as a function of sleep deprivation (Magill et al., 2003; Wiegmann et al., 1993), after extensive combat training (Deijen et al., 1999), and in a multitasking environment (Thomas et al., 1999). Tasks involving memory and attention particularly benefited by tyrosine supplementation. Additionally, relative to placebo, tyrosine may alleviate stress-induced decrements in performance of psychomotor skills such as marksmanship (O'Brien et al., 2007). Tyrosine might also reduce negative mood states including fatigue, confusion, and tension that accompany environmental stressors (Banderet and Lieberman, 1989).

Safety Concerns

Studies investigating the effects of tyrosine on cognitive behavior and psychomotor performance have examined doses of the amino acid ranging between 50 and 300 mg/kg body weight. The majority of these studies have used healthy, young military personnel of normal weight as participants. The number of participants in these studies ranges from 8 to 75. Participants reported no adverse consequences of tyrosine supplementation. However, it is important to note that in all of these studies, only a single trial of tyrosine supplementation was examined. There are no data on the effects of chronic tyrosine supplementation on cognitive function, or on the actions of tyrosine in individuals over the age of 35.

A review of the literature on the use of tyrosine supplements did not find any studies indicating significant interactions between tyrosine and medications.

Considerations Specific to the Military

There is no indication that tyrosine will impart benefits to military personnel *under normal garrison situations*. However, tyrosine could benefit military personnel experiencing stressful environmental conditions that are typically associated with decrements in cognitive behavior, such as intense combat, exposure to extreme heat or cold, high altitudes, and sleep deprivation. Additionally, tyrosine could potentially improve mental performance when military personnel are required to respond to multiple demanding cognitive and psychomotor tasks. The scientific evidence for these putative effects, however, is still preliminary and lacks confimation.

Relevant data and conclusions on efficacy and safety reviews and publications identified for tyrosine are shown in Table 4-14 on pages 288–293.

References

Ahlers, S. T., J. R. Thomas, J. Schrot, and D. Shurtleff. 1994. Tyrosine and glucose modulation of cognitive deficits resulting from cold stress. In *Food components to enhance performance*, edited by B. M. Marriott. Washington, DC: National Academy Press. Pp. 301-320.

Banderet, L. E., and H. R. Lieberman. 1989. Treatment with tyrosine, a neurotransmitter precursor, reduces environmental stress in humans. *Brain Res Bull* 22(4):759-762.

Chinevere, T. D., R. D. Sawyer, A. R. Creer, R. K. Conlee, and A. C. Parcell. 2002. Effects of L-tyrosine and carbohydrate ingestion on endurance exercise performance. *J Appl Physiol* 93(5):1590-1597.

Deijen, J. B., and J. F. Orlebeke. 1994. Effect of tyrosine on cognitive function and blood pressure under stress. *Brain Res Bull* 33(3):319-323.

Deijen, J. B., C. J. E. Wientjes, H. F. M. Vullinghs, P. A. Cloin, and J. J. Langefeld. 1999. Tyrosine improves cognitive performance and reduces blood pressure in cadets after one week of a combat training course. *Brain Res Bull* 48(2):203-209.

Magill, R. A., W. F. Waters, G. A. Bray, J. Volaufova, S. R. Smith, H. R. Lieberman, N. McNevin, and D. H. Ryan. 2003. Effects of tyrosine, phentermine, caffeine, D-amphetamine, and placebo on cognitive and motor performance deficits during sleep deprivation. *Nutr Neurosci* 6(4):237-246.

Mahoney, C. R., J. Castellani, F. M. Kramer, A. Young, and H. R. Lieberman. 2007. Tyrosine supplementation mitigates working memory decrements during cold exposure. *Physiol Behav* 92(4):575-582.

Neri, D. F., D. Wiegmann, R. R. Stanny, S. A. Shappell, A. McCardie, and D. L. McKay. 1995. The effects of tyrosine on cognitive performance during extended wakefulness. *Aviat Space Environ Med* 66(4):313-319.

O'Brien, C., C. Mahoney, W. J. Tharion, I. V. Sils, and J. W. Castellani. 2007. Dietary tyrosine benefits cognitive and psychomotor performance during body cooling. *Physiol Behav* 90(2-3):301-307.

Shurtleff, D., J. R. Thomas, J. Schrot, K. Kowalski, and R. Hardford. 1994. Tyrosine reverses a cold-induced working memory deficit in humans. *Pharmacol Biochem Behav* 47(4):935-942.

Thomas, J. R., P. A. Lockwood, A. Sing, and P. A. Deuster. 1999. Tyrosine improves working memory in a multitasking environment. *Pharmacol Biochem Behav* 64(3):495-500.

Wiegmann, D. L., D. F. Neri, R. R. Stanny, S. A. Shappell, A. H. McCardie, and D. L. McKay. 1993. *Behavioral effects of tyrosine during sustained wakefulness*. Pensacola, FL: Naval Aerospace Medical Research Laboratory.

VALERIAN

Background

Valerian[15] is an herbal product made from the roots of the plant *Valeriana officinalis* that has been used for hundreds of years as a mild hypnotic. Over 150 individual compounds can be found in valerian, and

[15]The monographs were developed in order to evaluate the review process outlined in Chapter 5. The monographs present scientific reviews of safety and efficacy, but do not attempt to provide a final assessment of safety or efficacy.

although the exact mechanism by which it works is unknown, valepotriates and valerenic acid have been proposed as active ingredients (Houghton, 1999). One study found that valerian extracts bind to benzodiazepine receptors in vitro (Holzl and Godau, 1989). It was subsequently reported that valerian extract increased gamma-aminobutyric acid (GABA) concentrations in the synaptic cleft, but this was complicated by the presence of endogenous GABA in the aqueous extract used (Gyllenhaal et al., 2000; Santos et al., 1994). Among the 31,044 people who completed the 2002 Alternative Health/Complementary and Alternative Medicine supplement to the National Healthy Interview Survey, 5.9 percent reported using valerian. Of those users, 29.9 percent reported insomnia as a reason for taking the supplement (Bliwise and Ansari, 2007). Women reported using it more than men (2.6:1 ratio), and 23.4 percent reported using it to treat anxiety and/or depression.

Putative Benefits

Despite published literature and widespread belief that valerian has positive effects on sleep, the lack of scientifically sound clinical trials and longer-term studies investigating valerian makes it inappropriate to attribute any sleep-promoting efficacy to valerian. The available evidence suggests, but does not clearly demonstrate, the possibility that valerian may improve sleep quality (Bent et al., 2006), but this is not an outcome recognized by the U.S. Food and Drug Administration (FDA). Recent reviews suggest that valerian generally produced decreased sleep latency, fewer nocturnal awakenings, and improved subjective sleep quality. However, in some studies the placebo effect was large, and in others the beneficial effects of valerian were not seen until after 2 to 4 weeks of therapy (Beaubrun and Gray, 2000). Five studies of valerian for sleep that included polysomnographic (PSG) recordings revealed no consistent, statistically significant changes in any PSG outcome measures (i.e., in sleep-onset latency, sleep efficiency index, sleep period time, time in each sleep stage, and number of arousals). Six randomized trials showed no difference between valerian and placebo groups in terms of sleepiness the next morning (Bent et al., 2006).

Safety Concerns

Despite recommended dosages for valerian, there may be significant differences in effective dose among the many commercially available products. First, the number and amount of active chemicals can vary greatly within individual species and between different species of plants used to produce a valerian dietary supplement (Hobbs, 1989), though most reputable distributors use the level of valerenic acid in their product for standardization

(Gyllenhaal et al., 2000). Second, since valerian is considered an over-the-counter supplement by the FDA, its contents and manufacturing process are not strictly regulated. Third, valerian products come in a variety of forms and dosages. Adult dosages for insomnia range from 1.5 to 3 g of actual herb or root, which roughly corresponds to 400–900 mg of an aqueous extract, taken 30–60 minutes before bedtime (Morin et al., 2007). Owing to the lack of comprehensive randomized, double-blind, placebo-controlled trials (Stevinson and Ernst, 2000), valerian is not recommended for subjects under the age of 18 years.

The FDA generally regards valerian as safe, but some studies have reported concerns about toxicity. One study reported hepatoxicity in four women using a combination of valerian and another herbal product called skullcap (*Scutellaria* spp.) (MacGregor et al., 1989). Concern has also been expressed about the cytotoxicity of valepotriates, constituents found in negligible amounts in most valerian preparations. Valepotriates contain an epoxide group and were found to act as alkylating agents in vitro. However, this property was not found in vivo, presumably because of the poor absorption and distribution of valepotriates (Tortarolo et al., 1982; Wagner et al., 1998).

Most studies reporting on the side effects of valerian found them to be mild and generally not more common than the placebo condition. In a placebo-controlled study of 128 subjects, one person experienced nausea and withdrew from the study. However, it was not possible to attribute the nausea definitively to valerian (Leathwood et al., 1982). Another placebo-controlled study found more adverse events with placebo than with valerian (Donath et al., 2000). Some evidence suggests that valerian does not have measurable hangover effects (Leathwood et al., 1982) or adverse effects on cognitive or psychomotor performance (Hallam et al., 2003), but further studies are needed to confirm these claims.

Considerations Specific to the Military

Valerian has the potential for unwanted synergy with other sedating agents that may be ingested. Therefore, people engaged in safety-sensitive activities that require alertness and quick responses should not take valerian in conjunction with other sedating substances, especially not in conjunction with prescription medications having sedating effects. Thirteen (12 percent) of the 109 medications most frequently prescribed for military personnel (e.g., hypnotics, anxiolytics, antidepressants, opioids) have sedating side effects.

Relevant data and conclusions on efficacy and safety reviews and publications identified for valerian are shown in Table 4-15 on pages 294–295.

References

Beaubrun, G., and G. E. Gray. 2000. A review of herbal medicines for psychiatric disorders. *Psychiatr Serv* 51(9):1130-1134.

Bent, S., A. Padula, D. Moore, M. Patterson, and W. Mehling. 2006. Valerian for sleep: A systematic review and meta-analysis. *Am J Med* 119(12):1005-1012.

Bliwise, D. L., and F. P. Ansari. 2007. Insomnia associated with valerian and melatonin usage in the 2002 National Health Interview Survey. *Sleep* 30(7):881-884.

Diaper, A., and I. Hindmarch. 2004. A double-blind, placebo-controlled investigation of the effects of two doses of a valerian preparation on the sleep, cognitive and psychomotor function of sleep-disturbed older adults. *Phytother Res* 18(10):831-836.

Donath, F., S. Quispe, K. Diefenbach, A. Maurer, I. Fietze, and I. Roots. 2000. Critical evaluation of the effect of valerian extract on sleep structure and sleep quality. *Pharmacopsychiatry* 33(2):47-53.

Gyllenhaal, C., S. L. Merritt, S. D. Peterson, K. I. Block, and T. Gochenour. 2000. Efficacy and safety of herbal stimulants and sedatives in sleep disorders. *Sleep Med Rev* 4(3):229-251.

Hallam, K. T., J. S. Olver, C. McGrath, and T. R. Norman. 2003. Comparative cognitive and psychomotor effects of single doses of *Valeriana officianalis* and triazolam in healthy volunteers. *Hum Psychopharmacol* 18(8):619-625.

Hobbs, C. 1989. Valerian: A literature review. *HerbalGram* 21:19-34.

Holzl, J., and P. Godau. 1989. Receptor binding studies with *Valeriana officinalis* on the benzodiazepine receptor. *Planta Medica* 55:642.

Houghton, P. J. 1999. The scientific basis for the reputed activity of valerian. *J Pharm Pharmacol* 51(5):505-512.

Leathwood, P. D., F. Chauffard, E. Heck, and R. Munoz-Box. 1982. Aqueous extract of valerian root (*Valeriana officinalis* L) improves sleep quality in man. *Pharmacol Biochem Behav* 17(1):65-71.

MacGregor, F. B., V. E. Abernathy, S. Dahabra, I. Cobden, and P. C. Hayes. 1989. Hepatotoxicity of herbal remedies. *Br Med J* 299(6708):1156-1157.

Morin, A. K., C. I. Jarvis, and A. M. Lynch. 2007. Therapeutic options for sleep-maintenance and sleep-onset insomnia. *Pharmacotherapy* 27(1):89-110.

Santos, M., F. Ferreira, A. T. Cunha, A. P. Carvalho, and T. Macedo. 1994. An aqueous extract of valerian influences the transport of GABA in synaptosomes. *Planta Medica* 60(3):278-279.

Stevinson, C., and E. Ernst. 2000. Valerian for insomnia: A systematic review of randomized clinical trials. *Sleep Med* 1(2):91-99.

Tortarolo, M., R. Braun, G. E. Hübner, and H. R. Maurer. 1982. In vitro effects of epoxide-bearing valepotriates on mouse early hematopoietic progenitor cells and human T-lymphocytes. *Arch Toxicol* 51(1):37-42.

Wagner, J., M. L. Wagner, and W. A. Hening. 1998. Beyond benzodiazepines: Alternative pharmacologic agents for the treatment of insomnia. *Ann Pharmacother* 32(6):680-686.

TABLE 4-2 Relevant Data and Conclusions on Efficacy and Safety Reviews and Publications Identified for Chromium

Review/ Clinical Trial Reference	Type of Study and Subjects	Indication	Control	Dose	Product Specification
Campbell et al., 1999	Double-blind, randomized n=18 men, 56–69 y	Increasing lean body mass and strength	Placebo	500 μg, 2×/d for 12 wk	Nutrition 21, San Diego, CA
Diaz et al., 2008	Randomized n=35 overweight women	Reducing body weight, increasing lean body mass, and improving aerobic fitness	Placebo	133 μg chromium picolinate and 0.59 g conjugated linoleic acid 3×/d for 3 mo in conjunction with dietary energy restriction and exercise program	None reported
Livolsi et al., 2001	Randomized n=15 female softball players	Increasing lean body mass and strength	Placebo	500 μg/d chromium picolinate for 6 wk	Nutrition 21, San Diego, CA
Lukaski et al., 2007	Double-blind, randomized n=83 females, age 19–50 y	Reducing body weight and altering body composition	Placebo	187 μg chromium for 12 wk	Nutrition 21, San Diego, CA
Martin et al., 2006	Double-blind, randomized n=37, age 25–75 y, with type 2 diabetes	Reducing body weight and adipose tissue, glycemic control, insulin sensitivity	Placebo	1,000 μg/d chromium picolinate for 6 mo	None reported
Nissen and Sharp, 2003	Meta-analysis of 12 studies involving chromium supplementation with weight training in healthy men and women	Increasing lean body mass and strength	Placebo	200 to 1,000 μg	None reported

Clinical Details and Outcomes Measured	Conclusions/Results	Adverse Events Profile	Interactions with Pharmaceuticals, Foods, or Other Dietary Supplements
Body composition, metabolic rate, muscle strength	High-dose chromium picolinate supplements did not influence body composition, strength, or power development.	None reported	None reported
Body composition measured by DEXA; aerobic fitness measured by heart rate and VO_2[b] maximum during exercise	No differences in heart rate, VO_2 maximum, or body composition between participants receiving chromium or placebo.	None reported	None reported
Body weight, percent body fat, lean body mass, strength	No differences in muscle strength or body composition.	None reported	None reported
Body weight; skin fold thickness; bone mineral content; fat mass; lean body mass; hematocrit	Participants given chromium and placebo lost similar amounts of weight and body fat; no differences in bone mineral content, fat-free or hematocrit as a function of supplementation or time.	None reported	None reported
DEXA measurement of body composition; glucose tolerance following a 75-g challenge; urinary chromium excretion; blood levels of triglycerides; free fatty acids, insulin, adiponectin, and C-peptide	Improved glycemic control, increased insulin sensitivity, attenuated body weight gain, changes in body fat distribution with chromium picolinate.	None reported	None reported
Body composition measured by skin folds, hydrostatic weighing, and DEXA[a]	Chromium supplementation associated with small, nonsignificant increases in lean body mass and strength.	None reported	None reported

continued

TABLE 4-2 Continued

Review/ Clinical Trial Reference	Type of Study and Subjects	Indication	Control	Dose	Product Specification
Pittler et al., 2003	Meta-analysis of 10 trials that met all inclusion criteria and 7 studies that were not suitable for statistical pooling Normal-weight and obese males and females engaged or not engaged in weight training	Reducing body weight	Placebo	200 to 400 µg/d for 6 to 26 wk	Various
Trumbo and Ellwood, 2006	Review of five studies assessing effect of chromium picolinate on the risk of type 2 diabetes in obese and normal-weight men and women. Studies included from 13 to 44 participants	Improving insulin sensitivity and glucose tolerance	Placebo	400 to 1,000 µg/d for 12 to 32 wk	Various

[a]Dual-energy X-ray absorptiometry (DEXA) is an enhanced form of X-ray technology that is used to measure bone loss. DEXA is the established standard for measuring bone mineral density.

[b]Oxygen uptake.

Clinical Details and Outcomes Measured	Conclusions/Results	Adverse Events Profile	Interactions with Pharmaceuticals, Foods, or Other Dietary Supplements
Body weight, body fat, lean body weight	Small effect of chromium picolinate compared with placebo for reducing body weight; however, difference due primarily to results of two trials.	None reported	None reported
Insulin resistance and oral glucose tolerance test (OGTT)	One intervention study showed a beneficial effect of chromium picolinate on insulin sensitivity; no studies showed a beneficial effect of chromium picolinate on OGTT.	None reported	None reported

TABLE 4-3 Relevant Data and Conclusions on Efficacy and Safety Reviews and Publications Identified for Creatine

Review/ Clinical Trial Reference	Type of Study and Subjects	Indication	Control	Dose	Product Specification
Bemben and Lamont, 2005	Review	Sport and exercise performance	Various	Various	None reported
Calfee and Fadale, 2006	Review	Effects of creatine use	None reported	None reported	None reported
Cornish et al., 2006	Double-blind, randomized, repeated measures n=17 men, competitive college ice hockey players	Athletic performance (sprint skating)	Placebo	0.3g/kg body mass/d creatine monohydrate for 5 d	Muscle Tech Research and Development Inc., Bramptom, ON, Canada

Outcomes Measured	Conclusions/Results	Adverse Events Profile	Interactions with Pharmaceuticals, Foods, or Other Dietary Supplements
Ergogenic effects related to sports and exercise performance (isotonic/dynamic peak force, isokinetic peak torque, isometric force production, muscle soreness and damage, jumping/sprinting, sprint power cycling, continuous and intermittent endurance)	Beneficial effects of creatine supplementation for repeated, short bouts of high-intensity exercises, particularly isotonic/dynamic peak force parameters. Benefits seen for males and females of all ages.	No strong scientific evidence to support any reported adverse effects; however, no well-controlled long-term studies available	None reported
Athletic performance	Some beneficial effects on athletic performance: increasing strength in outcomes of short-duration anaerobic activities. No improvement in endurance performance.	Weight gain (1.6–2.4 kg) Minor gastrointestinal discomfort and muscle cramps Possible adverse renal effects	None reported
Sprint skating performance (skating treadmill test, lactate analysis, isokinetic testing, and dietary analysis)	No differences between placebo and treatment group for skating treadmill test, blood lactate, isokinetic testing, dietary intake, or changes in body mass. Creatine monohydrate supplementation had no effects on sprint skating performance.	None reported	None reported

continued

TABLE 4-3 Continued

Review/ Clinical Trial Reference	Type of Study and Subjects	Indication	Control	Dose	Product Specification
Derave et al., 2003	Double-blind, randomized n=33 healthy adults (26 men, 7 women, age 18–30 y)	Glucose tolerance	Placebo (maltodextrin)	2 wk immobilization phase: 3 daily doses of 5 g creatine 6 wk retraining phase: 2.5 g/d creatine or 2.5 g/d creatine, 40 g/d protein, and 6.7 g/d amino acids	None reported
Doherty et al., 2002	Double-blind, randomized, crossover n=14 men, mean age (± SD) 22.7 ± 3.5 y	Exercise performance (treadmill running)	Placebo (200 mL artificially sweetened water drink)	0.3 g/kg creatine monohydrate for 6 d (given as 4 doses/d); caffeine abstinence 5 mg/kg caffeine in 200 mL artificially sweetened water drink taken 1 h prior to testing	Isotar Creatine Direct, Westcott and Westcott Ltd., Clevedon, UK
Glaister et al., 2006	Double-blind, randomized n=42 physically active male students	Exercise performance (sprint running)	Placebo (6 g maltodextrin for 4 d)	5 g creatine monohydrate and 1 g maltodextrin for 4 d	Starmax Nutrition, Hereford, UK

Outcomes Measured	Conclusions/Results	Adverse Events Profile	Interactions with Pharmaceuticals, Foods, or Other Dietary Supplements
Muscle GLUT-4[a] muscle glycogen, muscle creatine content, muscle fiber type composition, muscle force, and body weight	Changes in muscle GLUT-4 were not significantly different between groups during immobilization phase; significant increases in GLUT-4 and muscle glycogen after retraining for creatine and creatine plus protein groups; no treatment effects observed for body weight. Creatine supplementation stimulates GLUT-4 and glycogen content in human muscle only when combined with changes in habitual activity level.	None reported	None reported
Plasma caffeine concentration, body mass, MAOD,[b] treadmill run time to exhaustion, total VO_2 rating of exhaustion, and metabolic data	Body mass increased during creatine supplementation and was maintained during placebo and caffeine trials; no increase in MAOD between trials. Acute caffeine intake was ergogenic after creatine supplementation period and caffeine abstinence.	None reported	None reported
Body mass, mean sprint time, blood lactate	Increase in body mass relative to placebo (0.7 kg increase) and reduction in body fat (0.4% reduction). No significant between-group differences in fast sprint time, mean sprint time, fatigue, or posttest blood lactate concentration. Creatine supplementation has no benefit on multiple sprint running performance.	None reported	None reported

continued

TABLE 4-3 Continued

Review/ Clinical Trial Reference	Type of Study and Subjects	Indication	Control	Dose	Product Specification
Graham and Hatton, 1999	Review of literature on creatine published from 1966 to 1999	Safety and efficacy	Various	Various	None reported
Greenwood et al., 2003	Observational n=approximately 100 college football players, age 18–23 y	Muscle cramping and injury	Noncreatine-containing supplement	15.75 g/d creatine monohydrate for 5 d and an average of 5 g/d thereafter (5- to 10-g doses) over a 3-y period	Experimental and Applied Sciences, Degussa Bioactives/ Traco Labs, Champaign, IL, and MetaResponse Modifiers, San Clemente, CA
Groeneveld et al., 2005	Double-blind, randomized n=175 patients with ALS,[c] ages 18–75 y Patients taking 50 mg riluzole twice daily	Neuroprotective and adverse effects	Placebo (Polycose) for 310 d	5 g creatine monohydrate 2×/d for 310 d	DSM Fine Chemicals Inc., Heerlen, the Netherlands

Outcomes Measured	Conclusions/Results	Adverse Events Profile	Interactions with Pharmaceuticals, Foods, or Other Dietary Supplements
Various	As of 1999, no high-quality research on the effects of creatine exists. Little data on short-term and long-term safety of creatine. Limited evidence of benefits. May enhance the performance of high-intensity, short-duration exercise.	May be related to renal dysfunction	Studies on drug interactions are needed
Injury rates, number of missed practices	Incidence of cramping, heat/dehydration, muscle tightness, noncontact joint injuries, contact injuries, illness, number of missed practices due to injury, players lost for the season, and total injuries/missed practices were generally proportional or lower than the creatine use rate among players. Creatine supplementation does not appear to increase the incidence of injury or cramping in college football players. Supplement intake was not blinded or randomized and compliance was self-reported.	No evidence of significant adverse effects	None reported
Reported adverse effects, renal function, urinary creatine	Creatine supplementation was stopped in 3 patients due to complaints of diarrhea and nausea. No significant differences in occurrence of adverse effects between groups.	Severe diarrhea (n=2) and nausea (n=1) Water retention	None reported

continued

TABLE 4-3 Continued

Review/ Clinical Trial Reference	Type of Study and Subjects	Indication	Control	Dose	Product Specification
Gualano et al., 2007	Double-blind, randomized n=22 sedentary healthy men, mean age 24 y	Glucose tolerance and insulin sensitivity; non-insulin-dependent diabetes mellitus	Placebo (dextrose)	0.3 g/kg body weight per d creatine for 1st wk 0.15 g/kg body weight per d creatine for next 11 wk	None reported
Hespel et al., 2002	Double-blind, randomized, crossover n=10 students (9 men, 1 woman), age 21–24 y	Muscle relaxation; exercise performace	Placebo (maltodextrin)	4 × 5 g/d creatine monohydrate for 4 d 4 × 5 g/d creatine monohydrate and 5 mg/kg body weight per d caffeine 2 other protocols with just caffeine	Creatine Fuel, Twin Laboratories, New York, NY

Outcomes Measured	Conclusions/Results	Adverse Events Profile	Interactions with Pharmaceuticals, Foods, or Other Dietary Supplements
VO_2 max test, aerobic exercise training, plasma glucose, and plasma insulin	Significant decrease in oral glucose tolerance test compared to placebo. No differences in fasting insulin. Creatine supplementation in combination with moderate aerobic training over 3 mo improved glucose tolerance in healthy sedentary males but did not alter insulin sensitivity.	No adverse effects were reported in either treatment group	None reported
Maximal knee extension torque, contraction time, relaxation time	No significant differences in muscle contraction time. Caffeine intake increased relaxation time; creatine intake shortened relaxation time, compared to placebo. Combined intake of caffeine and creatine have opposing effects. Short-term caffeine intake inhibits muscle relaxation and conteracts the benefits of creatine supplementation in muscle relaxation.	None reported	Caffeine and creatine have opposing effect on muscle relaxation time

continued

TABLE 4-3 Continued

Review/ Clinical Trial Reference	Type of Study and Subjects	Indication	Control	Dose	Product Specification
Hoffman et al., 2006	Randomized n=33 men college football players	Endocrine changes, strength training performance	Placebo (10.5 g/d dextrose)	10.5 g/d creatine monohydrate or 10.5 g/d creatine monohydrate and 3.2 g/d β-alanine 10-wk program	None reported
Kilduff et al., 2004	Double-blind, randomized n=21 endurance-trained men, mean age 27 y	Cardiovascular, metabolic, and thermoregulatory responses and exercise performance in hot conditions	Placebo (160 g/d glucose polymer in warm/hot water for 7 d)	22.8 g/d creatine monohydrate and 35 g glucose polymer in warm/hot water for 7 d	None reported
Klivenyi et al., 2004	Animal study n=11–13 transgenic mice in each treatment group	ALS	Unsupplemented diet	Diet supplemented with 2% creatine, or 0.05% rofecoxib, or 0.012% celecoxib or combinations of all these	Avicena, Inc., Cambridge, MA

Outcomes Measured	Conclusions/Results	Adverse Events Profile	Interactions with Pharmaceuticals, Foods, or Other Dietary Supplements
Body composition, strength measures, biochemical and hormonal analyses, anaerobic power	No significant differences in change in body mass. Greater changes in lean body mass and percent body fat with combination β-alanine and creatine, than creatine alone. Increased strength improvement with creatine alone or with β-alanine. Resting testosterone was elevated with creatine intake, but no other significant endocrine changes. No significant changes seen in power performance for any group. Addition of β-alanine to creatine supplements enhanced strength performance more than creatine supplementation alone.	None reported	Additive benefit of β-alanine in strength and power training
ICW,[d] TBW,[e] thermoregulatory responses (heart rate, temperature), cardiovascular responses, time to exhaustion	Creatine supplementation increased ICW and TBW and reduced heart rate, temperature, sweat rate. No significant decrease in time to exhaustion. Creatine is beneficial for prolonged exercise in hot conditions.	No reports of gastrointestinal distress or muscle cramping	None reported
Survival, PGE_2[f] tissue content, motor performance, body weight	Significant improvement of survival rates in all mice except those with unsupplemented diet. An additive neuroprotective effect was seen in mice fed combination diets, compared to single supplements. Improved motor performance in supplemented mice, with additive effect for combination diets. Creatine used in combination with rofecoxib and/or celecoxib can be a useful strategy in the treatment of ALS.	None reported	Creatine used in combination with celecoxib and/or rofecoxib (COX-2 inhibitors) had an additive effect on motor performance and survival rate

continued

TABLE 4-3 Continued

Review/ Clinical Trial Reference	Type of Study and Subjects	Indication	Control	Dose	Product Specification
Korzun, 2004	Randomized n=16 healthy adults, age ≥19 y	Hyperhomo-cysteinemia	Daily multivitamin for 8 wk	Daily multivitamin for 4 wk Then, creatine monohydrate (equal to twice their daily creatinine excretion on a molar basis) and a daily multivitamin for 4 wk	Experimental and Applied Sciences, Golden, CO Centrum One-a-Day multivitamin
McMorris et al., 2006	Double-blind n=20 students (17 men, 3 women), mean age 21.1 y	Cognitive and psychomotor performance and mood state due to sleep deprivation	Placebo	5 g creatine monohydrate, 4×/d for 7 d	Creapure, Deguss AG, Dusseldorf, Germany
Mendel et al., 2005	Double-blind n=16 (15 male, 1 female), age 22–33 y	Thermoregulatory response to exercising in the heat (cycling)	Placebo (10 g Solka-flok in 60 g Gatorade) for 5 d	20 g creatine in 60 g Gatorade for 5 d	None reported

Outcomes Measured	Conclusions/Results	Adverse Events Profile	Interactions with Pharmaceuticals, Foods, or Other Dietary Supplements
Serum folate, erythrocyte folate, serum vitamin B_{12}, tHcy[g]	Significantly greater reduction in tHcy seen in creatine plus multivitamin group than multivitamin group. Modest doses of creatine supplements may lower tHcy in humans.	None reported	None reported
Cognitive tests (RMG,[h] verbal and spatial short-term memory tests), psychomotor tests, mood state, plasma catecholamines and cortisol	At 24 h of sleep deprivation, the creatine group had significantly less change in performance from 0 h in RMG, choice reaction time, balance, and mood state. No significant differences between groups in plasma concentrations of catecholamines and cortisol. Creatine supplementation has a positive effect on cognitive and psychomotor performance and mood state after 24 h sleep deprivation.	None reported	None reported
Body weight, temperature response to exercise in the heat	Significant increase in body weight for creatine group. Core temperature was lower after supplementation in both groups. No differences in mean body and mean skin temperatures. No significant effect of short-term creatine supplementation. Did not have a negative effect on thermoregulation during exercise in heat.	None reported	None reported

continued

TABLE 4-3 Continued

Review/ Clinical Trial Reference	Type of Study and Subjects	Indication	Control	Dose	Product Specification
Op't Eijnde et al., 2006	Animal study n=24 male Goto-Kakizaki rats with inherited type 2 diabetes	Type 2 diabetes	Unsupplemented diet	Diet supplemented with 2% creatine monohydrate	Creapure, Degussa, Freising, Germany
Pline and Smith, 2005	Review	Renal function	Various	Various	None reported
Pluim et al., 2006	Double-blind, randomized n=36 men, competitive tennis players, mean age 22 y	Tennis performance	Placebo (maltodextrose and dextrose)	Loading phase: 0.3 g/kg body weight/d for 6 d Maintenance phase: 0.03 g/kg body weight/d for 28 d	Podium, Synergen, Switzerland, and creatine monohydrate, MSD, the Netherlands
Pritchard and Kalra, 1998	Case report n=1 man, age 25 y with nephrotic syndrome taking cyclosporin	Renal dysfunction		15 g/d for 1 wk, then 2 g/d for 7 wk	None reported

Outcomes Measured	Conclusions/Results	Adverse Events Profile	Interactions with Pharmaceuticals, Foods, or Other Dietary Supplements
Body weight, food intake, blood D-glucose, blood insulin, insulinogenic index, muscle biochemistry	Creatine supplementation significantly increased muscle creatine content and lowered the insulinogenic index; this was mainly attributable to a lowering of plasma insulin concentration. Creatine supplementation may improve the sensitivity to insulin in extrapancreatic sites of young male rats.	None reported	None reported
Measures of renal function	In healthy, young adults, creatine supplementation does not have a negative effect on renal function.	Two cases of renal dysfunction	None reported
Speed of serve, ground stroke speed and precision, sprint test, strength measurements	No differences in performance or change in body weight during the loading phase. During maintenance phase, significant increase in body weight in creatine group. No differences in performance between groups. Creatine supplementation does not improve tennis performance and should not be recommended for tennis players.	No gastrointestinal complaints or muscle cramps	None reported
Serum creatinine, creatinine clearance	Serum creatinine levels increased (103 μmol/L to 180 μmol/L). One month after stopping supplementation, levels dropped to 128 μmol/L. In this case, there is strong circumstantial evidence that creatine is responsible for deterioration in renal function.	Renal dysfunction	None reported

continued

TABLE 4-3 Continued

Review/ Clinical Trial Reference	Type of Study and Subjects	Indication	Control	Dose	Product Specification
Reardon et al., 2006	Controlled n=17 healthy, active adults (11 men, 6 women), ages 18–27 y	Endurance training and performance (cycling)	Placebo (24 g/d maltodextrin for 7 d, then 6 g/d for 3 wk)	Load: 20 g/d creatine monohydrate and 4 g/d maltodextrin for 7 d Maintenance: 5 g/d creatine monohydrate and 1 g/d maltodextrine for 3 wk	Musashi Pty Ltd, Australia
Santos et al., 2004	Double-blind n=34 male athletes, ages 21–30 y, training for a marathon	Inflammation and muscle soreness associated with long-distance running	Placebo (60 g maltodextrine for 5 d)	20 g/d creatine monohydrate and 60 g carbohydrate (maltodextrine) for 5 d	None reported
Scheff and Dhillon, 2004	Animal study, randomized n=85 adult male Sprague-Dawley rats subjected to moderate controlled cortical contusions	Neuroprotection following traumatic brain injury	Unsupplemented diet	Diet supplemented with 0.5% or 1.0% creatine monohydrate for 2 wk	Sigma Chemical Co., St. Louis, MO

Outcomes Measured	Conclusions/Results	Adverse Events Profile	Interactions with Pharmaceuticals, Foods, or Other Dietary Supplements
Muscle total creatine and glycogen content, body weight, body fat, oxidative capacity, endurance performance	Muscle total creatine and glycogen contents were elevated in both groups. No significant anthropometric changes in either group, or changes in oxidative capacity. Both groups had significant reductions in carbohydrate oxidation; significant increases in lipid oxidation, total work, and average power output. No treatment effect of creatine supplementation on any parameter of endurance performance.	None reported	None reported
Cell death, inflammation markers, muscle soreness markers (CK,[i] lactate dehydrogenase, PGE_2,[j] and TNFα[k])	After running a 30 km race, increase of cell death and inflammation markers in placebo group. Increase of CK, PGE_2, TNFα in creatine group. No significant difference between groups in time to finish the race. Supplementation with creatine reduced cell damage and inflammation after an exhaustive 30-km running race.	None reported	None reported
Lactate and free fatty acid levels in cortex and hippocampus	Both lactate and free fatty acid levels were significantly increased in all tissues ipsilateral to the injury. Animals supplemented with creatine had significantly lower levels. Greater neuroprotection was seen in animals fed a 1% creatine diet than those fed a 0.5% creatine diet. In adult male rats, a diet supplemented with creatine can provide substantial neuroprotection in part by suppressing secondary brain injury.	None reported	None reported

continued

TABLE 4-3 Continued

Review/ Clinical Trial Reference	Type of Study and Subjects	Indication	Control	Dose	Product Specification
Shao and Hathcock, 2006	Review of randomized, controlled human studies that address safety of creatine or risk assessment		Various	Various	None reported
Smith and Dahm, 2000	Survey of creatine use n=328 student athletes (182 men, 146 women), age 14–18 y				
Sullivan et al., 2000	Animal study, randomized n=40 adult ICR mice and 24 adult Sprague-Dawley rats subjected to moderate, controlled cortical contusions	Neuroprotection following traumatic brain injury	Daily injections of 3 mg/g body weight olive oil for 1, 3, or 5 d before injury	Daily injections of 0.1 mL/10 g body weight of creatine monohydrate suspended in olive oil for 1, 3, or 5 d before injury	Sigma Chemical Co., St. Louis, MO
Thorsteinsdottir et al., 2006	Case report n=1 healthy man, age 24 y with acute renal failure and proteinuria			15 g/wk creatine monophosphate, multiple herbs, nonherbal supplements, and vitamins for 6 mo	

Outcomes Measured	Conclusions/Results	Adverse Events Profile	Interactions with Pharmaceuticals, Foods, or Other Dietary Supplements
	The Observed Safe Level risk assessment method indicates that the evidence of safety of creatine intake is strong at intakes up to 5 g/d for chronic supplementation. Although much higher levels have been tested under acute conditions without adverse effects and may be safe, the data for intakes above 5 g/d are not sufficient for a confident conclusion of long-term safety.		None reported
Adverse effects	8.2% of students surveyed reported creatine use.	Diarrhea, cramps, and loss of appetite were reported	None reported
Tissue damage, synaptic homeostasis	Less cortical damage found in mice (up to 36%) and rats (up to 50%) that were given creatine. Significant increases in mitochondrial membrane potential; significant decreases in intramitochondrial oxygen levels of reactive oxygen species and calcium. Based on this animal model, creatine may have effective use as a neuroprotective agent against acute and delayed neurodegenerative processes.	None reported	None reported
Adverse effects	Previously healthy male presented with acute abdominal pain, polydipsia, and polyuria. He was diagnosed with acute renal failure. Biopsy showed acute interstitial nephritis. Kidney function returned to normal after cessation of supplement intake.	Renal dysfunction	Patient was also taking a large number of other herbs, supplements, and vitamins

continued

TABLE 4-3 Continued

Review/ Clinical Trial Reference	Type of Study and Subjects	Indication	Control	Dose	Product Specification
Volek et al., 2001	Double-blind, randomized n=20 healthy men, mean age 23 y	Exercise performance in the heat (sprint cycling)	Placebo (powdered cellulose—equivalent amount to creatine intake)	0.3 g/kg body weight creatine monohydrate daily for 7 d	Creatine Fuel, Twin Laboratories, Inc., Hauppauge, NY
Volek et al., 2006	Review of the nutritional needs of female strength athletes	Efficacy of creatine supplementation for female athletes		Various	
Warber et al., 2002	Double-blind, randomized n=26 male soldiers, mean age 32 y	Performance of military training tasks (obstacle course, mood state, and marksmanship)	Placebo (sports bar without creatine)	4 sports bars/d containing 6 g creatine monohydrate per bar for 5 d	M&M Mars, Inc., NJ
Watsford et al., 2003	Double-blind, randomized n=22 healthy men, mean age 23.4 y	Musculotendinous stiffness and exercise performance	Placebo	20 g/d creatine for 7 d, then 10 g/d for 21 d	None reported

Outcomes Measured	Conclusions/Results	Adverse Events Profile	Interactions with Pharmaceuticals, Foods, or Other Dietary Supplements
Body mass, body water, cardiovascular responses, temperature responses, kidney function, and peak and mean power	Significant increase in body mass in creatine group. No differences between groups for heart rate, blood pressure, and sweat rate responses. Greater increase in peak power found in the creatine group after sprints. Creatine supplementation had a positive effect on repeated sprint cycle performance in the heat without changes in thermoregulatory responses.	No adverse effects were found	None reported
High-intensity exercise performance; leucine rate of appearance	Like men, women may also benefit from creatine supplementation for improving exercise performance.	None reported	None reported
Anthropometric data, body composition, maximal oxygen uptake, obstacle test performance, bench press performance, rifle marksmanship performance, and mood	No difference between groups on obstacle test performance, rifle marksmanship, or mood. Creatine group had significant increase in bench press repetitions. Creatine usage resulted in 1.4 kg increase in body mass and a 0.5% decrease in body fat, both significantly different than placebo. Short-term supplementation with creatine improved performance on strength tests, but did not significantly improve performance on a military obstacle course in male soldiers.	No reports of gastrointestinal distress or any other medical problems or symptoms	None reported
Body mass, isometric force, rate of force development, and musculotendinous stiffness	Significant gain in body mass, countermovement jump height, and drop jump height. No increase in musculotendinous stiffness. Creatine supplementation did not cause muscle strain injuries. Performance enhancement was found.	None reported	None reported

continued

TABLE 4-3 Continued

Review/ Clinical Trial Reference	Type of Study and Subjects	Indication	Control	Dose	Product Specification
Weiss and Powers, 2006	Double-blind, randomized, counter-balanced n=24 athletic, healthy men, mean age 22.9 y	Exercise performance in the heat (cycling)	Placebo	25 g/d creatine monohydrate for 5 d	Creatine Fuel, Twin Laboratories, Inc., Ronkonkoma, NY

[a]GLUT-4 is a factor in the regulation of blood glucose and the primary glucose transporter in skeletal muscle.
[b]Maximal accumulated oxygen deficit.
[c]Amyotrophic lateral sclerosis.
[d]Intracellular water.
[e]Total body water.

Outcomes Measured	Conclusions/Results	Adverse Events Profile	Interactions with Pharmaceuticals, Foods, or Other Dietary Supplements
Heart rate, blood pressure, core temperature, body water volumes and sweat loss, relative humidity, side effects	No differences in changes in heart rate, blood pressure, temperature, sweat loss, or relative humidity between groups. Creatine group had significant increase in body water volumes. Short-term creatine supplementation does not impair the thermoregulatory response during exercise in the heat.	None reported	None reported

[f]Prostaglandin E_2.
[g]Total plasma homocysteine.
[h]A random movement generation test.
[i]Creatinase kinase.
[j]Prostaglandin E_2.
[k]Tumor necrosis factor-alpha.

TABLE 4-4 Relevant Data and Conclusions on Efficacy and Safety Reviews and Publications Identified for DHEA

Review/ Clinical Trial Reference	Type of Study and Subjects	Indication	Control	Dose	Product Specification
Kroboth et al., 1999	Review of changes in DHEA in aging, disease, and with drug or vitamin use. Individual studies had 5–36 subjects			Oral doses from 50 to 1,600 mg/d	Various
Salek et al., 2002	Review of effects of disease and drugs on DHEA				

Clinical Details and Outcomes Measured	Conclusions/Results	Adverse Events Profile	Interactions with Pharmaceuticals, Foods, or Other Dietary Supplements
Effects of various drugs and disease states on DHEA; effects of DHEA supplementation on blood DHEA, behavior (mood, depression, cognition), body composition	Blood DHEA is lower in variety of clinical conditions including anorexia nervosa, renal disease, diabetes, and lupus. Acute, strenuous exercise increased DHEA in two studies. One study on U.S. Army Rangers during training observed an increase in morning DHEA that was interpreted as response to exercise, sleep, and energy balance stress. Blood DHEA increased from 1.7- to 14-fold depending on oral dose and gender. Inconsistent effects were reported on body composition.	The majority of studies showed an inverse relationship between DHEA/DHEA-S concentrations and cardiovascular disease Minimal serious side effects; some include changes in hormone concentrations, increased facial hair, nasal congestion, headache, fatigue, and mild insomnia	Some drugs reduced (e.g., dexamethasone, insulin) while others increased (e.g., benfluorex, diltiazem) blood DHEA
			Some drugs decrease DHEA by inhibiting ACTH (dexamethasone), including P450 (central nervous system agents). Some drugs increase DHEA by inhibiting sulfatase (danazol) or measure clearance rate (insulin) One epidemiological study showed that blood DHEA-S was inversely associated with multivitamin use and positively with retinol supplementation

continued

TABLE 4-4 Continued

Review/ Clinical Trial Reference	Type of Study and Subjects	Indication	Control	Dose	Product Specification
Allolio and Arlt, 2002	Review of epidemiological and clinical trial research in those with adrenal insufficiency as well as normal older adults	Reduce consequences of aging	Various	25, 50, 100 mg/d used in various studies	Various
Bahrke and Yesalis, 2004	Review of anabolic androgenic steroids and related substances	Performance, body composition, and health			
Mayer and Forstner, 2004	Review of rodent studies	Liver cancer		0.45–1% of the diet for 52–100 wk depending on study	

Clinical Details and Outcomes Measured	Conclusions/Results	Adverse Events Profile	Interactions with Pharmaceuticals, Foods, or Other Dietary Supplements
Hormone concentration, blood lipids, well-being and mood, body composition, and performance	Increase in testosterone and decreased HDL in women, increase in estrogen in men. Neuronal growth and development affected. Low DHEA in men (no association in women) associated with reduced longevity and higher incidence of cardiovascular disease (unclear whether marker of illness or predictor/contributor). Improved overall well-being, sexual satisfaction, and mood following months of treatment but no effect on cognitive performance. Some studies report increased lean body mass and muscle strength but none of the double-blind trials observed these effects. Use in clinical populations with adrenal insufficiency and chronic glucocorticoid treatment may be warranted as well as in individuals with impaired well-being, mood, or sexuality. Not enough evidence to recommend use for reducing normal effects of aging. Increase in testosterone or enhance adaptations to resistance training in young men; increases in testosterone and virilizing effects are noted in women. Not of benefit for male athletes and has masculinizing effects in women.	Mild and transient side effects: facial acne, increased sebum production; effect on promoting sex hormone-dependent cancer is still "unsettled" and requires more research	None reported
Liver metabolism, hepatocarcinogenesis, modulation of chemically induced hepatocarcinogenesis	Hepatic tumor promotion and inhibition effects depending on dose, rat strain, and duration of ingestion. Liver metabolism increases and becomes catabolic (e.g., reduction of glycogen).		

continued

TABLE 4-4 Continued

Review/ Clinical Trial Reference	Type of Study and Subjects	Indication	Control	Dose	Product Specification
Brown et al., 2006	Review of several prohormone supplements for athletes	Performance and body composition		Doses up to 1,600 mg/d	Various
Evans et al., 2007	Cochrane Collaboration review of randomized, placebo-controlled trials in people age >50 y without dementia who received DHEA of any dose for more than 1 d	Effect on cognitive function in elderly	Placebo	50 mg/d	Various
Raven and Hinson, 2007	Update on review previously performed in 2001, postmenopausal women	Chronic disease			

Clinical Details and Outcomes Measured	Conclusions/Results	Adverse Events Profile	Interactions with Pharmaceuticals, Foods, or Other Dietary Supplements
Serum hormone concentration, health and performance effects	Acute ingestion: Men—Increases serum DHEA, androstenedione, estrogen, but not testosterone. Women—Increases DHEA, androstenedione, testosterone. Chronic ingestion: Men—Dose-dependent increases in DHEA, androstenedione with no change in testosterone. Studies in young novice or older experienced weight lifters report no benefit on fat loss, muscle gain, or muscle function. Women—Increases serum testosterone, acne, facial hair, insulin resistance. Few studies evaluated effects on muscle size and strength concurrent with resistance training. Conclusion: No benefit of DHEA supplements for athletes.	DHEA may have some similar effects on androstenedione reduction in HDL. Speculation on possible effects on premature closure of epiphyseal plates during growth, hypertrophy of areas of the brain related to aggression, and prostate hypertrophy. No evidence of change in liver function markers	None reported
	No evidence of improvement in memory or other aspects of cognitive function in nondemented older people.	One trial reported reduced performance in the visual memory recall test with DHEA. No consistent adverse effects, none longer than 3 mo	None reported
	Supplementation is not recommended for majority of postmenopausal women. Only exceptions could be those with the lowest endogenous DHEA or those with low bone mineral density.		

continued

TABLE 4-4 Continued

Review/ Clinical Trial Reference	Type of Study and Subjects	Indication	Control	Dose	Product Specification
Morales et al., 1998	Double-blind, randomized, crossover n=9 men, 10 women	Aging-related reduction in muscle strength and hormones	Placebo for 6 mo	100 mg/d for 6 mo	Diosynth Corporation, Chicago, IL. Purity confirmed with HPLC
Baulieu et al., 2000	Double-blind, randomized n=280 healthy men and women, ages 60–79 y	Reduce consequences of aging	Placebo for 12 mo	50 mg/d for 12 mo	Prasterone
Percheron et al., 2003	Double-blind, randomized n=280 healthy men and women, ages 60–80 y	Muscle function change during aging	Placebo for 12 mo	50 mg/d for 12 mo	Akzo Laboratories, Diosynth, France
Missmer et al., 2004	Case-control nested within Nurses' Health Study n=322 women who developed breast cancer		None reported	None reported	None reported
Villareal and Holloszy, 2004	Double-blind, randomized n=52 elderly men and women, age 65–78 y	Abdominal fat and insulin action	Placebo	50 mg/d for 6 mo	Schering-Plough, Munich, Germany

Clinical Details and Outcomes Measured	Conclusions/Results	Adverse Events Profile	Interactions with Pharmaceuticals, Foods, or Other Dietary Supplements
Body composition (DEXA), serum hormones, muscle strength	Both genders: Increased serum DHEA to young adult range Women—Increase in body weight by 1.4 kg, increased testosterone to concentrations greater than normal range Men—Elevation of serum IGF-1,[a] reduction in body fat mass of 1.0 kg, increase in muscle strength. DHEA improved body composition.	None reported	None reported
Blood hormones, bone mineral density and turnover markers, libido parameters, skin integrity	Small increase in estrogen and testosterone (particularly in women), reduced bone turnover and increased libido, improved skin integrity in women over 70 y, reduced some effects of aging on bone, skin, and libido.	None reported	None reported
Muscle strength and cross-sectional area and serum DHEA	Serum DHEA restored to ranges for young adults (increase of >200%) but no effect on muscle strength or cross-sectional area. No benefits found.	None reported	None reported
Blood samples collected 8–9 y prior to development of breast cancer. Measured for concentration of endogenous sex hormones and stratified into quartiles	High DHEA was associated with higher risk of developing hormone-sensitive breast cancer. Relative risk for those in highest DHEA quartile was 2.3 compared to those in lowest quartile.	Risk of breast cancer	
Magnetic resonance imaging for visceral and subcutaneous abdominal fat, glucose and insulin response to oral glucose tolerance test	More reduction in visceral and subcutaneous fat area, and insulin area under the curve compared with placebo. Glucose area under the curve was unchanged. Could play a role in reducing abdominal fat and improving insulin sensitivity in aged individuals.	None reported	None reported

continued

TABLE 4-4 Continued

Review/ Clinical Trial Reference	Type of Study and Subjects	Indication	Control	Dose	Product Specification
Kaaks et al., 2005a	Case-control nested within the European Prospective Investigation into Cancer and Nutrition cohort n=370 premenopausal women who developed breast cancer	Endogenous hormones and breast cancer risk in premenopausal women	726 cancer-free matched controls	None reported	None reported
Kaaks et al., 2005b	Case-control study nested within the European Prospective Investigation into Cancer and Nutrition cohort n=677 postmenopausal women who developed breast cancer	Endogenous hormones and breast cancer risk in postmenopausal women	1,309 cancer-free matched controls	None reported	None reported
Nair et al., 2006	Double-blind, randomized n=87 men, 57 women, age ≥60 y	Prevention of age-related disabilities	Placebo	Men: 75 mg/d Women: 50 mg/d, placebo or testosterone patch 2-y treatment	Confirmed to be 95.5% pure upon analysis
Muller et al., 2006	Double-blind, randomized n=100 men, age ≥70 y	Prevention of frailty in elderly men	Placebo	50 mg/d DHEA (other arms included atamestane, atamestane and DHEA, or placebo)	Schering AG provided the tablets

[a]Insulin-like growth factor.

Clinical Details and Outcomes Measured	Conclusions/Results	Adverse Events Profile	Interactions with Pharmaceuticals, Foods, or Other Dietary Supplements
Blood concentrations of endogenous sex hormones	Highest quartile of blood DHEA had relative risk of 1.48 for breast cancer compared to those at lowest quartile.	Risk of breast cancer	
Blood concentrations of endogenous sex hormones	Highest quintile of blood DHEA had relative risk of 1.69 for breast cancer compared to those at lowest quintile.	Risk of breast cancer	None reported
Physical performance, body composition, bone mineral density, glucose tolerance, quality of life (Health Status Questionnaire), prostate imaging for size and PSA test	DHEA: Men—Increase in plasma DHEA and slight but significant increase in bone mineral density (femoral neck), but no effect on body composition, peak oxygen consumption (aerobic fitness), muscle strength, insulin sensitivity, or adverse events. Women—Modest increase in plasma testosterone and increase in DHEA, slight increase in bone mineral density at ultradistal radius. No improvement in muscle strength, aerobic fitness, quality-of-life indicators, or major adverse events. Testosterone and DHEA: Reduction in HDL, slight (<0.5 kg) but significant increase in fat-free mass. No evidence of benefit for physical performance. The modest effect on bone mineral density in one location for each gender is less than that for other pharmacological interventions, so is of limited value.	No effect on prostate size or blood PSA, liver function markers, electrolytes, or hemoglobin It was noted that 2 years of testing may not be sufficient to detect effects on prostate	None reported
Grip strength, leg extensor power	No effects of any treatment on any variable. No support for use of DHEA to reduce frailty in elderly men.	None reported	None reported

TABLE 4-5 Relevant Data and Conclusions on Efficacy and Safety Reviews and Publications Identified for Ephedra

Review/ Clinical Trial Reference	Type of Study and Subjects	Indication	Control	Dose	Product Specification
Andraws et al., 2005	Review of clinical trials	Weight loss and athletic performance and cardiovascular risk	Placebo	Doses of ephedrine and related compounds ranged from 60–150 mg/d	Various
Boozer et al., 2002	Randomized, double-blind n=167 BMI[a]= 31.8±4.1 kg/m^2	Weight loss	Placebo	Ephedra 90 mg/d, caffeine 192 mg/d, for 6 mo	None reported

Outcomes Measured	Conclusions/Results	Adverse Events Profile	Interactions with Pharmaceuticals, Foods, or Other Dietary Supplements
Efficacy and safety of ephedra and ephedrine for the treatment of obesity	Studies to date have examined small cohorts for relatively short periods of time (usually ≤6 mo), and have high attrition rates, and most studies have looked at ephedrine in combination with caffeine and, in several cases, aspirin. Weight loss due to these products, while statistically significant, may not be clinically relevant (1 kg) with anywhere from a 2- to 4-fold increase in side effects compared to placebo.	Modest incidence of cardiovascular side effects, including mild and transient increases in systolic and diastolic blood pressure, heart rate, and palpitations No major adverse cardiovascular events (i.e., stroke, myocardial infarction, or malignant arrhythmias) Adverse event profiles may be different in cohorts with preexisting cardiovascular disease	None reported
Changes in blood pressure, heart function, body weight, body composition, and metabolic changes	Body weight, body fat, and low-density lipoprotein cholesterol decreased significantly. Increased high-density lipoprotein cholesterol. Small changes in blood pressure variables (+3 to –5 mm Hg), and increased heart rate (4±9 vs. –3±9 bpm). No increase in cardiac arrhythmias. By self-report, dry mouth, heartburn, and insomnia were increased in the treatment group; the placebo group reported more diarrhea. Herbal ephedra/caffeine supplements promoted reduction in body weight and body fat and improved blood lipids without significant adverse events.	Reports of irritability, nausea, chest pain, and palpitations did not differ, nor did numbers of subjects who withdrew	None reported

continued

TABLE 4-5 Continued

Review/ Clinical Trial Reference	Type of Study and Subjects	Indication	Control	Dose	Product Specification
Coffey et al., 2004	Double-blind, randomized, multicenter n=102, ages 18–65 y, with 30<BMI≤39.9 kg/m^2	Weight loss	Placebo	Ephedra product containing 125 mg ma huang (10 mg ephedra at 8%), 250 mg kola nut (60 mg caffeine at 25%), 100 mg white willow bark (15 mg salicin at 15%), 12 wk	None reported
Hackman et al., 2006	Double-blind, randomized n=61 healthy premenopausal women, BMI 27–39 kg/m^2	Weight loss	Placebo	Ephedra/caffeine 9 mo study	Mixture providing 40 mg/d ephedra alkaloids, 100 mg/d caffeine, high-potency mixture of vitamins, minerals, omega-3 fatty acids

Outcomes Measured	Conclusions/Results	Adverse Events Profile	Interactions with Pharmaceuticals, Foods, or Other Dietary Supplements
Weight, percent body fat, fat mass, waist circumference, BMI, blood pressure, and pulse measured at 2 d, 1 wk, 2 wk, 4 wk, 8 wk, and 12 wk postrandomization	Additional weight loss (average=1.5 kg) and greater reductions in BMI and waist circumference in treatment group but may not be clinically significant. No differences observed in percent body fat, fat mass, diastolic or systolic blood pressure, pulse, the occurrence of any adverse event. Testing of the study product by two independent laboratories indicated that it only had approximately half the amount of ephedrine alkaloids and caffeine indicated on the label.	None reported	None reported
Changes in body weight, body composition, lipids, insulin, leptin, adiponectin, ghrelin, and self-reports of physical activity, diet, and quality-of-life indexes as well as well blood pressure, heart rate, electrocardiograms, urinalysis, blood histology, serum chemistry measures, and self-reported symptoms	The treatment group lost significantly more body weight (–7.18 kg) and body fat (–5.33 kg) than the control group (–2.25 and –0.99 kg, respectively), and showed significant declines in serum cholesterol, triglycerides, cholesterol to high-density lipoprotein ratio, glucose, fasting insulin, and leptin. Blood pressure, electrocardiograms, other clinical chemistry measures, blood histology, urinalysis, and self-reported physical activity were similar in both groups. The treatment group reported more energy and decreased appetite compared with placebo and scored higher on a quality-of-life domain assessing vitality. Low dose (40 mg/d) of ephedra alkaloids plus caffeine appeared safe and effective in causing loss of weight and body fat and improving several metabolic parameters, including insulin sensitivity and lipid profiles, when tested under physician supervision.	Dry mouth, insomnia, nervousness, and palpitations	None reported

continued

TABLE 4-5 Continued

Review/ Clinical Trial Reference	Type of Study and Subjects	Indication	Control	Dose	Product Specification
Keisler and Hosey, 2005	Review	Weight loss and athletic performance	Placebo	Various	Various
Shekelle et al., 2003	Meta-analysis 52 randomized clinical trials 65 case reports	Weight loss and athletic performance and safety analysis	Placebo/ none	10–20 mg/d low dose, 40–90 mg/d middle dose, 100–150 mg/d high dose, up to 6 mo	Various

Outcomes Measured	Conclusions/Results	Adverse Events Profile	Interactions with Pharmaceuticals, Foods, or Other Dietary Supplements
Athletic performance	Ephedra use showed a 0.6–0.8 kg/mo weight loss compared to placebo. Caffeine plus ephedra resulted in a 1.0 kg/mo weight loss compared to placebo, reported only over a 6-mo period. No long-term data exist. The majority of the studies published in the literature show no effect on athletic performance.	Myocardial infarction reported in two male athletes ages 16–19 y Cardiac arrhythmias, hemorrhagic stroke, and seizures have been reported in young athletes Development of psychotic symptoms including decreased sleep, increased agitation, hostility, paranoid delusions, and auditory hallucinations in men ages 19–33 y. Kidney stones have also been reported	None reported
Weight loss, heart palpitations, and psychiatric, autonomic, or gastrointestinal symptoms	Pooled results for trials with ephedrine (n=5), ephedrine and caffeine (n=12), ephedra (n=1), and ephedra and herbs containing caffeine (n=4) yielded estimates of weight loss of 0.6, 1.0, 0.8, and 1.0 kg/mo, respectively, greater than placebo. No trials of ephedra and athletic performance were found; seven trials of ephedrine were too heterogeneous to analyze. Ephedrine and ephedra promote modest short-term weight loss (approximately 0.9 kg/mo more than placebo) in clinical trials. No data regarding long-term weight loss and insufficient evidence to support use of ephedra for athletic performance.	Psychiatric disturbances, autonomic and gastrointestinal symptoms, and heart palpitations Data are insufficient to draw conclusions about adverse events occurring at a rate less than 1.0 per thousand	None reported

continued

TABLE 4-5 Continued

Review/ Clinical Trial Reference	Type of Study and Subjects	Indication	Control	Dose	Product Specification
Bell et al., 2001	Randomized, double-blind n=24 healthy, untrained men	Athletic performance	Placebo= Metamucil (bulk-forming laxative)	Caffeine (5 mg/kg body weight) and ephedrine (1.0 mg/kg body weight)	None reported

Outcomes Measured	Conclusions/Results	Adverse Events Profile	Interactions with Pharmaceuticals, Foods, or Other Dietary Supplements
The trials (3-, 5-, 10-min exercise) commenced 1.5 h treatment or placebo Anaerobic power and ATP production from anaerobic metabolism (MAOD[b]) Measurement of blood lactate, glucose, and catecholamines (postdrug ingestion just before exercise and 3-, 5-, and 10-min post exercise)	Ephedrine increased power output during the early phase of the Wingate test. Caffeine increased time to exhaustion and O_2 deficit during the MAOD test. Caffeine, ephedrine, and a combination increased blood lactate, glucose, and catecholamine levels. Improvement in anaerobic exercise performance may be caused by stimulation of the central nervous system by ephedrine and stimulation of skeletal muscle by caffeine. The outcomes and conclusions of this study were challenged by Goldberg et al. (2002) in a letter to the Editor-in-Chief, owing to clinical significance and statistical methods used to analyze the data.	None reported	None reported

continued

TABLE 4-5 Continued

Review/ Clinical Trial Reference	Type of Study and Subjects	Indication	Control	Dose	Product Specification
Bell et al., 2002	Controlled n=12	Athletic performance	Placebo (P) =300 mg Metamucil (bulk-forming laxative)	Caffeine (C) (4 mg/kg body weight) and ephedrine (E) (0.8 mg/kg body weight)	None reported

Outcomes Measured	Conclusions/Results	Adverse Events Profile	Interactions with Pharmaceuticals, Foods, or Other Dietary Supplements
VO_2,[c] VCO_2,[d] V_E,[e] heart rate, and ratings of perceived exertion measured during the run Blood lactate, glucose, and catecholamines	Run times in minutes were 46.0 for C, 45.5 for E, 45.7 for C&E, and 46.8 for P. The run times for the E trials (E and C&E) were significantly reduced compared with the non-E trials (C and P). Pace was increased for the E trials compared with the non-E trials over the last 5 km of the run. The E trials (E and C&E) produced significantly faster run times and rate of perceived effort), a reduction of 1.75% of the non-E trials (C and P). VO_2 was not affected by drug ingestion. Heart rate was elevated for the ephedrine trials (E and C&E). Caffeine increased the epinephrine and norepinephrine response associated with exercise and also increased blood lactate, glucose, and glycerol levels. Ephedrine reduced the epinephrine response but increased dopamine and free fatty acid levels. The additive nature of E and C was not evident, with the primary ergogenic effect being attributed to E.	None reported	None reported

continued

TABLE 4-5 Continued

Review/ Clinical Trial Reference	Type of Study and Subjects	Indication	Control	Dose	Product Specification
Jacobs et al., 2003	Double-blind n=13 healthy men	Athletic performance	Placebo= 300 mg Metamucil (bulk-forming laxative)	Caffeine (4 mg/ kg body weight) and ephedrine HCl (0.8 mg/kg body weight)	Anhydrous caffeine (Sandoz Canada) and ephedrine HCl (Roberts Pharmaceutical Canada)

Outcomes Measured	Conclusions/Results	Adverse Events Profile	Interactions with Pharmaceuticals, Foods, or Other Dietary Supplements
Muscular endurance	Ephedrine trials (C&E and E), indicated a transient but significant increase in the mean number of repetitions completed for both the leg-press and bench-press exercises compared with the non-ephedrine trials (C and P), but only during the first set of traditional resistance-training exercise. Total weight lifted during all three sets was greater for the trials involving ephedrine ingestion. Systolic blood pressure was significantly increased with both ephedrine treatment trials when compared with the other trials (C&E=156 mm Hg; E=150 mm Hg; C=141 mm Hg; P=138 mm Hg). Acute ingestion of E or C&E increases muscular endurance during the first set of traditional resistance-training exercise. The performance enhancement was attributed primarily to the effects of E; there was no additive effect of caffeine.	High blood pressure	None reported

continued

TABLE 4-5 Continued

Review/ Clinical Trial Reference	Type of Study and Subjects	Indication	Control	Dose	Product Specification
Magkos and Kavouras, 2004	Review	Athletic performance	Placebo	Various	Caffeine plus ephedrine
Abourashed et al., 2003	Review of adverse events	Weight loss, performance enhancements	Various	Various	Various

Outcomes Measured	Conclusions/Results	Adverse Events Profile	Interactions with Pharmaceuticals, Foods, or Other Dietary Supplements
Performance enhancement and metabolic parameters	Mixtures of caffeine and ephedrine HCl have been reported to confer a greater ergogenic benefit than either drug used alone. Data on increased performance are limited but consistent during submaximal steady-state aerobic exercise, short- and long-distance running, maximal and supramaximal anaerobic cycling, and weight lifting. Blood glucose and lactate concentrations were increased during exercise with ingestion of caffeine and ephedrine in combination; similar effects on lipid fuels (free fatty acids and glycerol) are less pronounced. Concentrations of epinephrine and dopamine are significantly increased though the effects on norepinephrine are less clear. No physiologically significant effects have been reported on pulmonary gas exchange during short-term intense exercise following ingestion of caffeine, ephedrine or their combination; during longer and/or more demanding efforts, some sporadic enhancements have been shown. Despite the type of activity being performed, caffeine and ephedrine combined are quite effective in decreasing the rating of perceived exertion.	Increase in heart rate	None reported
Weight loss, performance enhancements, and potential health risks	Of the 140 adverse events submitted to the FDA for dietary supplements between 1997 and 1999, 31% were probably related to ephedra and 31% were deemed possibly related.	Various	None reported

continued

TABLE 4-5 Continued

Review/ Clinical Trial Reference	Type of Study and Subjects	Indication	Control	Dose	Product Specification
Bent et al., 2003	Review of case series and case reports		None reported	Various	Various
Dhar et al., 2005	Review of adverse events		Various	Various	Various

Outcomes Measured	Conclusions/Results	Adverse Events Profile	Interactions with Pharmaceuticals, Foods, or Other Dietary Supplements
The relative risk and 95% confidence interval for experiencing an adverse reaction after ephedra use compared with other herbs. This risk was defined as the ratio of adverse reactions to ephedra versus other products, divided by the ratio of their relative use in the United States	Although products containing ephedra accounted for only 0.82% of sales of herbal products in the United States, they were associated with 64% of all adverse event reports for such products. The relative risks for an adverse reaction in persons using ephedra were extremely high compared with other herbs, ranging from 100 for kava to 720 for *Ginkgo biloba.* Use of ephedra is associated with a risk for adverse reactions that is greatly increased compared with other herbal products, and its use should be restricted.	Various	None reported
Cardiovascular adverse events related to ephedra use		Ephedra use is associated with ischemic and hemorrhagic stroke, cardiac arrhythmias including ventricular tachycardia, coronary vasospasm, acute myocardial infarction, tachycardia-induced cardiomyopathy, and sudden death. Increased coronary vasoconstriction, tachycardia, and hypertension due to ephedra may be the mechanism of induced myocardial ischemia and infarction. Hemorrhagic stroke is likely secondary to hypertension or cerebral vasculitis	None reported

continued

TABLE 4-5 Continued

Review/ Clinical Trial Reference	Type of Study and Subjects	Indication	Control	Dose	Product Specification
Haller et al., 2005	Review of 65 cases (4 MedWatch reports from 1993 to 1999)		None reported	Various	Ephedra/ caffeine
Kalman et al., 2002	Double-blind, randomized n=27 healthy overweight adults (ages 21–60 y)		Placebo	Ephedra 335 mg, guarana 910 mg, bitter orange 85 mg, for 14 d	Xenadrine

Outcomes Measured	Conclusions/Results	Adverse Events Profile	Interactions with Pharmaceuticals, Foods, or Other Dietary Supplements
Probability of causation based on temporal relationship, biological plausibility, and underlying risk factors in supplement-associated seizure cases Characterization of the patterns of use and types of supplements involved in cases of seizures Identification of trends that may explain potential risks factors for dietary supplement-related seizures	Of the 65 cases, 20 seizures were judged to be probably related, 13 possibly related, and 10 unrelated to use of dietary supplements; 5 cases were not seizures, and 17 cases contained insufficient information. In the 20 probably related cases, 19 involved ephedra, 14 involved herbal caffeine, and in 1 case, the supplement contained an array of elemental salts but no herbal constituents. Ephedra was also associated with 7 of the 13 possibly related cases, and caffeine was contained in 5 of these supplement products. Weight loss (45%) and athletic performance enhancement (30%) were the most often cited reasons for supplement use. Ephedra was implicated in 27 of 33 dietary supplementation-associated seizures reported to the FDA over a 7-year period.	None reported	None reported
Systolic and diastolic blood pressure, heart rate, serial electrocardiograms, and Doppler echocardiograms		No cardiovascular side effects observed No significant effects observed in heart rate, systolic blood pressure, diastolic blood pressure, left ventricular ejection fraction, heart valve function, or in cardiovascular physiology within the parameters measured compared to placebo	None reported

continued

TABLE 4-5 Continued

Review/ Clinical Trial Reference	Type of Study and Subjects	Indication	Control	Dose	Product Specification
Maglione et al., 2005	Review n=1,800 adverse events (from MedWatch reports through September 2001)			Various	Various
Miller, 2004	Review	Weight loss and athletic performances	Various	Ma huang, ephedra, ephedrine-type alkaloids, ephedrine, and dietary supplements (doses not reported)	None reported

Outcomes Measured	Conclusions/Results	Adverse Events Profile	Interactions with Pharmaceuticals, Foods, or Other Dietary Supplements
Serious psychiatric events: psychosis, mania or severe agitation, severe depression, hallucinations, delusions, suicide attempts, paranoia, or violent behavior	Of the almost 1,800 adverse events, 57 were classified as serious psychiatric events. Patients with preexisting psychological/psychiatric conditions and/or use of other mood-altering medications or illicit substances were involved in 2/3 of these psychiatric cases. There was insufficient documentation for the majority of case reports to make an informed judgment about a relationship between the specific adverse event and the use of ephedra. No definitive causal link could be drawn between ephedra and psychiatric complications from the case reports evaluated.	Psychosis	None reported
Weight loss, athletic performance, efficacy, safety	Few studies support the efficacy or safety of these supplements. Weight loss and athletic performance appear to be only modestly improved, for short durations, in the setting of large numbers of (sometimes serious) adverse event reports.	Seizures, myocarditis, myocardial infarction	None reported

continued

TABLE 4-5 Continued

Review/ Clinical Trial Reference	Type of Study and Subjects	Indication	Control	Dose	Product Specification
Vukovich et al., 2005	Double-blind, randomized, crossover n=8 healthy subjects (4 men, 4 women), mean age 23.4±0.8 y and 22.5±3.1% body fat		Placebo	20 mg ephedra alkaloids and 150 mg caffeine	Ephedra extract plus caffeine
Boerth and Caley, 2003	Case report n=1 women, age 21 y			Two supplements containing ephedra	None reported
Charatan, 2003	Case report n=1, healthy overweight male athlete, age 23 y			Ephedra (20 mg ephedrine) 3/d	Xenadrine RFA1

Outcomes Measured	Conclusions/Results	Adverse Events Profile	Interactions with Pharmaceuticals, Foods, or Other Dietary Supplements
REE[f] Heart rate and blood pressure Blood glucose, caffeine, ephedrine, and free fatty	After 3 h, heart rate was 22.7% higher than baseline for the caffeine/ephedra group compared with 8.9% higher for the placebo group. At 3 h, systolic blood pressure was 9.1% higher than baseline for the caffeine/ephedra trial compared with a difference from baseline of only 1.9% for the placebo trial. There was no effect of the caffeine and ephedra combination on diastolic blood pressure. During the last 30 min, REE was 4.5% higher in the placebo trial and 10.7% higher in the caffeine/ephedra trial; REE was 8.5% higher in the caffeine/ephedra trial compared with the placebo trial. Free fatty acids increased over time in both the placebo and caffeine/ephedra trials (from 0.5 to 0.63 mEq/L and from 0.48 to 0.8 mEq/L, respectively). Conclusion: Caffeine and ephedra, at doses of 150 mg and 20 mg ephedrine, respectively, result in a significant elevation in REE, heart rate, and blood pressure. Although significant, the increase in energy expenditure is negligible in terms of weight loss.	Increases in heart rate, blood pressure	None reported
Medical history	The patient's medical history was significant for familial bipolar disease. She remained hospitalized for 2 weeks and was treated for acute psychotic disorder; she was discharged with a diagnosis of schizoaffective disorder, bipolar type.	Potential minor role in exacerbating the mania	None reported
Organ failure	Patient died suddenly of heatstroke that resulted in multiorgan failure following a training workout after taking Xenadrine RFA1 for weight loss.	Sudden death due to heatstroke causing multiple organ failure	None reported

continued

TABLE 4-5 Continued

Review/ Clinical Trial Reference	Type of Study and Subjects	Indication	Control	Dose	Product Specification
Chen-Scarabelli et al., 2005	Case report n=1 woman, age 45 y			Ephedra plus other herbs	Xenadrin
Chen et al., 2004	Case report n=5 (2 men, 3 women), ages 19–45 y			Ephedra plus other herbs	Ripped Fuel, Metabolife 356, ma huang, Hydroxycut
Haller and Benowitz, 2000	Review n=140 case reports (from adverse events reported to the FDA from 1997 to 1999)		Various	Various	Shape-Fast Plus, Ripped Force, Ripped Fuel, Herbalife's Thermojetics, Metabolife 356, OmniTrim Extra Vitamin-Fortified tea, Ultimate Orange, Purple Blast, Diet Fuel, Fit America Natural Weight Control Aid, Per-Form Dieter's Natural tea, Diet-Phen, Ultimate Nutrition Product ma huang, Magic Herb

Outcomes Measured	Conclusions/Results	Adverse Events Profile	Interactions with Pharmaceuticals, Foods, or Other Dietary Supplements
Tissue analysis	Patient died of cardiovascular collapse after taking Xenadrin in combination with aspirin, Nicotrol, and Prozac. Tissue analysis revealed nonspecific degenerative alterations in the myocardium such as lipofuscin accumulation, caspase activation, and cleavage of myofibrillary proteins.	Cardiovascular collapse	Case confounded by concomitant ingestion of aspirin, Prozac, and Nicotrol, and possible marijuana use
Patient-reported symptoms (dizziness, headache, right- or left-side weakness, aphasia and/or slurred speech), MRI[g]	MRI scans showed single or multiple areas of infarction. Ephedra-containing products appear to have predisposed these five patients to both ischemic and hemorrhagic strokes.	Ischemic stroke	Multiple herbal and caffeine use
	Use of ephedra alkaloids was considered definitely or probably associated with 31% of cases, and another 31% possibly related. Of the events related to ephedra, 47% were cardiovascular and 18% were central nervous system events. Hypertension was the most frequent adverse event (17 reports); followed by palpitations, tachycardia, or both (13); stroke (10); and seizures (7). There were 10 events resulting in death, and 13 resulted in permanent disability; 63% of patients were under the age of 45 y. Serious events occurred in persons taking low doses of ephedra (12–36 mg/d), and 11 events occurred in healthy individuals; most of the cases were in individuals under the age of 45 y.	Cardiovascular events, hypertension, seizures	None reported

continued

TABLE 4-5 Continued

Review/ Clinical Trial Reference	Type of Study and Subjects	Indication	Control	Dose	Product Specification
Haller et al., 2005	Review n=65 case reports (adverse events reported to the FDA from 1993 to 1999)			Various	Formula 1, Amp II Pro Drops, Herbalife Thermojetics, Thermochrome 500, Shape–Fast, Power Trim, Metabolift, Victory Turbo Pump
Jacobs and Hirsch, 2000	Case report n=2 men, ages 27 and 20 y			Ephedra plus other herbs, creatine, DHEA, ginseng	None reported

Outcomes Measured	Conclusions/Results	Adverse Events Profile	Interactions with Pharmaceuticals, Foods, or Other Dietary Supplements
Hypoglycemia, secondary stroke, cardiac arrest, seizure	Of the 65 cases, 20 cases of seizures were judged as probably related, 13 as possibly, and 10 as unrelated; 5 cases were not seizures; and 17 cases did not contain enough information to be analyzed. Of the 20 probable cases, 19 were associated with ephedra, and 14 with herbal forms of caffeine. Of the 13 possible cases, ephedra was associated with 7 and caffeine with 5. Seizures were associated with hypoglycemia in 3 cases, secondary to stroke in 2 cases, and cardiac arrest in 2 cases. Of the 33 cases of probable and possible seizure associated with ephedra use, 18 were in subjects 18–39 y of age.	Seizures	None reported
Mood, psychosis, agitation	A 27-year-old man presented to the emergency room (ER) with suicidal ideation and irritable mood. He had a 2-year history of ephedra use. Once he stopped using ephedra, his mood returned to normal. A 20-year-old man presented with acute psychosis and agitation. He was taking ephedra-containing dietary supplements, ginseng, DHEA, and creatine with caffeine.	Psychosis	None reported

continued

TABLE 4-5 Continued

Review/ Clinical Trial Reference	Type of Study and Subjects	Indication	Control	Dose	Product Specification
Jordan et al., 2004	Case reports n=13 subjects with impaired baroflex function due to autonomic failure			Pseudoephedrine or phenylpropanolamine (12.5–25 mg)	None reported
Libman et al., 2005	Case report n=1 male bodybuilder, age 37 y			Ephedra	MuscleTech Hydroxycut used daily for 3 y and nandrolone and stanazol used weekly for 1 y

Outcomes Measured	Conclusions/Results	Adverse Events Profile	Interactions with Pharmaceuticals, Foods, or Other Dietary Supplements
Systolic blood pressure	Phenylpropanolamine increased systolic blood pressure by 21 mm Hg after 90 min. However, when ingested with 16 oz of room-temperature tap water, phenylpropanolamine increased systolic blood pressure by 82 mm Hg. When taken with 16 oz of water, 30 mg of pseudoephedrine increased systolic blood pressure 52 mm Hg on average and by as much as 88 mm Hg. Ephedra alkaloids increase blood pressure significantly in individuals with impaired baroreflex function. Concomitant ingestion of ephedra alkaloids and water produced a greater increase in blood pressure.	Increased blood pressure when taken with 16 oz of water	None reported
Cardiac function, visual disturbances	Patient presented with progressive headaches, blurred vision in left visual field, decreased exercise tolerance, and palpitations. Electrocardiogram (ECG) showed right atrial fibrillation, MRI scan confirmed a right middle cerebral artery territorial infarction with minor hemorrhagic transformation.	Visual disturbances and cardioembolic stroke. Case confounded by use of anabolic steroids	None reported

continued

TABLE 4-5 Continued

Review/ Clinical Trial Reference	Type of Study and Subjects	Indication	Control	Dose	Product Specification
LoVecchio et al., 2005	Case report n=1 healthy woman, age 20 y			Ephedra plus other herbs; Metabolife 356 contains ma huang (labeled 12 mg ephedrine), guarana extract (labeled 40 mg caffeine), chromium picolinate, and various herbal and vitamin ingredients per tablet Reported ingestion of 4 tablets of Metabolife 356, 30 min prior to episode and 6–15 tablets/d for 3 d prior	Metabolife 356, Metabolife International Inc., San Diego, CA
Morgenstern et al., 2003	Case-controlled study of hemorrhagic stroke between 1994 and 1999 n=702, ages 18–49 y		None reported	Ephedra and various other products	Various

Outcomes Measured	Conclusions/Results	Adverse Events Profile	Interactions with Pharmaceuticals, Foods, or Other Dietary Supplements
Family history, social history, review of systems	Patient experiencing symptoms of a transient ischemic attack (numbness to her left face, arm, and leg that began 1 hr before arrival, mild headache, and nausea). She denied any other similar episodes or prior medical problems. Family history, social history, and review of systems were otherwise negative. The patient's symptoms resolved within 4 hours and no rechallenge was performed.	Transient ischemic attack	None reported
Risk of hemorrhagic stroke	No association between the use of ephedra-containing products and increased risk for hemorrhagic stroke was observed.	None reported	None reported

continued

TABLE 4-5 Continued

Review/ Clinical Trial Reference	Type of Study and Subjects	Indication	Control	Dose	Product Specification
Naik and Freudenberger, 2004	Case report n=2 white male bodybuilders, ages 19 and 21 y			Ephedra plus other herbs, creatine	Stacker III, Ripped Fuel
Peters et al., 2005	Case reports n=6 (4 men, 2 women, ages 34–51 y)			Ephedra (unspecified)	Not reported

Outcomes Measured	Conclusions/Results	Adverse Events Profile	Interactions with Pharmaceuticals, Foods, or Other Dietary Supplements
Coronary artery disease, heart failure, adverse drug reaction (measured by a causality assessment probability scale)	A 19-year-old white man presented to the ER complaining of exertional shortness of breath and episodic chest pain radiating to the left arm. Left heart catheterization revealed no significant coronary artery disease, a dilated left ventricle, and global hypokinesis. He died 5 weeks later after returning to the hospital with recurring heart failure. A 21-year-old white man presented to the ER with recurrent chest pain and was diagnosed with myopericarditis. An ECG showed global hypokinesis with an ejection fraction of 40–50%. He was treated for myopericarditis with standard therapies for heart failure. An adverse drug reaction was possible between cardiomyopathy and ephedra use in these 2 patients.	Cardiomyopathy, heart failure, death, and disability due to long-term product use	None reported
Clinical and echocardiographic data, ejection fraction, New York Heart Association class	Patients attending an outpatient department with new onset heart failure were noted to have exposure to ephedra. All 6 patients had left ventricular dysfunction at presentation (mean ejection fraction 20±5%) and were treated with conventional heart-failure pharmacotherapy. All patients discontinued ephedra use as advised. New York Heart Association class improved from class III in 5 patients (class II in 1 patient) to class I, within a median of 6 mo (range 3–96). Ejection fraction improved to a mean of 47±6%.	Ephedra may be associated with left ventricular systolic dysfunction	None reported

continued

TABLE 4-5 Continued

Review/ Clinical Trial Reference	Type of Study and Subjects	Indication	Control	Dose	Product Specification
Simsek et al., 2006	Case report n=1 man, age 36 y			Ephedra plus other herbs, for 10 d	Xenadrine RFA1
Schweinfurth and Pribitkin, 2003	Case report n=1 woman, age 38 y, with no significant medical or medication history			Ephedra plus other herbs, dose not stated Taken 4–6 h prior to onset of symptoms	Ripped Fuel, Twin Laboratories, Hauppauge, NY
Moawad et al., 2006	Case report n=1 healthy man, age 29 y			Ephedra plus other herbs, dose not stated	Stacker 3 and Ripped Fuel Extreme

Outcomes Measured	Conclusions/Results	Adverse Events Profile	Interactions with Pharmaceuticals, Foods, or Other Dietary Supplements
Visual disturbances (measured by fundoscopy)	Patient had loss of lower half of visual field of his right eye, and a history of dyslipidemia. Fundoscopy of the right eye showed a branch retinal artery occlusion with cholesterol embolus at the upper nasal margin of the optic disk, diagnosed as ischemic optic neuropathy.	Visual disturbance in patient with dyslipidemia	None reported
Hearing loss	Patient had vertigo and sudden hearing loss in her right ear. Corticosteriod treatment failed to improve hearing. The patient was diagnosed with acute cochlear injury due to a drug-mediated vascular injury.	Hearing loss	None reported
Cardiac function, neurologic function, visual disturbances, liver function, renal function, blood pressure	Patient presented with generalized tonic-clonic seizure that occurred while playing basketball. He initially complained of the abrupt onset of a severe headache associated with confusion and lethargy. Initial laboratory values and ECG indicated acute myocardial infarction, fulminant liver failure, acute renal failure, rhabdomyolysis, and transient cortical blindness. Radiographic abnormalities and neurologic dysfunction subsequently resolved with correction of his systolic blood pressure. However, a week later he presented again at the ER with hypertensive crisis without an ephedra rechallenge. Hypertensive crisis may not have been related to ephedra.	Potential hypertensive crisis, posterior reversible encephalopathy syndrome, multiple organ failure	None reported

continued

TABLE 4-5 Continued

Review/ Clinical Trial Reference	Type of Study and Subjects	Indication	Control	Dose	Product Specification
Rakovec et al., 2006	Case report n=1 healthy woman, age 19 y			Ephedrine 50 mg once or twice a day for 10 d	None reported
Stahl et al., 2006	Case report n=1 man, age 21 y			Ephedrine 20 mg twice daily for 1 mo	Energel
Verduin and Labbate, 2002	Case report n=1 man, age 45 y, with schizophrenia, olanzapine-induced obesity, and hyperlipidemia			Ephedra (12 mg and 40 mg of caffeine) plus other herbs, several ephedra tablets per day for 2 wk	Metabolife

Outcomes Measured	Conclusions/Results	Adverse Events Profile	Interactions with Pharmaceuticals, Foods, or Other Dietary Supplements
Cardiac function	ECG revealed a typical pattern of idiopathic left ventricular tachycardia, with an heart rate of 170 beats per minute, narrow QRS complex, right bundle branch block, and left axis deviation. Ephedrine alone, or in combination with substances that increase its effects on the cardiovascular system, may also trigger paroxysms of nonischemic ventricular tachycardia. The use of ephedrine carries a risk of development of life-threatening arrhythmias.	Ventricular tachycardia	None reported
Muscle function, renal function	Patient had complete muscle failure after collapsing after a 2-mile run. Patient had tachycardia (heart rate 130+) and was hypotensive. Patient drank very little water over a 2-mo period.	Muscle failure likely due to dehydration	None reported
Psychosis, cognition	Patient was confused and agitated, actively hallucinating and incoherent. After a week of treatment he was able to go back to work. The temporal relationship between initiation of Metabolife and subsequent development of psychosis and delirium strongly suggests that ephedra was responsible for these symptoms.	Case confounded by antipsychotic medications	None reported

continued

TABLE 4-5 Continued

Review/ Clinical Trial Reference	Type of Study and Subjects	Indication	Control	Dose	Product Specification
Walton and Manos, 2003	Case reports n=3 men, ages 19, 21, and 33 y			Ephedra plus other herbs, dose not stated	Ripped Fuel, Twin Laboratories, Hauppauge, NY; Hydroxycut, MuscleTech Research and Development, Inc.; Metabolife

[a]Body mass index.
[b]Maximal accumulated oxygen deficit.
[c]Oxygen uptake.
[d]Rate of elimination of carbon dioxide.

Outcomes Measured	Conclusions/Results	Adverse Events Profile	Interactions with Pharmaceuticals, Foods, or Other Dietary Supplements
Psychosis, depressive symptoms	A 19-year-old man was referred for psychiatric evaluation due to decreased sleep, increasing aggressive and disorganized behavior, and paranoid delusions. A 21-year-old man experienced a brief psychotic episode after using Hydroxycut for 2 wk. A 33-year-old man presented with depressive symptoms, suicidal ideation, auditory hallucinations, and paranoid and grandiose delusions. The symptoms in all 3 cases were not abated after discontinuation of the source of ephedra, but did resolve after treatment with antipsychotic drugs, suggesting an underlying pathology.	Psychosis	None reported

[e]Pulmonary ventilation during exercise.
[f]Resting energy expenditure.
[g]Magnetic resonance imaging.

TABLE 4-6 Relevant Data and Conclusions on Efficacy and Safety Reviews and Publications Identified for Garlic

Review/ Clinical Trial Reference	Type of Study and Sample Size	Indication	Control	Dose	Product Specification
Ankri and Mirelman, 1999	Review of in vitro and animal studies	Antimicrobial	None reported	None reported	Pure allicin isolated from garlic bulbs
Ledezma and Apitz-Castro, 2006	Review of in vitro and human studies	Antifungal and anti-inflammatory	Terbinafine	Topical applications of ajoene for 7–15 d	Pure ajoene extracted from garlic
Martin and Ernst, 2003	Review 1 trial	Anti-*Helicobacter pylori* activity	None reported	Raw garlic	Raw garlic cloves
Rahman and Lowe, 2006	Review n=25 clinical studies	Cardiovascular disease	Matching placebo for some studies	None reported	Raw garlic, garlic powder tablets, garlic oil, aged garlic extract (20% ethanol)

Outcomes Measured	Conclusions/Results	Adverse Events Profile	Interactions with Pharmaceuticals, Foods or Other Dietary Supplements
Antibacterial, antifungal, and antiparasitic activities	The pure compound, allicin, inhibits the growth of a wide range of Gram-negative and Gram-positive bacteria, including multidrug-resistant enterotoxigenic strains of *Escherichia coli*. Allicin has shown antifungal activity against *Candida albicans* and antiparasitic activity against some major human intestinal protozoan parasites such as *Entamoeba histolytica* and *Giardia lamblia*. It has also has antiviral activity.	None reported	One study showed synergistic effects with antibiotics
Reduction in tinea pedis infections	Treatment produced a clinical cure in 79% of patients treated, with no recurrence 90 days after treatment.	None reported	None reported
Reduction in *Helicobacter pylori* load and urease activity	A study of garlic to treat *Helicobacter pylori* infections reported no significant effect on *Helicobacter pylori* load.	None reported Poor methodology	None reported
Reductions in serum cholesterol, platelet aggregation, blood pressure	A reduction in total cholesterol was indicated in 44% of clinical trials; the most profound effect was observed in garlic's ability to reduce platelet aggregation. Mixed results have been obtained for blood pressure and oxidative-stress reduction.	None reported	None reported

continued

TABLE 4-6 Continued

Review/ Clinical Trial Reference	Type of Study and Sample Size	Indication	Control	Dose	Product Specification
Ackermann et al., 2001	Review n=45 randomized trials and 73 additional studies reporting adverse events	Cardiovascular disease	Placebo	Raw garlic, garlic powder tablets, garlic oil, aged garlic extract (20% ethanol)	None reported
Pittler and Ernst, 2007	Review of three meta-analyses of various effects in double-blind, randomized, controlled clinical trials	Hypercholesterolemia	Placebo	None reported	Garlic (unspecified)

Outcomes Measured	Conclusions/Results	Adverse Events Profile	Interactions with Pharmaceuticals, Foods or Other Dietary Supplements
Reductions in serum cholesterol, low-density lipoprotein (LDL), platelet aggregation, blood pressure, triglyceride levels	Small reductions in the total cholesterol level at 1 mo (range of average pooled reductions, 0.03–0.45 mmol/L [1.2–17.3 mg/dL]) and at 3 mo (range of average pooled reductions 0.32–0.66 mmol/L [12.4–25.4 mg/dL]), but not at 6 mo. Changes in LDL and triglyceride levels paralleled total cholesterol level results. No statistically significant changes in high-density lipoprotein levels. Significant reductions in platelet aggregation and mixed effects on blood pressure outcomes.	Skin adverse effects: Dermatitis Allergic reactions: asthma, rhinitis Cardiovascular dysfunction: myocardial infarction Coagulation dysfunction: bleeding, epidural hematoma, increased international normalized ratio in persons taking warfarin Gastrointestinal tract dysfunction: small-intestine obstruction, esophageal and abdominal pain, and flatulence	None reported
Reduction in cholesterol levels	Modest reduction of 15.7 mg/dL compared to placebo over a treatment period of 8–24 wk. In an updated meta-analysis (n=971), including 3 additional trials, the effect was diminished to 13.6 mg/dL. In four new double-blind randomized clinical trials (n=3,670), no changes were reported in lipid levels for hypercholesterolemic patients.	None reported	None reported

continued

TABLE 4-6 Continued

Review/ Clinical Trial Reference	Type of Study and Sample Size	Indication	Control	Dose	Product Specification
Sengupta et al., 2004	Review of epidemiological studies	Reduced cancer risk	None reported	None reported	None reported
Milner, 2006	Review	Reduced cancer risk	None reported	Various	Various

Outcomes Measured	Conclusions/Results	Adverse Events Profile	Interactions with Pharmaceuticals, Foods or Other Dietary Supplements
Cancer risk reduction	Higher intake of *Allium* vegetables is associated with reduced risk of several types of cancers. These epidemiological findings correlate well with laboratory findings. Proposed mechanisms include inhibition of mutagenesis, modulation of enzyme activities, inhibition of DNA adduct formation, free-radical scavenging, and effects on cell proliferation and tumor growth.	None reported	None reported
Cancer risk reduction	Evidence indicates the anticancer properties of fresh garlic extracts, aged garlic, garlic oil, and a number of specific organosulfur compounds generated by processing garlic. These anticarcinogenic and antitumorigenic activities arise through both dose- and temporal-related changes in a number of cellular events involved in the cancer process, including those involving drug metabolism, immune competence, cell-cycle regulation, apoptosis, and angiogenesis. The ability of garlic and related allyl sulfur compounds to block growth of tumors in the colon, lung, breast, and liver suggests general mechanisms that are not tissue specific.	None reported	None reported

continued

TABLE 4-6 Continued

Review/ Clinical Trial Reference	Type of Study and Sample Size	Indication	Control	Dose	Product Specification
Hu et al., 2005	Review of drug interactions				Garlic extract containing 600 μg of allicin per 600 mg extract; garlic oil; aged garlic extract

Outcomes Measured	Conclusions/Results	Adverse Events Profile	Interactions with Pharmaceuticals, Foods or Other Dietary Supplements
Activity drug interactions with garlic products	Dextromethorphan and alprazolam: Administration of 1,800 mg of garlic extract twice a day (3 × 600 mg tablets) for 14 days increased the ratio of dextromethorphan to its metabolite; did not alter pharmacokinetics significantly. Chlorzoxazone: Oral administration of garlic oil to healthy volunteers for 28 days reduced CYP2E1 activity. No alterations were observed with midazolam. Protease inhibitors: Saquinavir—In 10 healthy volunteers, 3-wk administration of caplets containing 3.6 mg garlic powder extract twice daily decreased the plasma area under the curve by 51%, plasma concentrations by 49%, and C(max) by 54% of the protease inhibitor. These parameters did not return to baseline values after 10 d of washout. Ritonavir (400 mg single dose)—Administration of two capsules (10 mg Natural Source odorless garlic extract) for 4 days to 10 healthy volunteers did not significantly decrease the area under the curve of the protease inhibitor. Warfarin: Two case reports suggest that the combination of warfarin and garlic products may increase clotting time and potentially cause postoperative bleeding. Chlorpropamide: Possible interaction, causing hypoglycemia. Acetaminophen: Administration of aged garlic extract (~6–7 cloves of garlic) for 3 mo to 16 healthy volunteers did not alter its metabolism.	Severe gastrointestinal toxicity developed in two HIV-infected patients taking garlic supplements for more than 2 wk after beginning ritonavir (400 or 600 mg twice daily) therapy. The symptoms resolved after discontinuation of therapy. The symptoms reappeared after rechallenge with garlic, even at a low ritonavir dose of 100 mg twice daily	Dextromethorphan Saquinavir Warfarin Chlorpropamide

TABLE 4-7 Relevant Data and Conclusions on Efficacy and Safety Reviews and Publications Identified for *Ginkgo Biloba*

Review/ Clinical Trial Reference	Type of Study and Subjects	Indication	Control	Dose	Product Specification
Burns et al., 2006	Double-blind n=197 (93 adults ages 55–79 y and 104 adults ages 18–43 y)	Cognition, attention, executive function, and mood	Placebo	120 mg/d (40 mg 3×/d) for 12 wk	Ginkgoforte, Blackmores Ltd., Australia
Carlson et al., 2007	Double-blind, randomized, parallel design n=90	Cognitive function, quality of life, and platelet function	Placebo	160 mg/d (1×/d) for 4 mo	*Ginkgo biloba*-based product containing 160 mg *Ginkgo biloba*, 68 mg gotu kola (with caffeine), and 180 mg docosahexaenoic acid
Cieza et al., 2003	Double-blind, randomized, parallel group n=66 healthy adults ages 50–65 y	Mental function and quality of life	Placebo	720 mg/d (240 mg, 3×/d) for 4 wk	*Ginkgo biloba* special extract EGb 761, Schwabe-Germany

Clinical Details and Outcomes Measured	Conclusions/Results	Adverse Events Profile	Interactions with Pharmaceuticals, Foods, or Other Dietary Supplements
Cognitive abilities test, chronometric testing (speed of information processing), subjective well-being (mood)	Older adult group: significant trend for improvement of longer-term memory with ginkgo (d = 0.52). No statistically significant difference on any other measure. Young adult group: no statistically significant effects with ginkgo.	Headaches, sleep disturbances, gastrointestinal symptoms	None reported
Six standardized cognitive function tests, SF-36 Quality of Life questionnaire, platelet function, adverse events	One of six cognitive tests indicated significant protocol differences for placebo. No significant differences in quality of life, platelet function, or adverse events. High baseline scores may have contributed to the null findings.	No alterations in platelet function observed	None reported
Primary: subjects' judgment of their own mental health, general health, and quality of life based on three different visual analog scales. Secondary: motor performance and emotional evaluation	Significant improvements of self-estimated mental health, self-estimated quality of life with ginkgo extract. No differences of self-estimated general health. Better motor performance and emotional evaluation with ginkgo extract. Findings do not support the use of a ginkgo-containing supplement for improving cognitive function or quality of life in cognitively intact, older, healthy adults.	None reported	None reported

continued

TABLE 4-7 Continued

Review/ Clinical Trial Reference	Type of Study and Subjects	Indication	Control	Dose	Product Specification
Chow et al., 2005	Double-blind, randomized n=57 unacclimatized adults	High-altitude sickness	Placebo	240 mg/d of *Ginkgo biloba* for 5 d prior to ascent or acetazolamide	*Ginkgo biloba* product from NOW foods

Clinical Details and Outcomes Measured	Conclusions/Results	Adverse Events Profile	Interactions with Pharmaceuticals, Foods, or Other Dietary Supplements
AMS[a] symptoms graded based on the LLS[b]: Acute Mountain Sickness scoring system. Incidence of AMS was defined as LLS score ≥3 and headache	LLS scores: The median score of the acetazolamide group was significantly lower than that of the placebo group (effect size, 2), unlike that of the *Ginkgo biloba* group (effect size, 0). AMS frequency: Less frequently in the acetazolamide group than in the placebo group (effect size, 30%); similar between the ginkgo group and the placebo group (effect size, –5%). The study concluded that prophylactic acetazolamide therapy decreased the symptoms of AMS and trended toward reducing its incidence. No evidence of similar efficacy for *Ginkgo biloba* NOW product was found. This study was criticized because of small sample size and that ginkgo was not the primary constituent of the product (Betz and Costello, 2006). The products contain two additional plants, 125 mg *Eleutherococcus senticosus* (Rupr and Maxim) Maxim and 150 mg of *Centella asiatica* (L) Urb, and only 120 mg of *G. biloba* L extract.	None reported	None reported

continued

TABLE 4-7 Continued

Review/ Clinical Trial Reference	Type of Study and Subjects	Indication	Control	Dose	Product Specification
Cochrane review (Birks et al., 2002)	Review n=33 unconfounded, double-blind, randomized, placebo-controlled studies of patients with dementia or cognitive decline	Benefits for dementia or cognitive decline	Placebo	Various	Various

Clinical Details and Outcomes Measured	Conclusions/Results	Adverse Events Profile	Interactions with Pharmaceuticals, Foods, or Other Dietary Supplements
	Clinical Global Impression (CGI) scale: Dose less than 200 mg/d showed improvements compared with placebo at less than 12 wk (54/63 showed significant improvement compared with 20/63). Dose of 200 mg/d showed significant improvements at 24 wk (57/79 compared with 42/77). Cognition shows significant benefit for ginkgo as compared with placebo at 12, 24, and 52 wk, ginkgo (greater than 200 mg/d) at 12 wk, ginkgo (any dose) at 12 wk. Activities of daily living (ADL) shows significant benefit for ginkgo (dose less than 200 mg/d) as compared with placebo at 12 wk, at 24 wk, and at 52 wk. Measures of mood and emotional function show significant benefit for ginkgo (dose less than 200 mg/d) as compared with placebo at less than 12 wk and at 12 wk. The review concludes that *Ginkgo biloba* appears to be safe in use with no excess side effects compared with placebo, and there is promising evidence of improvement in cognition and function associated with ginkgo. However, the three most recent trials show inconsistent results.	Overall, there are no significant differences between ginkgo and placebo in the proportion of participants experiencing adverse events	None reported

continued

TABLE 4-7 Continued

Review/ Clinical Trial Reference	Type of Study and Subjects	Indication	Control	Dose	Product Specification
Cochrane review (Birks and Grimley Evans, 2007)	Review n=35 randomized, double-blind studies, subjects with acquired cognitive impairment, including dementia, of any degree of severity	Assessment of efficacy on cognition	None reported	Various	Various
Cochrane review (Hilton and Stuart, 2004)	Review n=12 clinical studies	Treatment of tinnitus	None reported	Various	Various

Clinical Details and Outcomes Measured	Conclusions/Results	Adverse Events Profile	Interactions with Pharmaceuticals, Foods, or Other Dietary Supplements
Various	Benefits associated with ginkgo (dose greater than 200 mg/d) at 24 wk (two studies), but not for a lower dose. Cognition shows benefit for ginkgo (any dose) at 12 wk (p=5 studies) but not at 24 wk. Results of five studies assessing ADLs showed benefit for ginkgo (dose less than 200 mg/d) compared with placebo at 12 wk (one study) and at 24 wk (three studies), but there are no differences at the higher dose. There are no data available on quality of life, measures of depression, or dependency. The evidence that ginkgo has predictable and clinically significant benefit for people with dementia or cognitive impairment is inconsistent and unconvincing.	No difference above placebo	None reported
	Limited evidence did not demonstrate that *Ginkgo biloba* was effective for tinnitus. Ten trials were excluded on methodological grounds. No trials reached a satisfactory standard for inclusion in the review.	Few side effects	None reported

continued

TABLE 4-7 Continued

Review/ Clinical Trial Reference	Type of Study and Subjects	Indication	Control	Dose	Product Specification
Elsabagh et al., 2005	Double-blind, randomized n=92 students, ages 18–26 y	Attention, memory, executive function, and mood	Placebo	120 mg/d (1x/d) and tested after 4 h (experiment 1) or 6 wk of treatment (experiment 2)	Ginkgo one-a-day tablets, Lichtwer Pharma UK, Mere Park, Marlow, Bucks, UK
Gertsch et al., 2004	Prospective, double blind, randomized n=614 healthy men and women	HAS[c]	Placebo	120 mg ginkgo, 250 mg acetazolamide, combination of 250 mg acetoazolamide and 120 mg ginkgo, or placebo, 2×/d	*Ginkgo biloba* extract GK 501, Pharmaton SA, Lugano, Switzerland

Clinical Details and Outcomes Measured	Conclusions/Results	Adverse Events Profile	Interactions with Pharmaceuticals, Foods, or Other Dietary Supplements
Mood rating scales, sustained attention, episodic and working memory, mental flexibility and planning	Experiment 1: Acute dose of ginkgo significantly improved performance on the sustained-attention task and pattern recognition memory task; however, there were no effects on working memory, planning, mental flexibility, or mood. Experiment 2: No significant effects on mood or any of the cognitive tests. Acute administration improved performance in tests of attention and memory. Tolerance to the effects may develop in young, healthy participants.	None reported	None reported
LLSR[d] score ≥3 with headache and one other symptom. Secondary outcome measures included blood oxygen content, severity of syndrome, incidence of headache, and severity of headache. Measured at the approach to Mount Everest base camp in the Nepal Himalayas at 4,280 m or 4,358 m and study end point at 4,928 m	Ginkgo at a dose of 240 mg/d, 3–4 doses prior to ascent, was not significantly different from placebo for any outcome. Acetazolamide group showed significant levels of protection. The incidence of acute mountain sickness was 34% for placebo, 12% for acetazolamide, 35% for ginkgo, and 14% for combined ginkgo and acetazolamide. The proportion of patients with increased severity of acute mountain sickness was 18% for placebo, 3% for acetazolamide, 18% for ginkgo, and 7% for combined ginkgo and acetazolamide.	Potential worsening of headaches associated with HAS. (Headaches usually resolve within 1 wk of daily use of the product.)	None reported

continued

TABLE 4-7 Continued

Review/ Clinical Trial Reference	Type of Study and Subjects	Indication	Control	Dose	Product Specification
Gertsch et al., 2002	Double-blind, randomized n=26 living at sea level	AMS[e]	Placebo	180 mg/d (60 mg 3×/d) for 48 h	*Ginkgo biloba* extract GK 501, Memfit, Pharmaton SA, Lugano, Switzerland
Kennedy et al., 2000	Double-blind, matching n=20, ages 19–24 y	Cognitive enhancement	Placebo	120 mg/d, 240 mg/d, and 360 mg/d	GK501 standardized *Ginkgo biloba* extract, Pharmaton SA, Lugano, Switzerland

Clinical Details and Outcomes Measured	Conclusions/Results	Adverse Events Profile	Interactions with Pharmaceuticals, Foods, or Other Dietary Supplements
The subjects received ginkgo or placebo starting 24 h before ascending Mauna Kea, Hawaii. Subjects were transported from sea level to the summit (4,205 m) over a 3-h period, including 1 hour at 2,835 m. LLSR Questionnaire was used as the primary outcome measure at baseline, 2,835 m, and after 4 h at 4,205 m. AMS was defined as a LLSR ≥3 with headache	Median LLSR at 4,205 m was significantly lower for ginkgo versus placebo (4, range 1–8 vs. 5, range 2–9). Ginkgo use did not reach statistical significance for lowering incidence of AMS compared with placebo (ginkgo 7/12, 58.3% vs. placebo 13/14, 92.9%). Twenty-one of 26 (81%) subjects developed AMS overall. The results suggest that pretreatment with ginkgo 60 mg three times daily may significantly reduce the severity of AMS prior to rapid ascent from sea level to 4,205 m.	None reported	None reported
Cognitive performance using the CDR computerized test battery immediately prior to dosing and at 1, 2.5, 4, and 6 h thereafter The primary outcome measures were: speed of attention, accuracy of attention, speed of memory, quality of memory	Ginkgo produced a number of significant changes in performance measures: Dose-dependent improvement of the speed of attention factor following both 240 mg and 360 mg of the extract, which was evident at 2.5 h and still present at 6 h. Other time- and dose-specific changes (both positive and negative) in performance of the other factors. The authors concluded that *Ginkgo biloba* is capable of producing a sustained improvement in attention in healthy young volunteers after acute dosing.	None reported	None reported

continued

TABLE 4-7 Continued

Review/ Clinical Trial Reference	Type of Study and Subjects	Indication	Control	Dose	Product Specification
Mattes and Pawlik, 2004	Double-blind, matched n=39, ages 23.6±5.4 y	Assessment of amelioration of the postlunch dip	Placebo	4 mg/kg/d for 13 wk	*Ginkgo biloba* extract
Roncin et al., 1996	Randomized n=44	AMS and vasomotor changes	Placebo	160 mg/d for 5 d	EGb 761
Solomon et al., 2002	Double-blind, randomized, parallel group n=230 adults, ages >60 y	Improvement of memory	Placebo	40 mg, 3×/d for 6 wk	Ginkoba, Boehringer Ingelheim Pharmaceuticals

Clinical Details and Outcomes Measured	Conclusions/Results	Adverse Events Profile	Interactions with Pharmaceuticals, Foods, or Other Dietary Supplements
Alertness, performance, affective state, chemosensory tests at wk 1, 5, 9, and 13	Subjects experienced the postprandial affective state decrement ("postlunch dip") but no performance decrement. Performance on the chemosensory tests improved over the 13-wk study for all subjects. *Ginkgo biloba* was ineffective at alleviating the symptoms of the postlunch dip or enhancing taste and smell function.	None reported	None reported
The primary outcomes assessment was based on the Environmental Symptom Questionnaire score and vasomotor changes measured by photoplethysmography and a specific questionnaire	No subject in the EGb 761 group developed AMS-cerebral versus 40.9% of subjects in the placebo group; this difference was very significant. Three subjects (13.6%) in the EGb 761 group developed AMS-respiratory versus 18 (81.8%) in the placebo group. Ginkgo also decreased vasomotor disorders of the extremities and improved circulation.	None reported above placebo	None reported
Standardized neuropsychological tests of verbal and nonverbal learning and memory, attention and concentration, naming, and expressive language Self-report on a memory questionnaire Caregiver clinical global impression of change	No significant differences between treatment groups on any outcome measure. Ginkgo did not facilitate performance on standard neuropsychological tests of learning, memory, attention, and concentration or naming and verbal fluency in adults ages 60 or older without cognitive impairment. There was also no difference between groups in self-reported memory function or global rating by spouses, friends, and relatives.	None reported	None reported

continued

TABLE 4-7 Continued

Review/ Clinical Trial Reference	Type of Study and Subjects	Indication	Control	Dose	Product Specification
Mix and Crews, 2002	Double-blind, randomized, fixed-dose n=262 adults, ages >60 y	Assessment of memory improvement in older adults	Placebo	180 mg/d	EGb 761
Stough et al., 2001	Double-blind, randomized n=61, ages 18–40 y	Memory and executive processing	Placebo	120 mg/d for 30 d	EGb 761

Clinical Details and Outcomes Measured	Conclusions/Results	Adverse Events Profile	Interactions with Pharmaceuticals, Foods, or Other Dietary Supplements
Change in performance scores on standardized neuropsychological measures (Selective Reminding Test [SRT], Wechsler Adult Intelligence Scale-III Block Design [WAIS-III BD] and Digit Symbol-Coding [WAIS-III DS] subtests, and the Wechsler Memory Scale-III Faces I [WMS-III FI] and Faces II [WMS-III FII] subtests) from pretreatment baseline to just prior to termination of treatment. Follow-up self-report questionnaire just prior to termination of the treatment phase	Significantly more improvement on spatial recognition tasks involving delayed (30 min) free recall and recognition of noncontextual, auditory–verbal material, compared with placebo. Significantly greater improvements in the WMS-III FII subtest assessing delayed (30 min) recognition of visual material (i.e., human faces), compared with placebo. However, the significant difference found between the two groups' pretreatment baseline scores on the WMS-III FII suggest this result should be interpreted with caution. Follow-up self-report questionnaire also revealed that significantly more adults in the EGb 761 group rated their overall abilities to remember as improved by treatment end compared with placebo. Overall, the results provided complementary evidence of the potential efficacy of *Ginkgo biloba* EGb 761 in enhancing certain neuropsychological/memory processes of cognitively intact adults 60 y of age and over.	None reported	None reported
A battery of validated neuropsychological tests before and after treatment to measure changes in memory and executive processing	Significant improvements in speed of information processing, working memory, and executive processing were attributable to the ginkgo extract.	None reported	None reported

continued

TABLE 4-7 Continued

Review/ Clinical Trial Reference	Type of Study and Subjects	Indication	Control	Dose	Product Specification
Subhan and Hindmarch, 1984	Double-blind, randomized, crossover n=8, ages 25–40 y	Central nervous system arousal, psychomotor performance, and short-term memory	Placebo	120, 240, and 600 mg	Tebonin (Germany) Tanakan (France)
Warot et al., 1991	Double-blind n=12	Assessment of vigilance, memory, reaction times	Placebo	600 mg/d	Tanakan (standardized ginkgo extract, France) and ginkgo extract
Bent et al., 2005	15 case reports between 1966 and 2004		None reported	Various	Various

Clinical Details and Outcomes Measured	Conclusions/Results	Adverse Events Profile	Interactions with Pharmaceuticals, Foods, or Other Dietary Supplements
Subjects completed a battery of psychological tests including CFF,[e] CRT,[f] subjective ratings of drug effects (LARS), and a Sternberg memory scanning test 1 h after treatment	No statistically significant changes from placebo were observed on CFF, CRT, or LARS. However, memory as assessed using the Sternberg technique was found to be significantly improved following treatment with ginkgo at a dose of 600 mg when compared to placebo, and results suggested a localized effect of the extract on the serial comparison stage of the reaction process. These results suggest a specific effect of the extract on central cognitive processes.	None reported	None reported
Objective measures of vigilance (CFF, CRT), memory tasks (pictures and Sternberg scanning tests), and self-rating evaluation (visual analogue scales). Test administered pre- and 1 h postdosing	No statistically significant changes from placebo were observed on CFF, CRT, or LARS. No differences between treatment were evident on Sternberg scanning test and picture recognition. Compared to baseline, free recall score, while decreasing under placebo and ginkgo extract, remained the same under Tanakan, indicating that the Tanakan product improved free recall.	None reported	None reported
Published case reports of bleeding events in persons using ginkgo were queried from MEDLINE, EMBASE, IBIDS, and the Cochrane Collaboration Database from 1966 to October 2004. Two reviewers independently abstracted a standard set of information to assess whether ginkgo caused the bleeding event	A temporal association between use of ginkgo and a bleeding event was described in the 15 published case reports, with most of the cases involving serious medical conditions (with 8 episodes of intracranial bleeding). Other risk factors for bleeding were identified in 13 of the case reports. Six reports clearly described cessation of ginkgo followed by lack of bleeding recurrence. In three reports, bleeding times were elevated when patients were taking ginkgo. The review concluded that a structured assessment of published case reports suggests a possible causal association between using ginkgo and bleeding events.	Potential bleeding due to chronic administration especially in combination with liver cirrhosis or use of nonsteroidal anti-inflammatory drugs or warfarin	None reported

continued

TABLE 4-7 Continued

Review/ Clinical Trial Reference	Type of Study and Subjects	Indication	Control	Dose	Product Specification
Hu et al., 2005	Review of case studies and clinical trials		None reported	Various	Various

Clinical Details and Outcomes Measured	Conclusions/Results	Adverse Events Profile	Interactions with Pharmaceuticals, Foods, or Other Dietary Supplements
A review of drug interactions with herbal products including ginkgo	One case report of an interaction with ginkgo and trazodone that resulted in coma. However, this case was confounded due to the numerous other drugs that were being taken by the patient. Interactions with warfarin, ticlopidine, and nonsteroidal anti-inflammatory drugs such as aspirin and ibuprofen have been reported. Changes in international normalized ratio (INR) and prolonged bleeding times have resulted when ginkgo was combined with these drugs. In healthy subjects, doses of ginkgo up to 480 mg/d did not alter bleeding times or INR. A small clinical trial demonstrated that administration of ginkgo (280 mg/d) for 14 d significantly decreased the plasma concentrations of omeprazole. A reduction in the efficacy of thiazide diuretics in one subject was indicated in one case report, and rodent studies have indicated that treatment with ginkgo in combination with diltazem inhibited the metabolism of the drug. Ginkgo did not alter the metabolism of midazolam or donepezil in clinical studies. Ginkgo (120 mg/d) decreased plasma insulin by 26% in hyperinsulinemic patients with type 2 diabetes mellitus taking antihyperglycemic drugs. Ginkgo may increase the hepatic clearance of insulin and antihyperglycemic drugs.	None reported	Trazodone, warfarin, aspirin, ibuprofen, ticlopidine, tolbutamide, chlorpropamide

continued

TABLE 4-7 Continued

Review/ Clinical Trial Reference	Type of Study and Subjects	Indication	Control	Dose	Product Specification
Wolf, 2006	Double-blind n=50 in each group, men, ages 20–44 y		Placebo	Aspirin (ASA) followed by aspirin + EGb 761 or aspirin + EGb 761 followed by aspirin 2×/d for 7 d Dose/d: 500 mg aspirin or 500 mg aspirin + 240 mg EGb 761®	EGb 761®

[a]Acute mountain sickness.
[b]Lake Louis Score.
[c]High-altitude sickness.

Clinical Details and Outcomes Measured	Conclusions/Results	Adverse Events Profile	Interactions with Pharmaceuticals, Foods, or Other Dietary Supplements
Bleeding time, coagulation parameters, and platelet activity in response to various agonists were determined. In addition, adverse events, laboratory variables, and vital signs were measured	ASA given alone prolonged bleeding time. ASA and the combination of ASA + EGb 761® exerted similar effects on all coagulation parameters measured: Bleeding time (ASA alone: 4.1 min before therapy, 6.2 min after therapy; ASA + EGb 761®: 4.2 min before therapy, 6.3 min after therapy Agonist-induced platelet aggregation (collagen-induced platelet aggregation—ASA: 84.5% before therapy, 81.0% after therapy; ASA + EGb 761®: 86.6% before therapy, 81.0% after therapy; adenosine diphosphate-induced platelet aggregation—ASA: 72.6% before therapy, 47.2% after therapy; aspirin + EGb 761®: 71.7% before therapy, 44.8% after therapy; ratio of means). Co-administration of aspirin and EGb 761® does not constitute a safety risk. No additive effect was observed.	In each group there was at least one adverse effect consisting mainly of coagulation disorders. The pattern of adverse effects matched the effects of aspirin on coagulation parameters. Mild to moderate gastrointestinal adverse effects were also reported in 12–18% of subjects	Bleeding in combination with aspirin, anticoagulants, alcohol

[d]Lake Louise self-report.
[e]Critical flicker fusion.
[f]Choice reaction time.

TABLE 4-8 Relevant Data and Conclusions on Efficacy and Safety Reviews and Publications Identified for Ginseng

Review/ Clinical Trial Reference	Type of Study and Subjects	Indication	Control	Dose	Product Specification
Cardinal and Engels, 2001	Prospective, double-blind, randomized n=40 healthy women and 43 men, mean age 25.7 y, with relatively normal psychological profiles	Enhancement of mental performance	Placebo (lactose)	200 or 400 mg/d (2 or 4 capsules/d) for 60 d	Standardized extract *Panax ginseng* G115, 100-mg capsules
Engels et al., 2001	Double-blind, randomized n=24 women	Exercise performance and short-term recovery	Placebo	400 mg/d (4 capsules/d) for 8 wk	Standardized extract *Panax ginseng* G115, 100-mg capsules
Engels et al., 2003	Double-blind, randomized n=38 active, healthy adults	Exercise performance and short-term recovery	Placebo	400 mg/d (4 capsules/d) for 8 wk	Standardized extract *Panax ginseng* G115, 100-mg capsules

Outcomes Measured	Conclusions/Results	Adverse Events Profile	Interactions with Pharmaceuticals, Foods, or Other Dietary Supplements
Positive affect, negative affect, and total mood disturbance. Measures were obtained pre- and post-intervention	No psychological benefits observed after 8 wk of chronic ginseng supplementation at its clinically recommended dose (200 mg/d) or at 400 mg/d compared to placebo.	None reported	None reported
Peak anaerobic power output, mean anaerobic power output, rate of fatigue (as measured by a Wingate ergonomic protocol), and recovery heart rates	No significant difference found for peak anaerobic power output, mean anaerobic power output, rate of fatigue, and immediate postexercise recovery heart rates. Prolonged supplementation with ginseng provided no ergogenic benefits during and in the recovery from short supramaximal exercise.	A single case of stomach upset associated with ginseng	None reported
Exercise performance (as measured by consecutive Wingate tests), absolute SIgA,[a] salivary protein concentrations, SIgA secretion rate (S-SIgA), the relation of SIgA to total protein, peak and mean mechanical power output, and heart rate during exercise recovery	Compared with resting levels, S-SIgA, SIgA:protein ratio, and saliva flow rate were significantly lower after exercise at baseline. Significant decline seen in both peak and mean mechanical power output across consecutive Wingate tests. Few changes seen in scores for salivary parameters, exercise performance, and exercise recovery heart rate between ginseng- and placebo-treated groups. Mucosal immunity was not affected as indicated by changes in SIgA at rest and after an exercise-induced state of homeostatic disturbance; neither did it improve physical performance or heart rate recovery for individuals undergoing repeated periods of exhausting exercise.	None reported	None reported

continued

TABLE 4-8 Continued

Review/ Clinical Trial Reference	Type of Study and Subjects	Indication	Control	Dose	Product Specification
Kennedy et al., 2001	Balanced crossover, double-blind, randomized n=20 healthy, young adults	Mood and cognitive performance	Placebo	320 mg (120 mg ginkgo, 200 mg ginseng), 640 mg (240 mg ginkgo, 400 mg ginseng), or 960 mg (360 mg ginkgo, 600 mg ginseng)	*Ginkgo biloba* standardized extract GK 501, 60-mg capsules; *Panax ginseng* standardized extract G115, 100-mg capsules
Kennedy et al., 2002	Balanced crossover, double-blind, randomized n=20	Mood and cognitive performance	Placebo	360 mg of ginkgo, 400 mg of ginseng, 960 mg of a product combining the two extracts	*Ginkgo biloba* standardized extract GK 501; *Panax ginseng* standardized extract G115
Lieberman, 2001	Review of 7 clinical trials	Physical performance and well-being	Placebo	Various	Various

Outcomes Measured	Conclusions/Results	Adverse Events Profile	Interactions with Pharmaceuticals, Foods, or Other Dietary Supplements
Effect on mood and aspects of cognitive performance (quality of memory, secondary memory, working memory, speed of memory, quality of attention and speed of attention)	A dose-dependent improvement in performance on the "quality of memory" factor was observed for the highest dose (960 mg). This effect was differentially targeted at the secondary memory rather than the working memory component. Also a dose-dependent decrement was seen in performance of the "speed of attention" factor for both the 320- and 640-mg doses.	None reported	None reported
Cognitive testing (using the CDR[b] computerized assessment battery and two serial subtraction mental arithmetic tasks) Mood testing (Bond-Lader visual analogue scales) Measured 1, 2.5, 4, and 6 h posttreatment dose	All three treatments were associated with an improvement of secondary memory performance on the CDR battery, with ginseng treatment showing some improvement in the speed of performing memory tasks and in accuracy of attention-related tasks. Ginkgo and the ginkgo/ginseng combination improved performance of the Serial Threes and Serial Sevens subtraction tasks. No modulation of the speed of performing attention tasks was evident. Ginkgo improved self-rated mood; lesser improvements with the combination product.	None reported	None reported
Physical performance, cognitive performance, immune function, disease state	No compelling evidence that ginseng had any positive effects on physical or cognitive performance, immune function, or any specific disease state.	None reported	None reported

continued

TABLE 4-8 Continued

Review/ Clinical Trial Reference	Type of Study and Subjects	Indication	Control	Dose	Product Specification
Reay et al., 2006	Balanced crossover, double-blind n=27 healthy, young adults	Cognition and glucose tolerance	Placebo	Standardized ginseng extract, 200 mg/d (2 capsules/day) 200 mg G115/0 mg glucose (ginseng); 0 mg G115/25 g glucose (glucose); or 200 mg G115/25 g glucose (ginseng/glucose combination)	*Panax ginseng* standardized extract G115, 100-mg capsules
Reay et al., 2005	Balanced crossover, double-blind n=30	Cognition and glucose tolerance	Placebo	Standardized ginseng extract, 100-mg capsules, 2 or 4/d	*Panax ginseng* standardized extract G115

Outcomes Measured	Conclusions/Results	Adverse Events Profile	Interactions with Pharmaceuticals, Foods, or Other Dietary Supplements
Cognitive function (as measured by Serial Threes subtraction task, Serial Sevens task, and RVIP[c] performance task), mental fatigue (visual analogue scale), blood glucose levels Measured 60 min posttreatment dose	*Panax ginseng* and glucose enhanced the performance of mental arithmetic tasks and ameliorated the increase in participants' subjective feelings of mental fatigue during performance of the sustained, cognitively demanding task performance. Glucose improved accuracy in performance of the RVIP. No evidence in any cognitive outcome measure of a synergistic relationship was found. A reduction in blood glucose levels was seen 1 hour following consumption of *Panax ginseng* without glucose. *Panax ginseng* may have glucoregulatory properties and can enhance cognitive performance. Conclusions from this study are limited due to poor methodology.	Not reported, poor methodology	Insulin and prescription medications to treat type 2 diabetes
Cognitive function (as measured by Serial Threes subtraction task, Serial Sevens task, and RVIP performance task), mental fatigue (as measured by a visual analogue scale), blood glucose levels Measured 60 min posttreatment dose, 6 times in immediate succession	Treatment with both 200-mg and 400-mg dosage led to significant reductions in levels of blood glucose levels at all three posttreatment measurements. Administration of 200 mg of ginseng significantly improved performance on the Serial Sevens subtraction task and significantly reduced subjective mental fatigue throughout all (with the exception of one time point in each case) of the postdose completions of the 10-min battery. *Panax ginseng* can improve performance and subjective feelings of mental fatigue during sustained mental activity. This effect may be related to the acute glucoregulatory properties of the extract.	None reported	None reported

continued

TABLE 4-8 Continued

Review/ Clinical Trial Reference	Type of Study and Subjects	Indication	Control	Dose	Product Specification
Scholey and Kennedy, 2002	Balanced crossover, double-blind n=20	Cognition	Placebo	320 mg (120 mg ginkgo and 200 mg ginseng) 640 mg (240 mg ginkgo and 400 mg ginseng) 960 mg (360 mg ginkgo and 600 mg ginseng) Given daily	*Ginkgo biloba* standardized extract GK 501; *Panax ginseng* standardized extract G115
Wesnes et al., 2000	Multicenter trial, double-blind n=256, ages 38–66 y	Memory-enhancement	Placebo	160 mg (60 mg ginkgo and 100 mg ginseng) 2×/d or 320 mg (120 mg ginkgo and 200 mg ginseng) 1×/d for 14 wk	*Ginkgo biloba* standardized extract GK 501; *Panax ginseng* standardized extract G115
Cheng, 2005	Review of interactions with warfarin n=3		None reported	Various	Various
Hu et al., 2005	Review of drug interactions with ginseng		None reported	Various	Various

Outcomes Measured	Conclusions/Results	Adverse Events Profile	Interactions with Pharmaceuticals, Foods, or Other Dietary Supplements
Cognitive function (as measured by Serial Threes and Serial Sevens subtraction tasks) Measured before treatment and 1, 2.5, 4, and 6 h thereafter	Ginseng: Dose-dependent improvement in speed of response during Serial Threes, depending on dosage. Ginkgo-ginseng combination (320 mg): Most significant and sustained increase in the number of Serial Sevens responses at all posttreatment testing times. Ginkgo-ginseng combination (640 and 960 mg): Improved accuracy on performance of the Serial Sevens and Serial Threes tasks with 640 and 960 mg, respectively.	None reported	None reported
Attention and memory (as measured by the CDR computerized cognitive assessment system) measured prior to receiving their first daily dose and repeated 1, 3, and 6 h later Mood states, quality of life, and sleep quality (as measured by questionnaire)	Ginkgo/ginseng combination significantly improved the Index of Memory Quality. Average improvement was 7.5%; this reflected improvements to different aspects of memory including working and long-term memory. Benefit was seen throughout the 12-wk dosing period as well as after a 2-wk washout.	None reported	None reported
Anticoagulant effects of warfarin	In three reports, ginseng reduced the anticoagulant effects of warfarin.	Reduced anticoagulant effects when used in combination with warfarin	Ginseng affects the anticoagulant properties of warfarin
Blood concentrations of alcohol and warfarin, mania, efficacy of the influenza vaccination	*Panax ginseng* was seen to reduce the blood concentrations of alcohol and warfarin, induce mania when used concomitantly with phenelzine, and increase the efficacy of the influenza vaccination.	None reported	Ginseng influences the effects of alcohol, warfarin, phenelzine, and influenza vaccine

continued

TABLE 4-8 Continued

Review/ Clinical Trial Reference	Type of Study and Subjects	Indication	Control	Dose	Product Specification
Jiang et al., 2004	Randomized, crossover n=12 healthy men		St. John's wort	Extract equivalent to 0.5 g *Panax ginseng* root and 8.93 mg ginsenosides as ginsenoside Rg1, given as 2 capsules 2×/d for 7 days 25 mg warfarin	Golden Glow Korean ginseng
Rosado, 2003	Case report n=1 male, age 58 y with a thrombosis on a mechanical bileaflet aortic valve prosthesis admitted to hospital with diagnosis of acute anteroseptal myocardial infarction and diabetic ketoacidosis				Ginseng product obtained overseas
Yuan et al., 2004	Double-blind, randomized n=20		Placebo	For 2 wk	*Panax quinquefolius* (American ginseng)

[a]Secretory immunoglobulin A.
[b]Cognitive Drug Research.
[c]Rapid visual information processing.

Outcomes Measured	Conclusions/Results	Adverse Events Profile	Interactions with Pharmaceuticals, Foods, or Other Dietary Supplements
Platelet aggregation, INR of prothrombin time, warfarin enantiomer protein binding, warfarin enantiomer concentrations in plasma, and S-7-hydroxywarfarin concentration in urine	No effect on INR and platelet aggregation by St. John's wort or ginseng. No effect on the apparent volumes of distribution or protein binding of warfarin enantiomers. St. John's wort significantly induced the apparent clearance of both S-warfarin and R-warfarin, which in turn resulted in a significant reduction in the pharmacological effect of warfarin. Co-administration of warfarin with ginseng did not affect the pharmacokinetics or pharmacodynamics of either S-warfarin or R-warfarin. *Panax ginseng* should not affect bleeding times during injury or in patients treated with warfarin.	None reported	Ginseng does not appear to affect the pharmacokinetics of warfarin
INR and coronary angiography	Thrombosis was thought to be caused through an interaction with ginseng and warfarin that produced a reduction in his INR.	Thrombosis	Ginseng interaction with warfarin
INR and plasma warfarin concentrations as measures of interactions of ginseng with warfarin	Peak INR significantly decreased compared to placebo (difference between ginseng and placebo. Significant reduction in the INR area under the curve (AUC), peak plasma warfarin level, and warfarin AUC. Peak INR and peak plasma warfarin level were positively correlated. Ginseng may reduce the efficacy of warfarin.	None reported	Ginseng interaction with warfarin

TABLE 4-9 Relevant Data and Conclusions on Efficacy and Safety Reviews and Publications Identified for HMB

Review/ Clinical Trial Reference	Type of Study and Subjects	Indication	Control	Dose	Product Specification
Slater and Jenkins, 2000	Review, included 84 references with at least 10 describing human clinical trials with HMB n=20–41	Muscle growth and strength	Placebo	Typically 3 g/d, a minority 1.5 or 6 g/d	Various
Nissen et al., 2000	Nine clinical trial studies that included safety data	Muscle growth and strength	Placebo	3 g/d for 3–8 wk	

Clinical Details and Outcomes Measured	Conclusions/ Results	Adverse Events Profile	Interactions with Pharmaceuticals, Foods, or Other Dietary Supplements
Total lean mass, strength gains, muscle protein breakdown, muscle soreness and damage indicators	Most studies with HMB supplementation of 3 g/d paired with resistance training observed enhanced lean tissue and strength gains; a minority of studies showed no effect. Evidence was reviewed suggesting that the benefits are primarily observed in untrained individuals with less response for trained subjects. The mechanism was suggested to be reduction in muscle protein catabolism.	Some studies performed routine blood screens for hepatic, renal, or immune effects or had surveys regarding adverse effects; none reported serious negative clinical effects. Similarly, none of the animal studies (most on lambs, chickens, and steers) have reported adverse effects with doses up to 100 g/d	None reported
Data provided on health-related blood measures, emotional profiles (Circumplex test of emotion), and adverse events reported via questionnaire	Emotional profiles: Only significant change was decrease in "unactivated unpleasant affect" (associated with reduced sensation of sluggish, bored, tired). Blood measures: Significant 3.7% decrease in serum cholesterol and 5.7% in low-denisty lipoproteins (effect was greater in subjects who began with elevated lipids). There was also less increase in high-denisty lipoproteins in response to exercise for HMB group, but this was eliminated when expressed relative to total cholesterol. Systolic blood pressure fell 3% more for the HMB than placebo group. None of the indicators of liver function or traditional blood chemistries were altered by HMB with the exception of a significant (2%) drop in blood potassium, a significantly greater increase in albumin/globulin ratio, and a significantly lower (0.5%) hematocrit in HMB.	No difference observed between placebo and HMB treatments	None reported

continued

TABLE 4-9 Continued

Review/ Clinical Trial Reference	Type of Study and Subjects	Indication	Control	Dose	Product Specification
Bohn et al., 2002	Review of several strength-enhancing supplements including HMB; four were not part of Slater and Jenkins (2000) review	Muscle growth and strength	Placebo	2–3 g/d	
Alon et al., 2002	Review of human studies; only additional clinical trial not included in reviews above was one on effect on body composition in cancer patients (May et al., 2002)	Body composition	Placebo	9 cancer patients received 3 g/d HMB+14 g/d arginine and 14 g/d glutamine	
Nissen and Sharp, 2003	Meta-analysis of nine HMB studies; two were not included in above reviews		Placebo	3 g/d (8 studies) or 38 mg/kg/d + resistance exercise	

Clinical Details and Outcomes Measured	Conclusions/ Results	Adverse Events Profile	Interactions with Pharmaceuticals, Foods, or Other Dietary Supplements
(See Slater and Jenkins above): Reduction in markers of muscle damage following 2-mile run reported in one study; beneficial effects on body composition observed in men and women 70 y of age and older	One study beyond Slater and Jenkins (2000) studied variety of markers of hematology as well as renal, hepatic function.	None reported	None reported
	Questionnaire on adverse events indicated no effect of HMB on adverse events in the patients; no effects on serum chemistries with exception of increase in blood urea nitrogen, sodium, phosphorus, and uric acid contrasted to reduction in placebo group. The treated cancer group had a greater increase in fat-free mass compared to placebo group over the 24-wk trial. Body fat was not different. There was no evaluation of HMB alone.	None reported	None reported
Net increase in lean mass gain of 0.28%/wk during resistance training with effect size of 0.15. Net increase in strength gain of 1.40%/wk and effect size of 0.19	HMB was one of few supplements reviewed that had anabolic effects when paired with resistance training.	None reported	None reported

continued

TABLE 4-9 Continued

Review/ Clinical Trial Reference	Type of Study and Subjects	Indication	Control	Dose	Product Specification
Palisin and Stacy, 2005	Review with 20 references; 6 were not included in above reviews	Various	Placebo	2 or 3 g HMB/d (depending on the study) alone or combined with creatine, arginine or lysine, or glutamine or arginine for 10 d to 12 wk	

Clinical Details and Outcomes Measured	Conclusions/ Results	Adverse Events Profile	Interactions with Pharmaceuticals, Foods, or Other Dietary Supplements
	Consensus of studies shows that HMB alone or in combination with other amino acids: – reduced loss of muscle mass and function in elderly, – improved fat-free mass gains in AIDS and cancer patients, – may improve fat-free mass and muscle strength gains in untrained better than in trained individuals, – is effective if consumed 4–8 wk but not briefly, and – does not cause adverse effects. The effect to reduce muscle damage is provocative but needs to be confirmed. The effects of longer treatments and higher doses need to be studied. Effect of HMB alone is not possible to determine in those studies that used it in combination with arginine and lysine (and the placebos in those cases were not isonitrogenous). Ransone et al., 2003: 35 football players consumed HMB or placebo for 4 wk; no difference in muscular strength or body composition. Crowe et al., 2003: 6 wk HMB (3 g) or HMB (3 g) + creatine (3 g) or control (received nothing) in 28 trained male rugby players; no effects were observed on health-related blood measures with exception of reduced bicarbonate and higher lymphocyte and monocyte counts in HMB (all still in normal range). Hoffman et al., 2004: No effect of 10 d of HMB in 26 players during preseason 2-a-day football practice on anaerobic power, hormones, or markers of muscle damage. *(continues)*	None reported	None reported

continued

TABLE 4-9 Continued

Review/ Clinical Trial Reference	Type of Study and Subjects	Indication	Control	Dose	Product Specification
Palisin and Stacy, 2005 *(continued)*					
Baxter et al., 2005		Dietary toxicity of calcium HMB (CaHMB)		0, 1, 2, 5% of diet as CaHMB for 91 days	CaHMB
van Someren et al., 2005		Effects on muscle damage caused by exercise	Placebo	3 g/d HMB + 0.3 g/d α-ketoisocaproic acid	Maximuscle HMB 1000, Maximuscle Ltd., Watford UK

Clinical Details and Outcomes Measured	Conclusions/ Results	Adverse Events Profile	Interactions with Pharmaceuticals, Foods, or Other Dietary Supplements
	Flakoll et al., 2004: 57 elderly women given 2 g HMB + 5 g arginine + 1.5 g lysine or placebo for 12 wk; supplement increased fat-free mass, whole-body protein synthesis, limb circumferences, strength, and functionality compared to placebo (not isonitrogenous placebo). Rathmacher et al., 2004: 3 studies, one on 34 healthy males, one on 43 HIV patients, one in 32 cancer patients; combination of 3 g HMB + 14 g arginine + 14 g glutamine; no adverse effects on blood chemistries (with exception that blood urea nitrogen increased), emotional profile, or adverse events; in fact, positive effects on emotional profile, reduced feeling of weakness, and increased red blood cells and lymphocytes.		
Mortality, clinical observations, body weight, food consumption, clinical and anatomic pathology evaluation	No effect on body weight, food intake, no meaningful hematological changes (some inconsistent effects on hematocrit), organ weights, micro- or macroscopic pathology. The only clinical chemistry measure changed was increase in inorganic phosphorus in 5% group. HMB was well tolerated up to 5% of the diet for 91 days.	None reported	None reported
Subjects consumed either HMB + α-ketoisocaproic acid or placebo for 14 days followed by performance of exercise designed to cause muscle damage	Combination supplement reduced the increase in marker of muscle damage, muscle soreness, percentage decrement in muscle strength, and increase in limb girth compared to placebo.	None reported	None reported

TABLE 4-10 Relevant Data and Conclusions on Efficacy and Safety Reviews and Publications Identified for Melatonin

Review/ Clinical Trial Reference	Type of Study and Subjects	Indication	Control	Dose	Product Specification
Arendt and Skene, 2005	Review of 14 studies	Jet lag and shift work	Various	1.8 mg sustained release or 5 mg fast release	
Brzezinski et al., 2005	Meta-analysis of 7 studies n=284 subjects	Insomnia	Placebo	Various	None reported
Buscemi et al., 2005	Meta-analysis of 14 randomized controlled trials	Insomnia and delayed sleep phase syndrome	Placebo	None reported	None reported
Buscemi et al., 2006	Meta-analysis	Secondary sleep disorders or sleep disorders accompanying sleep restriction	Placebo	Various; 0.5 mg to 7.5 mg	Various; mostly oral capsules and tablets

Clinical Details and Outcomes Measured	Conclusions/Results	Adverse Events Profile	Interactions with Pharmaceuticals, Foods, or Other Dietary Supplements
Sleep phase shifts	11 of 14 placebo controlled studies on the use of melatonin for jet lag found at least some benefit. The benefits included reduction in subjective jet lag, and improvements in sleep and alertness. The evidence for using melatonin to adapt to night-shift work was inconclusive.	Exogenous melatonin is a vasodilator—it lowers core body temperature, and it can affect skin blood flow. Therefore, if taken in a cold environment it may accelerate heat loss	None reported
Polysomnography and actigraphy used to measure sleep onset latency, total sleep duration, sleep efficiency	Melatonin treatment reduced sleep onset latency by an average of 4.0 minutes, increased sleep efficiency by 2.2%, and increased total sleep duration by 12.8 minutes.	None reported	None reported
Sleep onset latency, sleep efficiency, wakefulness after sleep onset, total sleep time, REM sleep percentage	Melatonin decreased sleep onset latency by an average of 7.2 minutes in insomniacs and by an average of 38.8 minutes in patients with delayed sleep phase syndrome. Some evidence that melatonin is not effective in treating primary sleep disorders over the short term (less than 4 wk).	No significant difference observed between melatonin and placebo	None reported
Sleep onset latency, sleep efficiency, wakefulness after sleep onset, total sleep time, REM sleep percentage	Change in sleep onset latency was not statistically significant. Although the increase in sleep efficiency in people with secondary sleep disorders was statistically significant with melatonin, the effect was small (1.9%) an increase of less than 10 min if the amount of time spent asleep for 8 h spent in bed.	The occurrence of adverse events was similar for melatonin and placebo. The most commonly reported adverse events were headaches, dizziness, nausea, and drowsiness	None reported

continued

TABLE 4-10 Continued

Review/ Clinical Trial Reference	Type of Study and Subjects	Indication	Control	Dose	Product Specification
Morin et al., 2007	Review	Insomnia, delayed sleep phase syndrome, jet lag	Various	Various; ranges from 0.3 mg to 5 mg	None reported
Wagner et al., 1998	Review	Insomnia and circadian disorders	Various	0.3 mg to 10 mg	Various
Bliwise and Ansari, 2007	Database evaluation n=31,044 adults (ages 18–61+); representative U.S. sample				

Clinical Details and Outcomes Measured	Conclusions/Results	Adverse Events Profile	Interactions with Pharmaceuticals, Foods, or Other Dietary Supplements
Sleep latency, sleep duration, sleep quality	Although there is some evidence supporting the use of melatonin in treating jet lag and sleep disturbance caused by shift work, more research is needed before melatonin can be recommended as a treatment for insomnia.	Common: fatigue, dizziness, headache, irritability, and drowsiness Less common: mood changes, hypotension, atherosclerotic plaques, hyperglycemia, mild gastrointestinal distress, increased intraocular pressure, fluctuations in reproductive and thyroid hormones	Potential synergy with other sedative hypnotics
Many, including sleep quality, sleep latency, EEG, sleep duration	The evidence may support melatonin use for circadian rhythm disorders and in patients with low melatonin levels such as the elderly; more evidence is needed before it can be recommended for insomnia in the general population.	Fatigue, headache, dizziness, irritability	None reported
	Data from 2002 Alternative Health/Complementary and Alternative Medicine supplement to the National Health Interview Survey: 5.2% of the survey sample used melatonin of which 27.5% (standard error=3.93) endorsed insomnia as one reason for use; 5.8% of the survey sample mentioned insomnia in association with valerian and melatonin use. Women used it more than men (5.5:1). Melatonin showed a 13.9% usage rate in association with anxiety/depression.	None reported	None reported

TABLE 4-11 Relevant Data and Conclusions on Efficacy and Safety Reviews and Publications Identified for Quercetin

Review/ Clinical Trial Reference	Type of Study and Subjects	Indication	Control	Dose	Product Specification
Lotito and Frei, 2006	Pharmacologic study	Inflammation and atherosclerosis			Quercetin
Nieman et al., 2007	Double-blind, randomized, controlled n=40 males	Upper respiratory infections and immune function after exercise	Placebo	1,000 mg/day twice daily for 3 wk prior and 2 wk after the 3-d period of exercise	Quercetin
Davis et al., 2007	Animal study			12.5 or 25 mg/kg body weight for 7 d	Quercetin
Okamoto, 2005	Review				Quercetin
IARC, 1999	Review				Quercetin
van der Woude et al., 2005	Tissue culture: breast cancer cells			10–80 μmol/L	Quercetin
Watjen et al., 2005	Tissue culture: hepatoma rat cells				Quercetin

Clinical Details and Outcomes Measured	Conclusions/Results	Adverse Events Profile	Interactions with Pharmaceuticals, Foods, or Other Dietary Supplements
Inhibition of endothelial molecule expression	Quercetin, among other hydroxyl flavones, was able to inhibit endothelial adhesion molecule expression.	None reported	None reported
Upper respiratory tract infections (URTI) and changes in immune function after cycling at high output for 3 h/d	No effects on natural killer cell activity, PHA-stimulated lymphocyte proliferation, polymorphonuclear oxidative burst activity, or salivary IgA output. Incidence of URTI during the 2-wk postexercise period differed significantly between groups. Quercetin might have antiviral effect.	None reported	None reported
Mitochondrial content in muscle and brain, endurance capacity	Significant increases in mitochondrial content in skeletal muscle and brain. Increased endurance capacity observed in the mice.	None reported	None reported
Carcinogenicity	Quercetin is not carcinogenic.	None reported	None reported
Carcinogenicity	Quercetin is not carcinogenic.	None reported	None reported
Cell proliferation	Biphasic effect: increase in cell proliferation at a low dose level (10–20 μmol/L) and decrease in proliferation at higher doses (40–80 μmol/L).	None reported	None reported
Effects on DNA	Biphasic effect: lower doses of 10–25 μmol/L protect against DNA strand breaks and induced apoptosis, but 50–250 μmol/L caused DNA damage.	None reported	None reported

TABLE 4-12 Relevant Data and Conclusions on Efficacy and Safety Reviews and Publications Identified for Sports Bars

Review/ Clinical Trial Reference	Type of Study and Subjects	Indication	Control	Dose	Product Specification
Burke et al., 2005	Crossover n=18 highly trained marathon runners	Athletic performance (marathons)	Placebo (426±227 mL) or water (386±185 mL)	Commercial gel providing 1.1±0.2 g/kg body mass carbohydrate	Powergel, Nestle Australia
Ebert et al., 2007	Randomized, crossover, not blinded n=8 well-trained male cyclists	Athletic performance (cycling in a warm environment)	None reported	0.4 L water and a sport gel or 2.4 L of a 7% carbohydrate-electrolyte drink Sports gel had same carbohydrate content as carbohydrate-electrolyte drink	Gu Energy Gel, Sports Street Marketing, Berkeley, CA
Rauch et al., 1999	2 random order trials n=6 male highly trained endurance cyclists, mean age 31	Ultra-endurance athletic performance (cycling)	None reported	Trial 1: 1.5 energy bars and 700 mL water every hr. Each bar has 19 g carbohydrate, 7 g fat, 14 g protein, 200 mg sodium, 50 mg potassium, <1 g fiber, and trace amounts of vitamins A, B, C, and E Trial 2: 700 mL of a 100 g/L glucose polymer solution every hr similar energy ingestion during both trials 330 min cycling per trial	None reported

Outcomes Measured	Conclusions/Results	Adverse Events Profile	Interactions with Pharmaceuticals, Foods, or Other Dietary Supplements
Body mass, performance on 2 half marathons	Mean body mass change of approximately 2.4%. Three runners reported gastrointestinal discomfort after consuming gel, which impaired marathon performance. The effect of gel on performance was insignificant (time was improved by 0.3% or 14 sec compared with placebo). No benefits of carbohydrate gel intake on half marathon performance.	Gastrointestinal discomfort	None reported
Maximal aerobic power, hydration status, body mass changes, sweat rate, blood glucose, blood lactose, rating of exertion, thermal sensation, and stomach fullness	No differences in bicycle treadmill speed, blood glucose, blood lactose, hydration status, perceived exertion, thermal sensation, or stomach fullness. Significantly lower absolute power output in water plus gel group to maintain same speed as carbohydrate-electrolyte drink group during treadmill test. Time to exhaustion was significantly shorter in water plus gel group. Ingestion of water and a sport gel reduced the exercise capacity of trained cyclists during laboratory cycling hill-climbing.	None reported	None reported
Maximal oxygen consumption, respiratory exchange ratio, heart rate, fat oxidation, perceived exertion	Fat oxidation rates were greater in subjects who ingested energy bar compared to those ingesting carbohydrate gel. Ingestion of a sports bar significantly enhanced fat metabolism during prolonged submaximal exercise. Ingestion of sports bar containing carbohydrate, fat, and protein during exercise, led to impaired performance on subsequent high-intensity exercise.	None reported	None reported

TABLE 4-13 Relevant Data and Conclusions on Efficacy and Safety Reviews and Publications Identified for Sports Drinks

Review/Clinical Trial Reference	Type of Study and Subjects	Indication	Control	Dose	Product Specification
Gibala, 2007	Review	Protein metabolism	Various	Various	None reported
Jeukendrup, 2004	Review	Exercise performance	Various	Various	None reported
Maughan and Murray, 2001	Review	Exercise performance	Various	Various	None reported
Nieman, 2007	Review	Immune function	None reported	None reported	None reported
Winnick et al., 1995	Double-blind, randomized, counter-balanced n=20 active adults (10 men, 10 women), mean age 23.9 y	Peripheral and central nervous system function	Placebo	6% carbohydrate solution: 5 mL/kg before exercise, 3 mL/kg after exercise, 8 mL/kg during exercise	Gatorade Sports Science Institute, Barrington, IL

Outcomes Measured	Conclusions/Results	Adverse Events Profile	Interactions with Pharmaceuticals, Foods, or Other Dietary Supplements
Endurance performance, repair and synthesis of muscle proteins, synthesis of muscle glycogen	One study found that ingestion of a sports drink with added protein provided no additional benefit on athletic performance. There is no established mechanism by which protein intake during exercise should improve acute endurance performance. Ingestion of protein with carbohydrate improves net protein balance during exercise and recovery compared with carbohydrate alone, but it remains to be determined whether this practice facilitates the adaptive response to chronic training.	None reported	None reported
Endurance capacity and performance	Ingestion of small amounts of carbohydrate (16 g/h) during exercise has positive ergogenic effects on performance. Larger amounts do not show any further benefits.	None reported	None reported
Various	Rehydration with sports drinks can restore the negative fluid balance caused by exercise. Sports drinks can also restore muscle glycogen after exercise. Ingestion of a sports drink at regular intervals during physical activity may enhance performance.		
Immune dysfunction	Ingestion of carbohydrate beverages during exercise is an effective countermeasure to exercise-induced immune suppression in marathon athletes. Carbohydrate supplementation decreases exercise-induced increases in plasma cytokines and stress hormones, but is largely ineffective against other immune components including natural killer cell function and salivary IgA, with an undetermined influence on incidence of upper respiratory tract infections.	None reported	None reported
Tests of peripheral and central nervous system function (sprints, jumping, mood evaluation, cognitive function, force sensation, motor skills tests, and target jumping accuracy)	Carbohydrate intake during exercise resulted in significantly faster 20-m sprint times and higher average jump height at the end of the exercise period. Carbohydrate intake also reduced force sensation, enhanced motor skills, and improved mood late in exercise. Carbohydrate intake during intermittent high-intensity exercise similar to that of team sports improved peripheral and central nervous system function late in exercise.	None reported	None reported

TABLE 4-14 Relevant Data and Conclusions on Efficacy and Safety Reviews and Publications Identified for Tyrosine

Review/ Clinical Trial Reference	Type of Study and Subjects	Indication	Control	Dose	Product Specification
Banderet and Lieberman, 1989	Double-blind, crossover n=23 male U.S. soldiers, ages 18–20 y	Mood, physical condition, and cognitive performance under environmental stress	Placebo	2 gelatin capsules adjusted to contain 50 mg/kg tyrosine	None reported
Wiegmann et al., 1993	Controlled n=20 male U.S. Marines, ages 21–27 y	Cognitive performance after sleep loss and sustained work	Placebo	2 doses of 75 mg/kg tyrosine	Ajinomoto Company, Inc.
Deijen and Orlebeke, 1994	Double-blind, randomized n=9 male and 7 female healthy subjects, ages 25–35 y	Cognitive performance	Placebo	100 mg/kg L-tyrosine	Country Life, Hauppauge, NY
Shurtleff et al., 1994	Controlled n=8 men	Cognitive performance	Placebo	Applesauce adjusted to contain 150 mg/kg tyrosine	Tysons & Assoc., Santa Monica, CA (crystalline tyrosine)
Neri et al., 1995	Double-blind n=20 male U.S. Marines, ages 21–27 y	Cognitive performance after sleep loss	Placebo	150 mg/kg tyrosine	None reported

Clinical Details and Outcomes Measured	Conclusions/Results	Adverse Events Profile	Interactions with Pharmaceuticals, Foods, or Other Dietary Supplements
Mood states, sustained attention, vigilance, processing spatial and verbal information, math skills, number coding, pattern recognition	Individuals were exposed to environmental stressors: Two levels of decreased temperature and reduced atmospheric pressure versus normal temperature and pressure. Relative to placebo, tyrosine significantly reduced symptoms of headache, coldness, distress, fatigue, muscular discomfort, and sleepiness in subjects who responded adversely to environmental stress. Tyrosine also reduced dizziness, feelings of confusion, unhappiness, hostility, and tension, and reversed the adverse effects of environmental stressors on cognitive performance on tasks measuring math skills, pattern recognition, vigilance, and coding.	None reported	None reported
Eye-hand coordination, short-term memory, dichotic listening, mood, sleepiness, blood pressure, heart rate	Participants tested under conditions with noise stressor. Across night performance on cognitive tasks decreased. However, tyrosine administration led to smaller decrements in performance in eye-hand coordination, and short-term memory than placebo. Additionally, participants reported being less sleepy after tyrosine than placebo.	None reported	None reported
Perceptual motor tasks, vigilance task, short-term memory test, Stroop task, and adjective checklist of mood	Relative to placebo, tyrosine improved performance on short-term memory and Stroop task.	None reported	None reported
Performance on delayed matching to sample test of working memory	Tested at ambient temperatures of 4°C and 22°C. Relative to placebo, tyrosine prevented cold-induced memory deficit.	None reported	None reported
Performance on psychomotor tasks and mood scales	Tyrosine prevented performance decline on a psychomotor task and exhibited reduction on lapse responses on a vigilance task in sleep-deprived participants.	None reported	None reported

continued

TABLE 4-14 Continued

Review/ Clinical Trial Reference	Type of Study and Subjects	Indication	Control	Dose	Product Specification
Deijen et al., 1999	Double-blind, randomized n=20 male and 1 female military cadets, ages 18–27 y	Cognitive performance	Carbohydrate-rich drink	2 g tyrosine in a protein-rich drink	PROTIFAR powder
Thomas et al., 1999	Double-blind, crossover n=10 male and 10 female active duty personnel and civilians, ages 20–38 y	Cognitive performance under stress condition	Placebo	Applesauce adjusted to contain 150 mg/kg tyrosine	None reported
Chinevere et al., 2002	Double-blind, randomized, counter-balanced n=9 male competitive cyclists	Endurance exercise performance	Polydextrose solution or aspartame solution	25 mg/kg tyrosine dissolved in a polydextrose solution or water	None reported
Magill et al., 2003	Double-blind, randomized n=76 men, ages 18–35 y	Cognitive performance when sleep deprived	Placebo	150 mg/kg	None reported
O'Brien et al., 2007	Double-blind n=15 soldiers (14 men, 1 women)	Cognitive and psychomotor performance after cold water immersion	Placebo	2 energy bars adjusted to each contain 150 mg/kg tyrosine	None reported

Clinical Details and Outcomes Measured	Conclusions/Results	Adverse Events Profile	Interactions with Pharmaceuticals, Foods, or Other Dietary Supplements
Memory, perceptual, motor, vigilance tasks, and mood scales	Tyrosine supplementation reduced cognitive deficits associated with psychosocial stress and fatigue associated with combat training. Tyrosine did not affect mood. Study design does not eliminate the possibility that other amino acids contributed to the observed results.	None reported	None reported
Simple task battery measuring working memory and multiple task battery consisting of four simultaneously occurring tasks measuring memory, math skills, visual monitoring, auditory monitoring	Tyrosine improved performance on multiple task battery, but not on simple task battery. Tyrosine might be beneficial to memory under conditions of increased cognitive stress (e.g., multiple cognitive demands placed on military personnel).	None reported	None reported
Time trial performance test on a stationary bicycle	Tyrosine, either alone or with carbohydrates did not improve cycling time trial performance.	None reported	None reported
Visual scanning, memory, logical reasoning, mathematical processing, reaction time, vigilance, pursuit tracking	Tyrosine showed positive effects for overcoming performance deficits due to prolonged sleep deprivation. Effects most pronounced for deficits in tasks measuring memory and mathematical processing.	None reported	None reported
Skin folds, U.S. Special Operations Command standardized tests of cognitive and physical performance evaluating short-term spatial memory and pattern recognition, complex reaction time, visual vigilance, mathematical reasoning, logical reasoning, psychomotor performance, marksmanship, grip strength, pull-ups, cycle ergometer, step ups	Tyrosine mitigated cold-induced decrements in performance on tasks measuring short-term memory, pattern recognition, and marksmanship.	None reported	None reported

continued

TABLE 4-14 Continued

Review/ Clinical Trial Reference	Type of Study and Subjects	Indication	Control	Dose	Product Specification
Mahoney et al., 2007	Double-blind n=19 military members	Cognitive performance and mood after acute cold stress	Placebo	2 energy bars adjusted to each contain 150 mg/kg tyrosine	None reported

Clinical Details and Outcomes Measured	Conclusions/Results	Adverse Events Profile	Interactions with Pharmaceuticals, Foods, or Other Dietary Supplements
Visual vigilance, reaction time, short-term memory, mood state, muscle discomfort, alertness	Tyrosine reduced cold-induced decrements in working memory and mitigated cold-induced increased score on tension subscale of mood test.	None reported	None reported

TABLE 4-15 Relevant Data and Conclusions on Efficacy and Safety Reviews and Publications Identified for Valerian

Review/ Clinical Trial Reference	Type of Study and Subjects	Indication	Control	Dose	Product Specification
Leathwood et al., 1982	Randomized, controlled n=128	Improvement of sleep quality and latency	Placebo	400 mg	Valerian aqueous extract
Donath et al., 2000	Randomized, double-blind, crossover n=16 (4 men, 12 women), ages 22–55 y, with psychophysiological insomnia	Sleep quality and structure	Placebo	600 mg/d for 8 d	Valerian extract (300 mg) pills as Sedonium
Beaubrun and Gray, 2000	Review	Sleep latency, nocturnal awakenings, and subjective sleep quality	Placebo	400 mg to 900 mg	Valerian extract
Bent et al., 2006	Review n=16 studies	Improving sleep quality	Placebo	Variable	Variable
Diaper and Hindmarch, 2004	Double-blind, crossover n=16 (5 men, 11 women) sleep-disturbed patients	Insomnia and improving sleep quality	Placebo	300 mg and 600 mg for 1 d	Valerian extract (300 mg) Sedonium
Hallam et al., 2003	Randomized, double-blind, crossover n=9 (5 men, 4 women) healthy subjects	Cognitive and psychomotor effects of valerian	Placebo	500 mg and 1,000 mg for 1 d	Valerian extract (500 mg) Herb Valley

[a]Electroencephalography is the technique of using electrodes placed on the scalp to measure electrical activity of the brain.

[b]Electro-oculography is a technique for measuring the resting potential of the retina.

Outcomes Measured	Conclusions/Results	Adverse Events Profile	Interactions with Pharmaceuticals, Foods, or Other Dietary Supplements
Subjective ratings of sleep quality, sleep latency, night awakenings, dream recall, next morning sleepiness	The aqueous extract of valerian produced a significant improvement in sleep quality in young, poor sleepers as well as a significant improvement in sleep quality in women who were poor sleepers. There were no differences between placebo and valerian in dream recall, night awakenings, or next morning sleepiness.	One person withdrew from the study because they experienced nausea. However, it was not possible to attribute the nausea definitively to valerian	None reported
Sleep structure changes as measured by EEG,[a] EOG,[b] EMG,[c] and ECG[d] Subjective sleep quality	In insomnia patients, valerian had positive effects on sleep structure and sleep perception. It can be recommended for the treatment of patients with mild psychophysiological insomnia.	More adverse events were seen under the placebo condition (18 vs. 3)	None reported
Sleep latency, nocturnal awakening, subjective sleep quality	Valerian generally produced decreased sleep latency and nocturnal awakenings and improved subjective sleep quality. However, in some studies the placebo effect was large and in others the beneficial effects of valerian were not seen until after 2 to 4 wk of therapy.	Rare, but may include headache, restless sleep, allergies, gastrointestinal problems, and mydriasis	Potential interaction with other sedative hypnotics
Sleep quality	Valerian may be an effective treatment for insomnia; larger studies needed.		
Time in bed, total sleep time, sleep latency, number of awakenings, total slow-wave sleep	No significant difference was found between either dose of valerian and placebo. Valerian is ineffective as an acute treatment for sleeping problems at these doses.	None reported	None reported
Critical flicker fusion, choice reaction time, digit symbol substitution test, symbol search test, digit span test, and visual analogue scales of mood	Valerian was without effect on either cognitive or psychomotor performance at the doses used in this study.	None reported	None reported

[c]Electromyography is a technique for evaluating physiologic properties of muscles.
[d]Electrocardiogram is a recording of the electrical activity of the heart over time.

5

Framework to Review the Safety of Dietary Supplements for Use by Military Personnel

BACKGROUND

The increasing popularity of dietary supplements among civilians and military personnel has raised questions about their safety and efficacy for both populations. In the United States, various government agencies are charged with ensuring the safety of consumable products by developing and implementing policy according to their legal authority. In the United States, decisions regarding the safety of ingested substances are made using three models, based on the nature and intended use of each substance. The basic models are the food model (based on the assumption, derived from historic consumption, that all foods are safe and therefore, no premarket safety assessment is necessary), the food additive model (based on premarket safety assessments submitted to the U.S. Food and Drug Administration [FDA] by manufacturers), and the drug model (based on risk-benefit assessments submitted to the FDA by manufacturers).

The Dietary Supplement Health and Education Act (DSHEA) of 1994 designated the FDA as the agency responsible for determining whether a marketed dietary supplement is unsafe (*Dietary Supplement Health and Education Act of 1994*, Public Law 103-417, 108 Stat 4325, 103rd Congress, October 25, 1994). The unique nature of dietary supplements (i.e., they are legally categorized as foods but are used to enhance health) and their history of use (i.e., some have been used as medicines for centuries by other cultures) have resulted in difficulty and confusion in establishing and implementing policies to address their safety. Despite wide concurrence that, given the nature of these products, a premarket approval process would be appropriate to address their safety, there is no such process in place. While DSHEA mandates that manufacturers wishing to market new dietary supplement ingredients inform the FDA of their intention, this notification is often not accompanied by a safety profile of the product.

The FDA relies on a postmarket adverse event surveillance system to monitor adverse effects and, along with other supporting scientific data, to take action against any dietary supplement identified as unsafe after it has been marketed. However, the voluntary nature of reports by consumers or others to the FDA presents important limitations, such as low reporting rate or poor data quality (see Chapter 6). The 2007 Dietary Supplement and Nonprescription Drug Consumer Protection Act represents a step forward in ensuring safety by mandating that companies report to the FDA any serious adverse event derived from the use of dietary supplements, but the success of this act in establishing an effective signaling system to identify supplement ingredients particularly in need of safety evaluation is still unknown. The act defines the term *serious adverse event* as an adverse event that

> (A) results in (i) death; (ii) a life-threatening experience; (iii) inpatient hospitalization; (iv) a persistent or significant disability or incapacity; (v) a congenital anomaly or birth defect; or (B) requires, based on reasonable medical judgment, a medical or surgical intervention to prevent a previously listed outcome described under subparagraph (A).

Also, in 2007, the FDA published the final rule, stipulated under DSHEA, establishing the minimum current good manufacturing practices (cGMPs) required for activities related to manufacturing, packaging, labeling, and storing dietary supplements to ensure their quality. This rule ensures consistency in product composition, but not the safety or efficacy of that product. The FDA is empowered to initiate regulatory action (e.g., banning a dietary supplement, taking an enforcement action [e.g., seizure or injunction] against a product or firm, or alerting the public) when the agency has evidence a product violates a provision of the Federal Food, Drug, and Cosmetic Act (FFD&C Act). Evidence that a product may be unsafe could include postmarket reports of severe adverse events, reports in the scientific literature of harm associated with exposure to a particular product or ingredient, or evidence of the presence of an adulterant such as an unforeseen contaminant or a purposeful adulterant.

In light of the growing use of dietary supplements, the FDA requested in 2002 that the Institute of Medicine (IOM) provide a process or framework for evaluating the safety of dietary supplement ingredients. Highlights of the IOM report *Dietary Supplements: A Framework for Evaluating Safety* (2005) were presented at the February 2007 workshop (see Jeffery in Appendix B).

The 2005 IOM report recognizes that the potential for a significant or unreasonable risk resulting from consumption of a dietary supplement varies depending on the specific circumstances of its use (e.g., under temperature extremes) or for specific populations (e.g., military personnel; see also Chapter 9 of the 2005 IOM report for a discussion of vulnerable groups). Thus, a vulnerable group may be at far greater risk from adverse effects of a given supplement than the general public. An example would be persons operating motor vehicles, who should not take sedative supplements such as valerian. Because neither federal dietary supplement policies nor the safety framework outlined in the 2005 IOM report was created with the specific needs (e.g., unique policies, behaviors, environmental stresses, and performance requirements) of the military population in mind, the U.S. Department of Defense (DoD) requested that this committee assess the applicability of the 2005 IOM report framework to a military setting and establish how it could be modified to determine which supplements need active management by the military.

The committee concluded that the 2005 IOM report's framework for the general population is not directly applicable to military personnel for reasons that include the military's need for optimal health and performance as well as the high demands for readiness and success in military operations. Benefits and/or risks to military personnel from use of a particular dietary supplement might also differ from those of the general population owing to specific unit missions and environments; for example, the thermoregulatory effects of some dietary supplements could be critical for military personnel operating in extreme temperatures, while they would be less important for the general population or for military personnel deployed to a more temperate area. Some groups of military personnel might experience risks and benefits from the use of dietary supplements different from those of other military personnel because of their unique responsibilities and tasks (e.g., aviators, those with access to nuclear weapons, or those conducting special operations).

The U.S. regulatory model to manage the use of dietary supplements may also be inadequate for certain military populations (see Chapter 1, Box 1-3). For example, because of the potentially life-threatening consequences of being in suboptimal mental or physical health while conducting military operations, military leadership might need to develop an active monitoring system, rather than basing decisions only on the passive system of voluntarily reported adverse events now in use (see Chapter 6). Furthermore, the potential gains in health or performance from the use of some dietary supplements need to be considered in managing their use. For instance, if dietary supplement X causes slight dehydration but substantially improves alertness, the management of X by military leadership might be different from that of dietary supplement Y, which induces a similar level of dehydration but imparts little benefit.

To summarize, this IOM committee was asked to review the 2005 IOM report's framework for evaluating the safety of dietary supplements and assess whether modifications are necessary for its application to the military.

This chapter does not enumerate the specific series of in vitro and in vivo toxicological and clinical tests that would be required to evaluate the safety of a dietary ingredient; these will vary with the specific ingredient(s), the users, and other factors. Instead, the chapter includes a framework to review the available scientific evidence and determine the level of concern; this is to be used as a tool to help military decision makers establish policies on the use of dietary supplements. In contrast to the 2005 IOM report framework, which—in accordance with the FDA's mandate—focused only on safety, this committee has provided general guidance for the military on integrating considerations of efficacy and safety when making policy on dietary supplement use.

The development of a framework to perform a complete risk-benefit analysis is beyond the scope of this report. It is also beyond the scope of this report to recommend definitive management actions. Examples are provided of possible actions (e.g., restricting or recommending the use of specific dietary supplements, developing educational programs) based on the level of concern (and the potential for benefit). To demonstrate application of the framework recommended, the committee reviewed a number of dietary supplements on the basis of published safety and efficacy reports (see Chapters 3 and 4) and identified those that might pose concerns or be of benefit. In addition, the committee's overall approach (i.e., including application of the framework and recommendations for action) was applied to a subset of those dietary supplements (Appendix D); it was outside the committee's task to provide a review of all dietary supplements. These monographs and case studies should be considered as examples; as recommended below, determining the specific actions to take in response to a dietary supplement review should be the prerogative of military leadership.

SAFETY FRAMEWORK FOR DIETARY SUPPLEMENTS: MODIFICATIONS FOR MILITARY USE

The committee's recommended approach to manage the use of dietary supplements in a military context comprises four related components: (1) improving monitoring of the use of dietary supplements by military personnel, (2) using a framework to determine the level of concern for dietary supplements in a military context, (3) implementing a system to report adverse events associated with dietary supplements, and (4) expanding education on dietary supplements.

This section describes the second component, that is, elements of the safety framework outlined in the 2005 IOM report that are particularly useful to the military in its need to understand the safety (and possible benefits) of the use of dietary supplements by military personnel. (For greater detail on the regulatory background and the statement of task of the 2005 IOM Committee on the Framework for Evaluating the Safety of Dietary Supplements, see Jeffery in Appendix B.)

The 2005 IOM report framework consists of a process for prioritizing, evaluating, and describing available information to establish risk of harm, together with a second, supportive component: a set of science-based principles that serve as guidelines for evaluating risk to human health (see Jeffery, Figure B-24, in Appendix B). It characterizes the nature of the scientific evidence that is likely to be available to the FDA and describes a process for organizing this evidence to assess the level of concern for a dietary supplement ingredient. A "significant or unreasonable risk of illness or injury" is the standard that warrants regulation by the FDA under the FFD&C Act, as amended by DSHEA. The process outlined in the 2005 IOM report is divided into three steps: signal detection, initial signal review to determine a preliminary level of concern, and integrated safety evaluation of dietary supplements. This process provides a basis for determining whether a dietary supplement is unsafe and for translating a serious concern into safety management actions. For example, a high level of initial concern based on a signal that leads to a high potential for a "significant or unreasonable risk of illness or injury" warrants a full evaluation of safety.

Proving that a dietary supplement presents an unreasonable risk is a substantial undertaking requiring valuable time and resources. The FDA, which bears responsibility for the safety of all dietary supplements on the market, is presently limited to responding to reports of serious adverse events as the primary signal for action. The DoD could take a more proactive stance, choosing to evaluate the effects of a dietary supplement and take management actions based on criteria pertinent to the demands of military service. Thus, the military may choose to focus attention on determining the safety of those dietary supplements with the highest volume of sales, even if there have been no adverse events reported for the general population. Furthermore, the scientific basis for concern may be more stringent and may include evidence of more subtle effects than those causing concern for the general public. For these reasons, the 2005 IOM report framework has been adapted to meet the specific needs of the military.

Described below are the three steps (i.e., signal detection, initial review of signals, and integrated safety evaluation) described in the 2005 IOM report, followed by their adaptation for the military.

Signal Detection

The 2005 IOM Safety Framework for Dietary Supplements: Adverse Event Monitoring

The 2005 IOM report suggested that, given the limited resources available to the FDA, a supplement should undergo a safety review only when the signal of a serious adverse event indicates the need. However, should resources permit, it was proposed that the FDA's attention should focus on signals that indicate a serious health problem may result from ingestion of a dietary supplement ingredient.

The 2005 IOM report framework suggested that if the FDA were able to operate proactively, review of a dietary supplement ingredient should be initiated on the basis of either a high prevalence of use in the general population, or a high level of use by a particularly vulnerable population.

As Modified for the Military: Adverse Events and Frequency of Use Monitoring

The military should proactively concern itself not only with dietary supplements associated with an adverse event but also with those most commonly sold on base, and with consideration for the safety of those military personnel who, because of their duties, would be particularly vulnerable to the adverse effects of specific supplements. For example, pilots might be susceptible to effects including hypoxia, cognitive decrements, or loss of spatial orientation. Similarly, those on active duty in adverse environments might be particularly vulnerable to supplements causing loss of thermal regulation (see Chapter 1, Box 1-3 for a list of special military populations). Conversely, if there were supplements that could aid in prevention of these adverse effects, this information might be of considerable benefit to the military.

Initial Review of Signals

The 2005 IOM Safety Framework for Dietary Supplements: Severity of Adverse Events

The second step in the process outlined in the 2005 IOM framework is the initial review of available information on the signal (i.e., adverse event reports). First, the nature of the signal information is examined to determine the preliminary level (low, moderate, or high) of concern about a potential risk to human health. This is not a detailed analysis of data, but rather an assessment to determine whether further evaluation of the supplement is indicated. If review of the reports shows an isolated case lacking reliable evidence that the supplement was likely to be a cause, the resulting low level of concern would indicate no further need for action at that time. If signal review results in even a moderate level of concern traced directly to the supplement, then other criteria, such as prevalence of use or potential to adversely affect vulnerable subpopulations, should be considered, which might result in elevation of the signal concern level to high. Signal review would typically be triggered by an adverse event report of medium or high concern.

As Modified for the Military: Severity of Adverse Events and Frequency of Use

> **Recommendation 4: The decision to initiate a review of a dietary supplement should be based on two criteria: severity and number of adverse events, and prevalence of use. The selection of dietary supplements for review should consider the particular vulnerabilities of the military subpopulations, which would depend on their missions and mission environments.**

Severity and number of adverse events As with the general population, one set of criteria relies on adverse event(s) reported by military or nonmilitary personnel. (See Chapter 6 for recommendations on a system to monitor adverse events for the military.)

Military health care professionals should identify any adverse events associated with dietary supplement use that might compromise the performance or survivability of military personnel. Such adverse events would include those that affect vigilance; have a significant adverse impact on alertness, mood, or cognitive performance; cause hypoxia; or affect balance or spatial orientation. They would also include impairment of clotting, hydration, immune function, or thermoregulation. Conditions to help categorize adverse events as high, moderate, low, and minimal are listed in Box 5-1. Summaries of adverse event reports should be submitted to the military committee or entity designated to oversee dietary supplements (herein referred to as the designated oversight committee; see Chapter 6), who will identify a signal of concern for a dietary supplement and determine whether a review is appropriate.

When the adverse event reported is serious or might compromise performance or survivability, the committee proposes a two-part response. The first step is to determine whether urgent action (e.g., new policies; see Figure 5-1) is warranted. Second, in conjunction with policy implemention and enforcement, a safety and efficacy review should be conducted. Adverse events of moderate concern might not signal the need for new policy, although the military should initiate a safety review (Figure 5-1). If no adverse effects are being noted from the use of a specific supplement and its safety review reveals no concern, then the determination would be made that the dietary supplement is of minimal concern and no further evaluation would be needed. Nevertheless, due to low reporting rates of adverse events,[1] the lack of such reports does not necessarily mean that the dietary supplement is safe. Further, the committee believes that because these products are bioactive, high frequency of use calls for a review of safety, unless the dietary supplement has already been declared to be of minimal concern.

The committee cautions that the linking of an adverse event to a dietary supplement ingredient might be confounded if the product contains multiple ingredients, or adulterants or adventitious contaminants. In the case of multiple ingredients, determination of causation for a particular substance requires careful review of all the individual ingredients in a product or the combination product itself. If contamination is the issue, then attribution of the source of the event is even more challenging. In either case, and until the cause of the adverse event is determined, the military might need to apply policies for the use of the suspect product as well as for any other product containing any of the ingredients found in the suspect product.

Prevalence of use A second criterion to commence a review relies on a proactive initiative by military leadership in response to the use of a new supplement similar to a drug or supplement that has previously caused safety concerns (e.g., bitter orange contains synephrine, closely related to ephedrine, the active component in ephedra); the high frequency of use of a supplement; or an increase in frequency of use in the general military population or specific subpopulations. To make such decisions, data from dietary supplement sales and survey data on dietary supplement use within the military would be required (see Chapter 2). For example, the military should review data on sales of dietary supplements from outlets located on base (e.g., Army and Air Force Exchange Service/Navy Exchange Service [AAFES/NEX], fitness centers) annually to determine which supplements have become popular. Because of the low reporting rates for adverse events, the lack of data on adverse events does not necessarily show that a dietary supplement is safe. Also, because these products are bioactive, a review of the safety of widely used dietary supplements is warranted unless the dietary supplement has been declared to be of minimal concern. If no ad-

---

[1]The 2007 Dietary Supplement and Nonprescription Drug Consumer Protection Act defines the term "serious adverse event" as an adverse event that (A) results in (i) death; (ii) a life-threatening experience; (iii) inpatient hospitalization; (iv) a persistent or significant disability or incapacity; (v) a congenital anomaly or birth defect; or (B) requires, based on reasonable medical judgment, a medical or surgical intervention to prevent a previously listed outcome described under subparagraph (A).

BOX 5-1
Description of Concern Levels Specific to Use of Dietary Supplements by Military Personnel

High concern

- Human epidemiological studies or adverse effects signaling:
  - Product has been found responsible for a serious adverse event
  - Performance degradation (e.g., for those deployed, in training, or in combat settings):
    - Product significantly affects vigilance
    - Product has significant adverse impact on alertness/drowsiness, mood alteration, cognitive performance
    - Product significantly induces hypoxia
    - Product significantly affects balance and spatial orientation
  - A decrease in survivability (e.g., for those deployed, in training, or in combat settings):
    - Product significantly inhibits clotting time
    - Product significantly promotes dehydration
    - Product significantly inhibits immune system
    - Product significantly disrupts body's ability to maintain thermal regulation
- Animal data signaling:
  - Serious adverse events as described above for human data, seen in animals at doses 10× recommended exposure for humans
  - Neoplasia
  - Severe organ toxicity (necrosis/dysplasia)
  - Reproductive failure/developmental effects
  - Severe neurological/behavioral changes
- In vitro data signaling:
  - Multiple different assays suggest the same pathological condition related to serious adverse events described for human data above
  - Concentrations of the dietary supplement causing severe adverse effects in vitro are similar to reported blood or plasma levels in humans following consumption of this dietary supplement
  - Chemical or plant species is similar to known toxic compound and/or banned dietary supplement, or similar to products having adverse effects described above in humans

verse effects are noted from the use of a specific supplement and its safety review reveals no concern, then the determination would be made that the dietary supplement is of minimal concern and no further evaluation would be needed.

Many factors need to be taken into consideration in determining a level of concern from adverse events reported, including the strength of the

Moderate Concern

- Human epidemiological studies or adverse events signaling:
  - Performance degradation (e.g., for those deployed, in training, or in combat):
    - Product has moderate impact on hydration, gastrointestinal function (e.g., diarrhea, nausea), thermal regulation, alertness/drowsiness, mood, or cognitive performance or may induce shortness of breath or syncope
  - A decrease in survivability (e.g., for those deployed, in training, or in combat):
    - Product has moderate impact on clotting time
    - Product has moderate or low ability to inhibit immune system
- Animal data signaling:
  - Moderate organ toxicity (atrophy, hyperplasia)
  - Reduced reproductive capacity/mild developmental effects
  - Altered clinical chemistry outside the reference range
  - Those adverse effects listed above as serious in humans, occurring at 100× the recommended dose range

Low Concern

- Human epidemiological studies or adverse events signaling:
  - Performance degradation:
    - Product has low impact on hydration, gastrointestinal function (e.g., diarrhea, distress, nausea), alertness/drowsiness, thermal regulation, mood, or cognitive performance
  - No decrease in survivability (product has no known impact on immune response or bleeding/clotting time)
- Animal data signaling:
  - Reduced food intake
  - Enzyme changes
  - Reversible degenerative changes

Minimal Concern

- Human epidemiological studies or adverse events signaling:
  - No serious adverse events
  - No performance degradation (product has no known impact on hydration, gastrointestinal function, thermal regulation, alertness/drowsiness, mood, or cognitive performance)
  - No decrease in survivability (product has no known impact on immune response or bleeding/clotting time)

evidence (e.g., how many adverse events were associated with the dietary supplements, the strength of the association, level of intake, intake of other medications or supplements, actual circumstances of use, characteristics of the individual user). The committee recommended that the evidence be reviewed and that the level of concern be determined by taking into consideration not only the the strength of the evidence but also the tasks

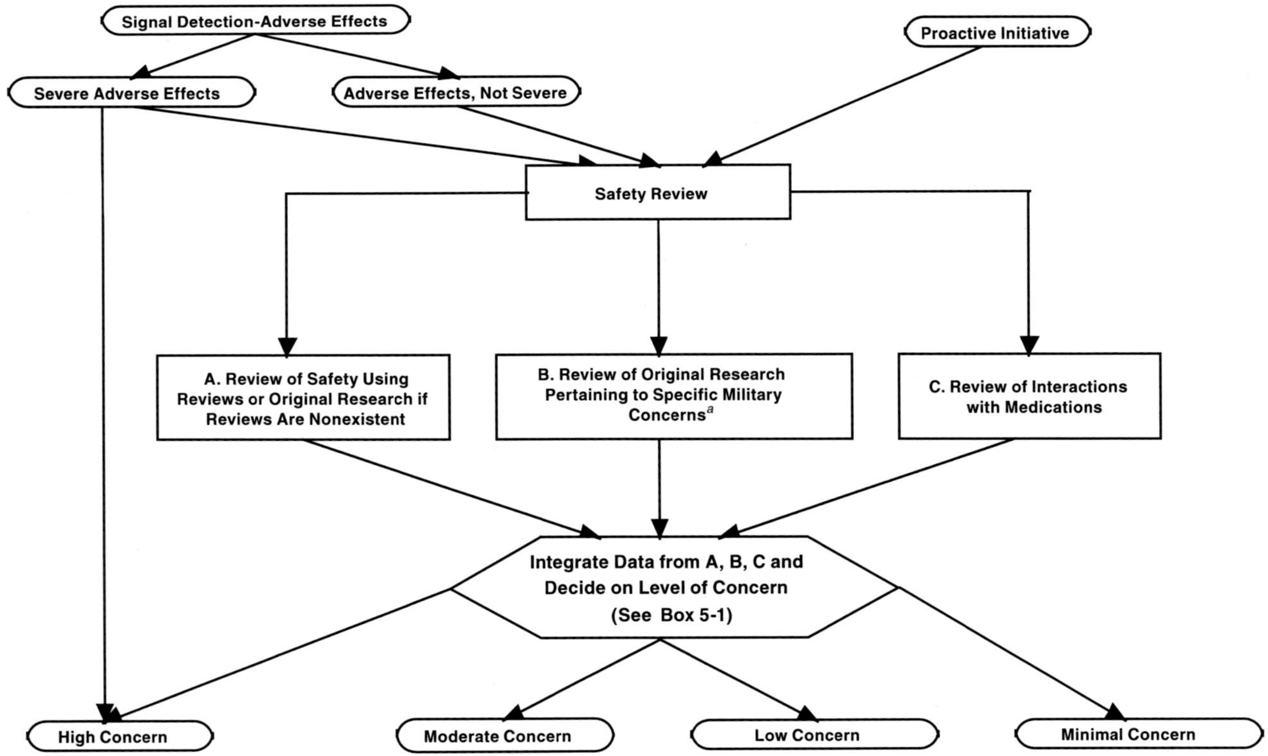

FIGURE 5-1 Framework to review the safety of dietary supplements.

[a]High physical activity, calorie restriction, hydration, gastrointestinal tract (diarrhea/nausea), liver health/function (xenobiotic clearance), cardiovascular health, mood/behavior altering, alertness/drowsiness, extreme heat/cold, injury/bleeding.

of the specific military subpopulation and the environment in which it will be conducting them (e.g., extreme temperatures or altitudes). As described further in Chapter 6, the designated oversight committee should review adverse events reported by the general population and by the military (as recorded in summaries submitted by the Medical Treatment Facilities' [MTF] Pharmacy and Therapeutics [P&T] Committees), as well as surveys of supplement use by military personnel, on an annual basis. As a result of these examinations, the designated oversight committee might recommend to the military leadership immediate action and/or conducting a review of published, science-based safety reviews by the review panel. The designated oversight committee may call a special meeting or conference call if adverse events are serious or frequent, as judged by the MTF P&T Committees.

Integrated Safety Evaluation

2005 IOM Framework: Integrated Safety Evaluation

The third step of the 2005 IOM report framework is a fully integrated safety evaluation (conducted by a panel of experts) of those dietary supplement ingredients that warrant further investigation based on the concern level raised by initial signal review. There are four components to an integrative evaluation (Figure B-25 in Appendix B): in-depth search and review of literature, drafting of a safety monograph, integrating this information into an analysis to complete the monograph, and review of the draft monograph by an expert advisory committee. In accordance with the FDA's designated function, the 2005 IOM report did not address any potential benefit of a dietary supplement.

Safety reviews of dietary supplements can be performed at various levels, depending on factors such as urgency and the availability of human and economic resources to conduct the review. The 2005 IOM report recommends that four categories of safety data be collected for evaluation following the detection of a signal: human data, animal data, data on related substances, and in vitro data. In conducting the safety review, the panel of experts would also consider possible interactions between a dietary supplement and medications or other xenobiotics. (Examples of monographs and evidence models are available online at http://www.iom.edu/CMS/3788/4605/19578.aspx.) A focused evaluation reviewing only one key ingredient or single area of concern such as cardiac health or renal health might also be appropriate. Both the comprehensive and the focused evaluation might include consultation with an expert committee, FDA personnel, or both, depending on the quality and clarity of the available data.

The integration of the available data using evidence-based principles is the final exercise in establishing a risk level for the dietary supplement, using a causal model diagram that integrates human, animal, in vitro, and even chemical information. Scientific principles for weighting and integrating data from these different categories were described in the 2005 IOM report (see also Jeffery, Box B-14, and Figures B-24 and B-25 in Appendix B).

As Modified for the Military: Integrated Safety Evaluation

Recommendation 5: The military should use the framework (Figure 5-1) to review the dietary supplements that raise safety concerns (per criteria above). The framework consists of the integrated evaluation of results from current, authoritative reviews (or, if no reviews are available, original research conducted over the previous 10 years) analyzing bioactivity and potential for drug interactions.

Efforts to review and summarize information to determine the concern level about a dietary supplement should consider not only individual ad-

BOX 5-2
Approach to Data Collection

The committee developed the following process to characterize the concern level (and efficacy) of a dietary supplement used by military personnel: (1) identify the dietary supplement that warrants review, (2) conduct literature searches, and (3) summarize conclusions about safety (and efficacy).

A proposed search process that is both cost-effective and valuable is summarized in Figure 5-2 as a stepwise decision-making tree. The committee believes that although an evidence-based review of original journal articles might provide a more comprehensive evaluation of safety, an evaluation from well-conducted, authoritative reviews could serve the purpose of alerting the military to potential problems (or benefits) and the need for active management.

In evaluating the safety of dietary supplements, data are needed on two basic attributes: bioactivity (negative or positive) of the ingredients and effects derived from synergistic or antagonistic interactions with other active substances (i.e., in foods, medications, or other active substances).

Bioactivity: Literature searches for systematic reviews of safety and efficacy of the dietary supplement of interest should be carried out in the appropriate databases (primarily PubMed, but also other databases [Napralert, Toxline, SciFinder, or other]). The focus should be on health concerns and unique environmental circumstances of military life. Some areas of particular interest to the military for safety (or efficacy) include specific conditions such as high level of physical activity; restriction of caloric intake; high altitude; extreme heat or cold; health issues such as dehydration, function of gastrointestinal tract, immune, cardiovascular, biliary, or renal systems; and neurobehavioral health. Medical Subject Headings

verse events reported but also integrate all other data pertinent to its safety. The scientific principles outlined for the FDA are expected to be used by the military to evaluate the data (see Box B-12 in Appendix B). For the integrated evaluation, the committee recommends an approach less expensive and time-consuming than the full evidence-based review described in the 2005 IOM report: an initial review of safety reviews authored by other reputable scientists (see Box 5-2). Evidence of the effect of interaction of dietary supplements with medications, focusing on medications frequently used by service members, should be taken into consideration. A military review panel should write a monograph for a dietary supplement that raises concerns (see models in Chapters 3 and 4). This review panel will be provided oversight by the U.S. Army Research Institute of Environmental Medicine, an Army medical research laboratory that investigates military nutrition issues. The review panel would include nutritionists, epidemiologists, toxicologists, clinicians, and pharmacognosists. Although contracting performance of the reviews out to a nonmilitary group might be feasible,

(MeSH) terms for the area of interest could help identify key search terms. Original research articles for safety (and efficacy) should be reviewed from the publication date of the last well-conducted review, or for the previous 10 years if no systematic reviews exist.

Interactions with food, medications, or other bioactive substances: Data on interaction with other bioactive compounds are scarce. For identifying interaction with medications, two online databases are particularly recommended: PubMed Plus and Clinical Pharmacology. If the dietary supplement of interest is not included, it may be necessary to search the complete listing of reviews for medication interactions. To enable this, a list should be created of the 100 medications most frequently prescribed for active duty personnel, including mechanism of action and indications for use. This listing should be updated by the military on a regular basis, but initially at least annually. Some of the potential warnings against the use of dietary supplements in combination with medications would be apparent from this list (e.g., the committee cautions against the use of melatonin in combination with other sedative substances). Because of the severe lack of data in the area of interactions, the committee suggests that hypothetical effects from interactions should be based on mechanistic rationale. Likewise, in the absence of clinical data, animal or in vitro data or chemical similarity to ingredients with known interactions can provide suggestive information about potential interactions. Conclusions from these latter approaches are uncertain though, as clinical research data have on occasion refuted initial speculations about synergistic effects. Once information is acquired on a potential interaction, further searches should be done specifically for possible interactive effects of the medication/dietary supplement combination, whether in review articles or original research and using the same databases as above.

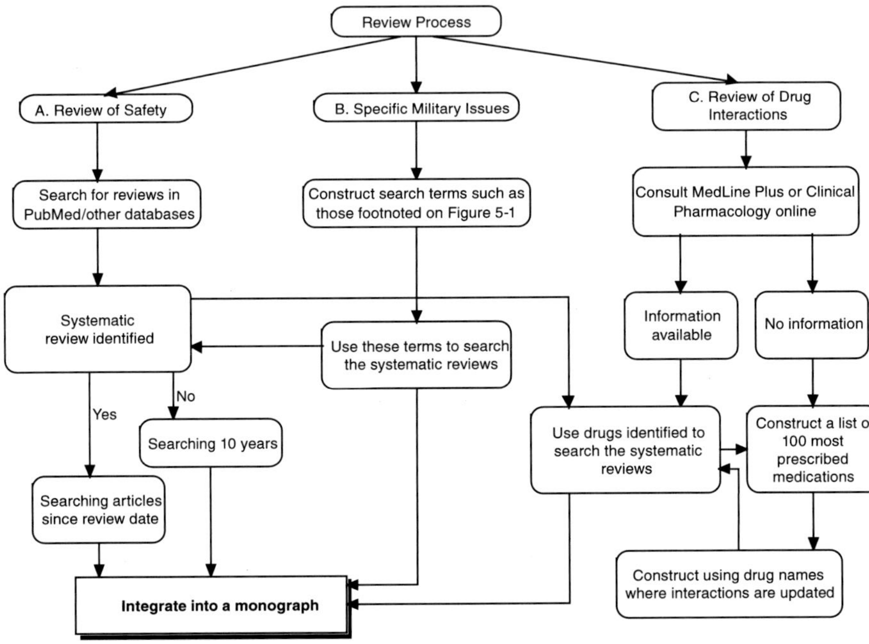

FIGURE 5-2 Stepwise algorithm depicting search strategy to review the safety of dietary supplements.

the safety and efficacy evaluation as it applies to military situations would be best conducted by a military review panel because they will be more cognizant of the demands and conditions unique to military operations and more experienced in identifying safety concerns relevant to military performance and survivability than a nonmilitary group.

In special cases, this activity could be followed by a more comprehensive safety review of original research, focused on performance and survivability as well as the particular health and environmental situations characteristic of military personnel. Some of these would be related to external situations (e.g., high-intensity physical activity, high altitude, temperature extremes) while some would reflect health concerns for individuals (e.g., injury or bleeding; dehydration; function of the gastrointestinal, immune, renal, hepatic, or cardiovascular system; altered behavior, alertness or drowsiness). This focused approach would not only shorten the length of time necessary for the review, but might also reduce the types of expertise required and ultimately result in information that is more useful. Original research from the time of the last review or, where current reviews are not available, original research conducted over the preceding 10 years, should also be surveyed. As a complement to database searches, a forum or coalition should be established to share data on adverse events and other information on dietary supplements (see Chapter 6).

Once the reviews of the individual dietary supplement are concluded, the review panel should declare its level of concern. The committee developed criteria on which to base the level of concern that use the same principles as the 2005 IOM framework but with a focus on survivability and performance issues (see Box 5-1). The concerns are classified from minimal to high, reflecting the level of performance degradation and survivability and taking into account the special circumstances (environment, hazards, stresses, and performance requirements) of concern to military personnel. If the data are insufficient to establish a level of concern, then the review panel could leave the review incomplete, awaiting further research on safety (and efficacy) or, depending upon the level of military concern, could request that the additional research be performed. It may or may not be appropriate for the military commander to recommend that the substance not be used by military personnel until the determination of concern level has been made.

The committee recognizes that owing to the potential for synergistic or antagonistic effects among ingredients, there are important challenges to applying this framework to products with multiple ingredients. However, because of safety concerns derived from these supplements and ingredient interactions, the committee's approach should also be applied to them. Two approaches to determining level of concern are offered below. In addition, the committee recommends focusing attention on signals from adverse event reporting and data on military usage of these products.

The committee did not provide a framework to evaluate efficacy; however, information on efficacy should also be collected and included in the monograph, since the potential for benefits of a dietary supplement will be factored into the final level of concern.

Decision to Take Action

2005 IOM Framework: A Safety Model for Decision Making

The 2005 IOM report recommends that the results of the safety evaluation should play a pivotal role in the FDA's determination of whether a supplement ingredient is unsafe. Furthermore, because an important component of DSHEA is public education about dietary supplements, it was anticipated that any monograph developed might be made publicly available on the FDA website.

Evidence that results in a high level of concern indicates the need for further investigation to determine whether a "significant or unreasonable risk of disease or injury" (the FDA basis for action) exists. Conversely, the 2005 IOM report suggested that when review of information (either at the initial review stage or as a result of an integrated safety evaluation) indicates a lower level of concern, the FDA should continue to monitor information about the dietary supplement ingredient. Monitoring could consist of passively receiving new signals of concern and/or maintaining routine searches of the scientific literature to gather data about specific existing or new concerns.

As Modified for the Military: Integrating Safety and Efficacy

Recommendation 6: The military's decisions on dietary supplement policy (e.g., rules, education, monitoring of use) should be based on conclusions about both safety and efficacy derived from the available published, authoritative scientific literature and considering conditions associated with a specific type of mission, location, and environment.

Although the development of a detailed process to establish a dietary supplement's level of efficacy was not within the scope of the current task and this committee was not constituted to address the question of efficacy, the committee concluded that considerations of safety and efficacy should be integrated to make decisions about policy on the use of dietary supplements in a military context. A more general description of benefit levels (Table 5-1) was developed by the committee to classify present and future

TABLE 5-1 Guide to Determine Level of Concern and Benefit to Formulate Decisions on Managing Dietary Supplement Use Among Military Personnel, Based on Science and Physiological Effects

Level of Concern or Benefit	Level of Science Documenting an Effect (Concern or Benefit)	Concern or Benefit Specific to Military Mission for Subpopulation of Interest
High	High level of science (large number of consistent high-quality studies)	High concern (or benefit)
Moderate	High level of science (large number of high-quality studies)	Moderate concern (or benefit)
	Moderate level of science	Moderate or high concern (or benefit)
Low/ Minimal/ Uncertain	Any level of science	Low, minimal, or no concern (or benefit)

dietary supplements by potential benefit. The determination of level of benefit is dependent on the number and quality of studies that demonstrate the benefit (or lack thereof) of interest to the military. It is advised that a road map to assess benefits be developed, similar to the framework for safety evaluation.

Because the determination of benefit and concern for a subpopulation is often specific to its mission, location, and environment, decisions on managing the use of dietary supplements should be made by the Office of the Assistant Secretary of Defense (Health Affairs) and by military commanders who will consider these factors along with the scientific evaluation recommended in this chapter. Considerations of the level of concern, potential benefit, and specific military population, tasks, and environments should be integrated in order to decide on appropriate action. The committee has developed the attached matrix (Table 5-2) as a guide to assist the military in making decisions on the use of dietary supplements. The potential actions suggested by the committee can be grouped into three different categories: policy, education, and monitoring. Any decisions for action should be made in consultation with the review panel of experts and the designated oversight committee, who will have a deep understanding of the scientific data.

The framework developed should help the military make decisions regarding the risks and benefits of dietary supplement use by carefully examining the science-based evidence, and should point to research gaps. Making decisions to recommend or restrict the use of a dietary supplement based on the limited data available is difficult. Also, recommendations to use a dietary supplement should be made carefully and only after clear evaluation of risks and benefits, since these recommendations will raise questions related to the personal choice of service members as well as financial and logistical implementation of the recommendation.

The committee recognizes the limitations on making decisions based on balancing risks and benefits; these limitations are related to the availability of data and the evaluation of risks and benefits. For example, for many products, lack of data on safety might preclude the military from determining the concern level. In these cases, the military might decide to support research and restrict the use of the supplement until a concern level can be determined. Furthermore, balancing considerations of benefits and concerns will present difficulties that derive from differences in strength of the evidence for safety and efficacy, lack of suitable indicators to compare the potential benefits and concerns, and the need to weigh the benefits and risks for different subpopulations. Other considerations will also need to enter into the decisions, such as the availability of other methods or supplements to achieve a similar beneficial effect without the risks.

TABLE 5-2 A Guide to Formulating Decisions on Managing Dietary Supplements for Military Personnel, Based on Safety Concerns and Modified by Potential for Benefit

		Suggested Actions Based on Level of Concern/Benefit[a]			
Benefit	Type of Action	High Concern	Moderate Concern	Low Concern	Minimal Concern
High	Policy	2	3	5	6
	Monitoring	7	7	7	7
	Education	8	8	8, 9	8, 9
Moderate	Policy	2	3	—	—
	Monitoring	7	—	—	—
	Education	8, 9	9	9	9
Low	Policy	1	4	—	—
	Monitoring	7	—	—	—
	Education	8, 9	9	9	9

[a]The determination of benefit and concern level for a military subpopulation is often specific to its task, environment, and location. Decisions on managing the use of dietary supplements should be made by the Office of the Secretary of Defense (Health Affairs) and military commanders who will consider these factors along with the scientific evaluation recommended in this chapter.

Policy:

1. DoD, service, and Surgeon General implement policy to prohibit use of product.
2. DoD, service, and Surgeon General specify parameters of use.
3. Unit & MTF commanders make decision on policy based on mission and subpopulation.
4. Posting of warning/educational labels (e.g., at military installation outlets and exercise facilities).
5. Commanders, health care personnel, and fitness center and unit trainers recommend that its use be considered for specific relevant personnel and circumstances.
6. Commanders, health care personnel, and fitness center and unit trainers recommend its use for specific relevant personnel and circumstances.

Monitoring:

7. Monitor for adverse events and frequency of use.

Education:

8. Educate commanders, health care personnel, and fitness center and unit trainers on risks and benefits of specific dietary supplements to enable them to make management decisions.
9. Educate all service members on risks and benefits of dietary supplements in general.

Policy This committee believes that whereas the conclusions about the level of concern and benefit (parallel to the "risk assessment" concept in a risk analysis model) should be determined by scientists (i.e., nutritionists, epidemiologists, and/or toxicologists), the decisions about implementing military policy (paralleling the "risk management" concept in a risk analysis model) should be pursued by commanders at the appropriate level in the military organizational structure. The specific actions taken in response to a dietary supplement review should be the prerogative of military commanders who are knowledgeable about the demands of a particular military subpopulation and its tasks. This model can be successful only when the scientists in the review panel and the designated oversight committee (see Chapter 6) consult and communicate with military leadership and decision makers.

Monitoring Surveillance (generally passive, but also active where there is a high level of concern or high level of potential benefits coupled with low concerns) is a potential management action to assess trends in supplement use, particularly the use of dietary supplements of high concern, multi-ingredient products, or products with high potential for benefit and low concern. Surveys can include questions about the use of any specific dietary supplement of high concern, particularly multi-ingredient products (see Chapter 2). An additional source of information on the use of dietary supplements is on-base (e.g., from AAFES/NEX and fitness centers) sales data. Such data could be gathered on an annual basis for all supplements; such collection is especially advisable for those of high concern level, those containing multiple ingredients, or those with high potential for benefit and low concerns. In addition to providing use trends, data from surveillance are vital to assess the strength of the adverse event signals and serve to complement data from adverse event reports (see Chapter 6).

Education Because members of the military obtain information about dietary supplements from many sources that often have no scientific authority, education based on objective analysis of the efficacy and safety data should be provided on which to make a decision to take supplements not restricted by military policy. Furthermore, educating the commanders, health care providers, and physical trainers about the safety and benefits of dietary supplements of interest or concern will permit these individuals to appropriately exercise leadership and provide guidance to military members. This educational component should be initiated as part of these leaders' formal training and should continue throughout their military careers (see also Chapter 6).

Communication between those responsible for the education of military service members and the designated oversight committee is critical. One way of providing information on dietary supplement safety and efficacy would be to develop a summary table showing both benefits and safety, together with an integrated concern level for the general military population and specific subpopulations (e.g., Table 5-3). Such a table could be used as a basis to develop educational materials for commanders, fitness or

TABLE 5-3 Summary of Risks and Putative Benefits for Selected Dietary Supplements Used by Military Personnel[a]

Dietary Supplements[b]	Potential Detrimental Effects to Military Performance[c]	Potential Detrimental Effects to Military Survivability[d]	Other Health Risks[e]
Performance enhancers			
Caffeine	Elevation of core body temperature by restriction of peripheral heat loss Elevation of circulating catechol-amines at high dosages	Moderate caffeine intake of 400 mg/d has not been associated with adverse effects in most people Mild to moderate locomotor agitation, tachycardia, diuresis, and anxiety. Sleep disturbance can occur if ingestion is within a few hours of sleep time	No data found[i]
Garlic	No data found	Méniere's disease, asthma, bleeding, gastrointestinal disorders	Epidural hematoma, increased international normalized ratio (INR)

Interactions with Medications[f] or Other Bioactive Substances	Withdrawal Effects	Putative Benefits[g]	Concern Level[h]
Sympathomimetic stimulant that may have synergy with other psychostimulants An increasing number of dietary supplements, performance-enhancing foods, and sports drinks contain caffeine, even if it is not listed on the label. This can further increase the amount of caffeine being ingested and add to detrimental effects, tolerance, and adverse events	Limited data indicating headache and caffeine craving	Substantial evidence that 100–600 mg caffeine can improve many aspects of cognitive and psychomotor performance during periods of sleep deprivation, and 200–600 mg can enhance physical endurance **High potential for benefit** (substantial evidence of beneficial effects for performance during sleep deprivation)	**Moderate**
Saquinavir: Clinically substantial reduction of AUC Ritonavir: No effect on AUC but increased incidence of gastrointestinal side effects Warfarin: Increased clotting time and INR, additive effect Chlorpropamide: Increased hypoglycemic effect Acetaminophen: Altered metabolism but not clinically substantial	No data found	No clinical studies for mental or physical performance Evidence of antimicrobial effects **Low potential for benefit** (substantial evidence of minimal beneficial effects)	**High** due to potential impact of chronic use on blood clotting

continued

TABLE 5-3 Continued

Dietary Supplements[b]	Potential Detrimental Effects to Military Performance[c]	Military Survivability[d]	Other Health Risks[e]
Ginkgo biloba	No data found	Transient headaches, gastrointestinal disturbances, sleep disturbances, bleeding with Warfarin and aspirin	No data found
Ginseng	No data found	Gastrointestinal effects	No data found
Tyrosine	No data found	No data found	No data found
Quercetin	No data found	No data found	No data found

Interactions with Medications[f] or Other Bioactive Substances	Withdrawal Effects	Putative Benefits[g]	Concern Level[h]
Warfarin, NSAID, alcohol: Theoretical interactions but studies do not support interactions Omeprazole: Reduced plasma concentrations of dietary supplement Thiazide diuretics: Reduced efficacy of diuretic	No data found	Little evidence of cognitive benefits in healthy, young individuals **Low potential for benefit** (substantial evidence of minimal beneficial effects)	**High** due to potential impact of chronic use on blood clotting
Warfarin: Three case reports reporting reduction in the INR Phenelzine: Induced mania Influenza vaccine: Increased the efficacy of vaccine when given in combination Alcohol: Reduced blood alcohol concentration	No data found	No benefits to physical performance in healthy, young individuals Some evidence of memory improvement and reduction in mental fatigue **Low potential for benefit** (substantial evidence of minimal beneficial effects)	**Low**
Theoretical with monoamine oxidase inhibitors	No data found	Evidence of improvement of cognitive function, mood states, and psychomotor functions especially under stressful situations **Moderate potential for benefit** (moderate level of science but high desirability)	**Minimal**
No data found	No data found	Some evidence of immune system improvement and antiviral properties **Moderate potential for benefit** (some level of science but high desirability)	**Minimal**

continued

TABLE 5-3 Continued

	Potential Detrimental Effects to		
Dietary Supplements[b]	Military Performance[c]	Military Survivability[d]	Other Health Risks[e]
Anabolic supplements (reported as "bodybuilding supplements" in surveys)			
Steroids			
Dehydroepiandrosterone (DHEA)	No data found		Neoplasia in rat studies, correlation to breast cancer in epidemiological studies, androgenizing effects in women
Nonsteroids			
Beta-hydroxy-beta-methylbutyrate	No data found	No data found	No data found

Interactions with Medications[f] or Other Bioactive Substances	Withdrawal Effects	Putative Benefits[g]	Concern Level[h]
Some drugs decrease DHEA blood levels (ACTH inhibitors and P450 inducers); caution when used concurrently with hormonal therapies	No data found	No effect on body composition, muscle, or cognitive function Some evidence for improvement in bone health and mood in older women **Low potential for benefit** (some evidence of minimal beneficial effects)	**High**
No data found	No data found	Some evidence of increase in lean tissue and muscle strength of untrained individuals **Moderate potential for benefit for untrained individuals or those in catabolic states such as negative energy balance** (moderate level of science but high desirability)	**Minimal**

continued

TABLE 5-3 Continued

	Potential Detrimental Effects to		
Dietary Supplements[b]	Military Performance[c]	Military Survivability[d]	Other Health Risks[e]
Creatine	Consider possibility of dehydration or renal effects	Case reports of renal failure No dehydration or gastrointestinal problems	No data found
Weight loss			
Ephedra (Ma huang)	No data found	Case reports of psychosis, vision impairment, muscle failure	Two- to fourfold increase in adverse effects: increased blood pressure, palpitations, heart rate. Case reports of cardiovascular adverse effects, stroke, psychosis, heart failure, seizure, vision impairment, transient ischemic attacks, muscle failure, and death
Chromium picolinate	No data found	Only isolated adverse effects reported (changes in cognitive behavior, allergic skin disorders, renal failure, and liver dysfunction)	Only isolated adverse effects reported

Interactions with Medications[f] or Other Bioactive Substances	Withdrawal Effects	Putative Benefits[g]	Concern Level[h]
Caffeine: Synergistic effect and opposing effects reported NSAID and some vitamins: Theoretical interactions	No data found	Substantial evidence of improvement in physical performance Substantial evidence of increase in muscle mass Some evidence of improvement in cognitive and psychomotor performance Potential for protection against traumatic brain injury **Moderate potential for benefit** (moderate evidence of benefits and high desirability)	**Low**
Interactions with other sympathomimetic drugs such as caffeine	Palpitations	Few studies show a small but substantial effect for weight loss Clinical studies show no evidence for performance enhancement **Moderate potential for benefit** (for weigh loss) (moderate level of science but high desirability)	**High**
Absorption reduced with phytates and medications that alter acidity of stomach	No data found	Some evidence of small effects on weight loss and body composition **Low potential for benefit** (substantial evidence of minimal beneficial effects)	**Low**

continued

TABLE 5-3 Continued

	Potential Detrimental Effects to		
Dietary Supplements[b]	Military Performance[c]	Military Survivability[d]	Other Health Risks[e]
Sleep aids			
Melatonin	Drowsiness/ sedation effects	Loss of core body heat Drowsiness/ sedation effects Gastrointestinal effects	No data found
Valerian	Drowsiness/ sedation effects	Drowsiness/ sedation effects Gastrointestinal effects	No data found
General health[j]			
Energy supplements[k]			
Sports bars	No data found	No data found	Could contribute to superfluous calories for inactive personnel

Interactions with Medications[f] or Other Bioactive Substances	Withdrawal Effects	Putative Benefits[g]	Concern Level[h]
Sedative hypnotics and anesthetics: Theoretical synergy	No data found	Some evidence of improvement of sleep Substantial evidence of circadian reentrainment under controlled conditions **Moderate potential for benefit** (evidence of circadian benefits and some sleep benefits)	**Moderate**
Sedative hypnotics and anesthetics: Theoretical synergy	No data found	Inconclusive evidence that valerian improves sleep **Low potential for benefit** (evidence of minimal beneficial effects)	**Moderate**
Unknown but unlikely, depending on individual ingredients	No data found	Evidence of improved exercise performance Supplement essential nutrients **High potential for benefit** (substantial evidence of benefits and high desirability)	**Minimal**

continued

TABLE 5-3 Continued

	Potential Detrimental Effects to		
Dietary Supplements[b]	Military Performance[c]	Military Survivability[d]	Other Health Risks[e]
Sports drinks	No data found	Hyponatremia (with excessive use)	Could contribute unnecessary calories for inactive personnel
Vitamins and Minerals			
Calcium	No data found	Minimal when below Tolerable Upper Intake Level (UL)	Minimal when below UL

Interactions with Medications[f] or Other Bioactive Substances	Withdrawal Effects	Putative Benefits[g]	Concern Level[h]
Unknown but unlikely, depending on individual ingredients	No data found	Evidence of improved exercise performance Some evidence of increased muscle protein synthesis, superior hydration, and reduction in muscle damage after strenuous exercise when drinks contain protein; requires further substantiation Plasma level better maintained during sweating when electrolytes are provided **High potential for benefit** (substantial evidence of benefits and high desirability)	**Minimal**
May reduce absorption and/ or efficacy of some medications	No data found	To reach adequate levels by supplementing the diet Sustain bone health and mood states; potential for further benefits with supplemental amounts **High potential for benefit** (substantial evidence of benefits and high desirability)	**Minimal** when below UL

continued

TABLE 5-3 Continued

	Potential Detrimental Effects to		
Dietary Supplements[b]	Military Performance[c]	Military Survivability[d]	Other Health Risks[e]
Iron	No data found	Minimal when below UL	Minimal when below UL
Selenium	No data found	Minimal when below UL	Minimal when below UL
Zinc	No data found	Minimal when below UL	Minimal when below UL
Multivitamins/ multiminerals	No data found	Minimal when below UL	Minimal when below UL

Interactions with Medications[f] or Other Bioactive Substances	Withdrawal Effects	Putative Benefits[g]	Concern Level[h]
	No data found	To reach adequate levels by supplementing the diet Sustain physical and cognitive performance **High potential for benefits** (substantial evidence of benefits and high desirability)	**Minimal** when below UL
	No data found	To reach adequate levels by supplementing the diet Maintain immune function; potential for further benefits with supplemental amounts **High potential for benefits** (substantial evidence of benefits and high desirability)	**Minimal** when below UL
	No data found	To reach adequate levels by supplementing the diet **High potential for benefit** (substantial evidence of benefits and high desirability)	**Minimal** when below UL
	No data found	To reach adequate levels by supplementing the diet **High potential for benefit** (substantial evidence of benefits and high desirability)	**Minimal** when below UL

continued

TABLE 5-3 Continued

	Potential Detrimental Effects to		
Dietary Supplements[b]	Military Performance[c]	Military Survivability[d]	Other Health Risks[e]
Vitamin C	No data found	Minimal when below UL	Minimal when below UL
Vitamin D	No data found	Minimal when below UL	Minimal when below UL
Vitamin E	No data found	Minimal when below UL	Minimal when below UL

[a]The monographs used to produce this table were developed in order to evaluate the review process outlined in Chapter 5. The monographs present scientific reviews of safety and efficacy, but do not attempt to provide a final assessment of safety or efficacy.

[b]Composition of dietary supplements varies widely; these are general categories and many include other ingredients or a combination of ingredients.

[c]Causing detriments to performance during military tasks (e.g., physical endurance, muscle strength, alertness, memory, stress, sleep patterns).

[d]Causing detriments to military survivability (e.g., bleeding or injury, dehydration, malfunction of gastrointestinal tract, stress, or altered behavior).

[e]Causing risks to health, excluding those in note 2 above.

[f]Refers to the 100 medications most prescribed for military personnel.

[g]Improvements of performance during military tasks (e.g., physical endurance, muscle strength, alertness, memory, stress relief, sleep patterns) based on level of desirability of the benefit to the military and level of science documenting a benefit (see details in Table 5-2).

[h]High, moderate, low, or minimal as described in Box 5-1 and modified based on putative benefits.

Interactions with Medications[f] or Other Bioactive Substances	Withdrawal Effects	Putative Benefits[g]	Concern Level[h]
	No data found	To reach adequate levels by supplementing the diet Maintain immune function **High potential for benefit** (substantial evidence of benefits and high desirability)	**Minimal** when below UL
	No data found	To reach adequate levels by supplementing the diet Maintain bone health **High potential for benefits** (substantial evidence of benefits and high desirability)	**Minimal** when below UL
Aspirin: Antithrombotic effects Warfarin	Unknown but unlikely	To reach adequate levels by supplementing the diet Maintain immune function **High potential for benefit** (substantial evidence of benefits and high desirability)	**Minimal** when below UL

[i]"No data found" means that there were no data found in the subject area showing an effect, either because the studies reviewed did not investigate this subject area or because, when investigated, there was no effect (i.e., health risk). Absence of evidence of risk, a frequent reality, does not necessarily indicate that there is no risk. Even if a study reported a lack of adverse effects, if the study is not adequately designed to identify risk (e.g., it is insufficiently powered, incompletely reported, does not include positive controls, or otherwise has inadequate mechanisms for detecting adverse events), its scientific validity is reduced or even null.

[j]Immune function enhancers, antioxidants, energy supplements, enhance recovery or performance.

[k]Refers to supplements containing macronutrients for energy or essential nutrients below the UL to meet physiological needs level, or electrolytes to replenish those lost during exercise. If energy supplements contain other ingredients (e.g., creatine), then an evaluation of each individual ingredient and interaction is warranted.

military unit trainers, and health care providers to inform service members. The committee cautions that such a summary table could be misinterpreted and therefore is not to be used as a sole source of information; it is meant to be used by those with sufficient scientific expertise as a tool to develop educational materials. Communication with service members should not establish a presumption that using dietary supplements is the norm or the expected behavior.

CHALLENGES OF THE PROPOSED FRAMEWORK FOR MILITARY PERSONNEL

The three types of challenges in evaluating the safety or efficacy of dietary supplements with the framework proposed by this committee are outlined in this section.

Insufficient Scientific Data

The practical value of the proposed framework depends on publicly available data. One critical challenge is acquisition of sufficient scientific data from literature searches to support an informed decision about the safety and efficacy of a dietary supplement within the military. Although there is an abundance of data for a few supplements, such as ephedra, the dearth of data for others hinders the determination of any definitive conclusion and further decision making. In Chapter 7, the committee provides its recommendations on the military undertaking research to address data gaps in areas of significant concern.

The committee emphasizes that absence of evidence of risk, a frequent reality, does not necessarily indicate that there is no risk. Even if a study reported a lack of adverse effects, if the study is not adequately designed to identify risk (e.g., it is insufficiently powered, incompletely reported, does not include positive controls, or otherwise has inadequate mechanisms for detecting adverse events), its scientific validity is reduced or even null.

Multi-Ingredient Dietary Supplements

Dietary supplements commonly contain multiple ingredients, and their compositions are frequently altered (e.g., they are reformulated with different proportions, amounts, and even ingredients) without any product name change. Finding data on the safety (or efficacy) of the myriad multi-ingredient products in the market is yet a bigger challenge than finding data on single-ingredient products. The committee concluded that these products merit special attention by frequent monitoring of their use, sales, and adverse event reports. The following are two potential approaches to determining the safety (or efficacy) of these products. Recognizing that both of these approaches (i.e., determining the safety of a total product or determining the safety of individual ingredients) have advantages and disadvantages, the application of either approach to evaluate the safety (and efficacy) of multi-ingredient products should be the prerogative of the military. Among other factors, the military should consider the strength of detected signals, prioritization of research gaps, and availability of resources. For either approach, there will be additional staff support required to maintain continuous surveillance of multi-ingredient products, including all the possible interactions.

Determining total product safety Given the virtual absence of data on multi-ingredient products, the military could decide to conduct research with study designs addressing military subpopulations and environments of interest, an approach that would be both expensive and time-consuming. In addition, the rapid turnover of products in the market may make it difficult or impractical to keep such research current.

Determining ingredient safety The level of concern (or efficacy) associated with the consumption of a multi-ingredient product could be determined by examination of each individual ingredient and of each potential interaction using the approach recommended in this chapter. The challenges in this case relate not only to the ingredients themselves but to the potential interactions among ingredients in the product. Furthermore, safety data on ingredient interactions are typically unavailable.

Presence of Contaminants

The linking of an adverse event to the use of a dietary supplement ingredient might be confounded if the product contains adulterants or contaminants. Attribution of the source of the adverse event becomes a formidable task. If enforced, the newly adopted cGMP rule should minimize the potential for inclusion of adulterants or contaminants. Because this rule will not be implemented until June 2008, its effectiveness remains to be evaluated.

OVERALL RECOMMENDATIONS

The committee recommends that the military use the proposed framework, modified from the 2005 IOM report framework, to determine whether a dietary supplement requires that military leadership take specific management actions to ensure optimal readiness and health protection of military personnel. This framework provides a methodology with a preestablished search strategy for generating a safety monograph for a dietary supplement, and a consistent format that provides key information which can be used to assist military policy makers. It also provides criteria to initiate safety reviews based on signals generated from an adverse event; or proactively, based on significant changes in dietary supplement consumption by military personnel. The following are overall recommendations related to the application of the framework:

- Determination of the level of concern for a dietary supplement should be based on published reviews of general safety concerns and on adverse effects and/or benefits specific to the military; the final integrated concern level should be predicated on safety concerns, modified by potential benefits, and based on special mission requirements and environments.
- The final, integrated concern level and the need for dietary supplement management should be determined in the context of specific subpopulations of the military and based on their special mission requirements, environments, and locations. This analysis should pay particular attention to military subgroups of interest for whom benefits and safety are of operational concern.
- Dietary supplement management should be predicated on safety concerns, modified by any proven benefits.
- A future task force or committee should more fully describe the process and framework to characterize the efficacy of dietary supplements of interest to the military and describe a detailed process to monitor the emergence of dietary supplements that could provide benefits to the military.
- To determine whether the level of concern for a dietary supplement should be reclassified as future research unfolds, research should be monitored on an annual basis, especially for those supplements for which a concern level could not be established due to lack of data. Based on recommendations of the designated oversight committee, the military might also decide to support or conduct research on a specific dietary supplement depending on its relevance to the military. For example, dietary supplements of military interest that are classified as being of high concern based on equivocal animal data could be referred to the research community to more fully characterize the level of concern in humans. It may or may not be appropriate for the military commander to recommend that the dietary supplement not be used by military personnel until that determination has been made.

REFERENCE

IOM (Institute of Medicine). 2005. *Dietary supplements: A framework for evaluating safety.* Washington, DC: The National Academies Press.

6

Monitoring Adverse Health Effects Associated with Dietary Supplement Use by Military Personnel

BACKGROUND

Making definitive declarations about the safety of drugs, foods, or dietary supplements is a challenging task, even with the most robust premarket studies. Among the multiple strategies (pre- and postmarketing) available, postmarket monitoring of adverse effects associated with these products becomes a very important tool to assess their safety. Often, a postmarket monitoring system serves as a complement to a risk or safety assessment to identify adverse effects that are not recognized in a laboratory or a small clinical study. In the case of food ingredients (i.e., additives and generally recognized as safe [GRAS] substances), the standard of safety is a "reasonable certainty of no harm" as indicated by either the food additive petition approval, GRAS notification, or GRAS self-affirmation process. For example, prior to marketing food additives, a petition that includes a safety assessment (i.e., available data on safety of the product) is sent to the U.S. Food and Drug Administration (FDA). Upon review of the petition, the FDA may issue a safety declaration. Once on the market, there is no established system to monitor adverse events from foods; however, if a new ingredient is introduced to a previously available food product, the FDA might informally ask the manufacturer to conduct postmarket monitoring of adverse events. Receipt of a sufficient number of complaints from consumers or consumer organizations might also prompt the FDA to investigate the safety of an ingredient.

In contrast, for drugs, a premarket risk-benefit analysis is conducted, followed by a postmarket safety evaluation that includes a passive, voluntary surveillance system. The premarket risk-benefit analysis is composed of three types of studies: animal toxicology and pharmacological studies, proof-of-principle studies for the disease or condition being addressed, and confirmatory studies of safety and efficacy (FDA, 2007). As a result of this required risk-benefit review, by the time a medication is on the market there are multiple well-conducted studies available that can later be used in support of an alleged association with an adverse event. Under the Federal Food, Drug, and Cosmetic Act, as amended by the Dietary Supplement Health and Education Act (DSHEA) of 1994, the law that regulates dietary supplement safety, the FDA does not have the authority to require a premarket safety assessment, yet bears the burden of proof to determine that a dietary supplement is unsafe before or after introduction in the marketplace. Because there are no premarket assessments required for dietary supplements, there is a paucity of laboratory safety studies; hence, postmarket monitoring of adverse events becomes even more significant for ensuring public health. DSHEA provided the FDA with the authority to develop monitoring systems and to take necessary actions when it has sufficient evidence that a product is unsafe (*Dietary Supplement Health and Education Act of 1994*, Public Law 103-417, 108 Stat 4325, 103rd Congress, October 25, 1994). The FDA has established a program called MedWatch to provide and elicit information on safety issues; reports from either health care professionals or consumers can be submitted voluntarily to the FDA or manufacturers via a standard form, form FDA 3500 (see Appendix E). The Dietary Supplement and Nonprescription Drug Consumer Protection Act made the reporting of life-threatening events to the FDA by manufacturers mandatory after December 2007 (the MedWatch 3500A form is used for this purpose) (*Dietary Supplement and Nonprescription Drug Consumer Protection Act*, Public Law 109-462, 109th Congress, December 22, 2006). Reports from both consumers and manufacturers are submitted through a passive monitoring system, that is, the FDA does not actively seek the adverse event reports. There are four steps to follow in such a system: (1) detect adverse events, (2) generate signals of public health concerns, (3) assess signals, and (4) take appropriate action.

As with medications and food ingredients, health risks from dietary supplement use are derived mainly from a consumer's individual susceptibility, or from the dietary supplement's inherent biological activity or interactions with medications. For the majority of dietary supplements, inherent toxicity might be expected to be less than that of medications because of the lower concentrations and potency per unit. Nevertheless, there are factors (i.e., the lack of composition standardization or a product compendium, multi-ingredient products, biased consumer attitudes, and a potential of overuse by some consumers) that increase the risks to health from the use of dietary supplements. Because dietary supplements are regulated as foods and many have a history of traditional use, there is a perception that they are safe and do not need a premarket approval process. However, it should be noted that products with a history of safe use may now be used in a different manner (e.g., with different solvents used for extraction, alternative plant parts used, longer duration of use) from traditional uses. Many consumers are also unaware that there is no requirement for federal approval of dietary supplements or advertisements promoting them, mistakenly assuming that dietary supplements must conform to the same regulations as drugs (Ashar et al., 2008). The differences in perception of risk between dietary supplements and drugs should be considered when attempting to model a surveillance system for dietary supplements.

There are many activities critical to the evaluation of risk-benefit profiles, such as adverse event surveillance, confirmatory laboratory safety studies, and data on use. Data from adverse event monitoring are complementary to data on use from dietary supplement surveys: survey data typically focus on the use of a specific dietary supplement within the population, whereas monitoring collects the numbers and types of adverse events resulting from its use. Both estimates are critical when making decisions about the safety of a product because their ratio (i.e., reporting proportion) may provide a rough estimate of the magnitude of a problem; in the case of dietary supplements, low reporting of adverse events and scarce information on dietary supplement use limit the utility of these data. Also, an association of use with an adverse event does not imply the demonstration of causality; rather, it intends to alert decision makers of potential concerns possibly requiring corrective actions. Determining causation requires rigorous clinical trials or research designs performed with animal models, not just analysis of adverse-event report data (IOM, 2005). Associations identified from adverse-event monitoring must be viewed as hypotheses regarding possible causal relationships between the substance and event, recognizing that there may be many possible reasons other than a direct causal relationship for the observed association (Almenoff et al., 2005).

Based on the heightened risks and the absence of an internal military process to report adverse events, this chapter discusses the need for the military to add dietary supplements to its current adverse-event monitoring system for medications so that this system responds to the unique risks and demands of military service. The chapter reviews the adverse-event monitoring efforts for the general population and for the military population, highlights challenges, and recommends improvements that build upon the current military system. Challenges might be categorized as related to the process of adverse event monitoring itself or related to the analysis of the data. Since those relating to data analysis (e.g., data mining statistical methods, identification of trends) are not unique to the military system, the committee discussed them briefly and refers to the published literature for further reading. The committee focused its deliberations on process-related challenges (e.g., low reporting rate; quality of data; use of integrated, electronic data). Taking the current system and policies as its foundation, this chapter makes recommendations for a collaborative approach in which appropriate institutions share data and lessons learned from their respective monitoring systems. The proposed approach will alert the military of potential concerns derived from using specific dietary supplements, particularly when performance might be compromised, and will serve as a signal to initiate appropriate actions by military leadership, as described in Chapter 5.

THE FDA'S PROCESS TO MONITOR ADVERSE EVENTS FROM DIETARY SUPPLEMENTS

To make recommendations about approaches to monitoring military personnel for adverse health events that might indicate a concern associated with consumption of dietary supplements, the committee reviewed the FDA's systems for both medications and dietary supplements. A more detailed description of the monitoring system for products regulated by the FDA is included in Appendix B (see sections by Dal Pan and Frankos and Mozersky). As mentioned above, to gauge the safety of dietary supplements, the FDA relies in part on evaluation of reports of adverse events possibly associated with their use. The FDA uses these evaluations to analyze trends and to detect a signal (i.e., a strong relationship between a dietary supplement and adverse events). However, a determination that a dietary supplement or dietary ingredient is unsafe would be based on a thorough assessment of not just reports of adverse events, but also of the scientific peer-reviewed literature on the safety of the dietary supplement or dietary ingredient.

Adverse events are most often reported via the submission of FDA's MedWatch 3500 form (see Appendix E), which is used to provide information from clinical trials, health care personnel, and consumer reports. To summarize the process, an individual (health care provider or consumer) communicates a description of the event and the patient to the FDA's Center for Drug Evaluation and Research, where the source of the event is categorized by origin (i.e., drug, dietary supplement, devices, biologics). The initial submission might be electronic or via telephone, standard mail, or fax; all reports are transcribed, regardless of the reporting mechanism. Reports are often submitted over the phone by a health care provider and received and transcribed verbatim by an FDA officer who typically does not probe for more information or details about the adverse event. By contrast, some manufacturers hire interviewers or facilitators trained to ask relevant questions of those submitting information on adverse events for entry in the

MedWatch form to be sent to the FDA. When potentially associated with a dietary supplement, reports are redirected to the FDA's Center for Food Safety and Applied Nutrition for evaluation.

For processing, MedWatch 3500 forms require only an identifiable reporter, a patient (anonymized), the suspect product, and a description of the adverse event. The information is reported regardless of the quality of the data, which is not validated. Apart from the patient's personal data and medical conditions, the form includes fields for entry of important information about the product (type, brand name, lot number, expiration date) and use (dose, frequency, date of initiation of use, consistent or inconsistent use, reason for use, last time of use before adverse event). Critical in identifying a signal is the section of the form referring to the event itself: event description, actions taken in response to event (e.g., sought medical attention), and documented diagnosis. FDA officials consider it advantageous to format this section as open-ended questions, offering the possibility of acquiring valuable information about the event circumstances (personal communication, Vasilios Frankos, Center for Food Safety and Applied Nutrition, May 30, 2007). The concomitant use of a drug and a dietary supplement or of a combination of dietary supplements might cause synergistic or antagonistic effects; the section in the form addressing the use of other medications and supplements is also therefore critical in evaluating the signal.

Once information is collected and distributed to the FDA's safety officers, analysis and signal detection follow. If an event is serious or uncommon, further steps are expeditiously taken: (1) a follow-up is requested, (2) other federal agencies are consulted, (3) a review of the literature is initiated, and (4) prior FDA reports on adverse events from similar products are consulted to identify trends. There is, however, no automatic signaling mechanism, and the weight of the evidence is considered case by case; the experience and consensus of safety officers usually dictate the decisions taken.

Until recently, these voluntary submissions and resultant MedWatch 3500 forms provided the only system to obtain information on postmarket adverse events associated with dietary supplements. To strengthen this system, the Dietary Supplement and Nonprescription Drug Consumer Protection Act mandates that after December 2007, serious adverse events[1] voluntarily reported to dietary supplement manufacturers by consumers and others must be submitted by the manufacturer to the FDA via the MedWatch 3500A form (see Appendix D). The form is slightly different from

[1]The 2007 Dietary Supplement and Nonprescription Drug Consumer Protection Act defines the term "serious adverse event" as an adverse event that (A) results in (i) death; (ii) a life-threatening experience; (iii) inpatient hospitalization; (iv) a persistent or significant disability or incapacity; (v) a congenital anomaly or birth defect; or (B) requires, based on reasonable medical judgment, a medical or surgical intervention to prevent a previously listed outcome described under subparagraph (A).

MedWatch 3500 in that it also solicits composition information from the product label as well as the manufacturer's contact information. Although this is a clear enhancement of the dietary supplement regulatory system and there is an expectation that the amount of data collected on adverse events will improve in both quality and quantity, the actual benefits from the act are still to be realized.

The potential misinterpretation of reports has resulted in some reluctance to make adverse event monitoring data available to others (see Kingston in Appendix B). Given the low reporting rate for dietary supplement-related adverse events, and the absence of a well-established system to monitor adverse events, it seems essential for organizations and manufacturers to collaborate to understand the limitations and uses of the current systems for reporting adverse events associated with dietary supplements. For example, the 2007 Institute of Medicine (IOM) report *The Future of Drug Safety* emphasized the importance of partnerships and the need for a concerted effort to make effective use of both public and private resources to address drug safety (IOM, 2007). Efforts to incorporate information from other sources, such as poison control centers (PCCs), have not, for various reasons, always been successful. The PCCs are private organizations whose purpose is to provide medical advice on how to treat an adverse outcome, not to assess the safety of substances. Calls received by PCCs include those prompted by nontoxic or unintended exposures to dietary supplements, medications, or other substances by children. Direct comparison of data from PCCs and MedWatch forms is not appropriate, since the same adverse-event data elements are not collected. The FDA therefore reviews PCC reports only when follow-up is necessary. The FDA has also been working with the University of California at San Francisco to monitor the PCC reports received by the San Francisco Center for Drugs and Dietary Supplements. Through this collaboration, it was determined that most adverse events in the PCC reports that were linked to dietary supplement use were associated with the use of stimulants (caffeine, ephedra-like products) and multi-ingredient dietary supplements, especially weight-loss products, and that these events were often associated with cardiac symptoms (personal communication, V. Frankos, Center for Food Safety and Applied Nutrition, FDA, May 30, 2007; Haller et al., in press).

Challenges in Adverse Event Data Collection Process and Analysis

Many experts and organizations have discussed challenges related to various aspects of monitoring adverse events from dietary supplements (see Kingston in Appendix B; LSRO, 2004; OIG, 2001; Woolf, 2006). For example, a 2001 report from the U.S. Department of Health and Human

Services (HHS) Office of the Inspector General (OIG) provides a detailed analysis of the effectiveness of the FDA's adverse event reporting system for dietary supplements in protecting the consumer (OIG, 2001). Although underreporting and suboptimal data quality are both attributes of a passive and voluntary system of surveillance, there are well-known advantages to a voluntary system, such as its nationwide character and the ability to distinguish at-risk groups and to generate safety signals.

This section highlights some of the challenges of the FDA's current system, many of which also apply to military reporting efforts (see below).

Data Collection Process

Low reporting rate When reported by the patient, adverse events are frequently described not directly to the FDA but to a health care provider. Receiving such information via the health care provider has obvious advantages in providing quality data, including the use of standardized medical terminology (e.g., symptoms, medications) and the opportunity to acquire additional information from the patient's medical records. Unfortunately, under the current voluntary system, the report rate is low—the OIG estimated in 2001 that less than 1 percent of all adverse events are reported to the FDA—for any of the following possible reasons. First, there is generally little consumer awareness of the importance of reporting adverse events from dietary supplements or even about the availability of a reporting system; if an individual is aware of the system, lack of familiarity with the form or lack of clarity in questions might deter submission. Second, patients are often reluctant to report the use of alternative treatments to their health care providers (IOM and NRC, 2005). Third, for some consumers, dietary supplements might be regarded as inherently safe since they are "natural," and consumers therefore fail to make a connection between use of a dietary supplement and the adverse effect, and do not report it (Ashar et al., 2008; IOM, 2005). Fourth, there is no clear common knowledge of what constitutes an adverse event (e.g., for some, only death or permanent disability would qualify, while others would include discomfort leading to absence from work, or admission to an emergency room for treatment of a symptom such as dehydration). Finally, recording the dietary history or asking about dietary supplement use is not a routine part of the medical history in either emergency room or follow-up ambulatory visits (except for ambulatory visits with some registered dietitians). While health care providers should, in theory, be sensitive to the importance of adverse event reporting, surveys have shown that even in the case of medications, physicians' beliefs and attitudes about the value of reporting adverse events contribute to low reporting rates (Figueiras et al., 1999). Other factors that might indirectly affect the report rate are the recency of introduction of the dietary supplement, media attention, and the level of educational or regulatory activity recently presented.

Quality of data collected The quality of information reported by phone or MedWatch 3500 form depends on the reporter's bias or beliefs as well as familiarity with medical reporting, signs, and symptoms. Forms filled by consumers often include incomplete or inaccurate information regarding an adverse event. For example, few consumers will be aware of how to code adverse events using standard codes for data entry (i.e., as found in the online Medical Dictionary for Regulatory Activities, which provides the coding of standard medical terminology [signs, symptoms, diagnosis, syndromes, laboratory and physiological data related to medical conditions] used by the FDA and others). To add to this difficulty, FDA safety officers do not typically probe for additional relevant information (e.g., brand name, dose, and other products or medications being taken concomitantly), nor is there much follow-up with the initial reporter to obtain more information (personal communication, V. Frankos, Center for Food Safety and Applied Nutrition, FDA, May 30, 2007).

The analysis of data from reports of adverse events related to dietary supplements is complicated by numerous unknowns about the product ingested, including the following: (1) potential product adulteration, (2) lack of identification of the part of the plant (e.g., root, seed) from which the botanical product is derived, (3) broad variation in plant nomenclature and geographical origin of plant, (4) unknown product composition due to lack of manufacturing and labeling requirements and continual product reformulation, and (5) patients' inability to accurately recall the types or number of dietary supplements being taken. The establishment of an association of an adverse event with a dietary supplement then becomes a significant challenge. An additional obstruction to data analysis is uncertainty of the duration of use or length of time between the exposure and the adverse effect.

The 2001 OIG report highlighted the difficulties presented by poor data quality. Adverse event report data were categorized as suboptimal, specifically providing limited medical information, limited information on products and manufacturers, limited information about the consumer, and limited ability to analyze trends. The report found that in 1999, the FDA recorded only 400 adverse events from dietary supplements via submission of MedWatch 3500 forms. Of those, medical records were unavailable in 58 percent of the cases, ingredients could not be determined in 32 percent, and there was no patient follow-up information available for 27 percent (OIG, 2001). The user guidance recently issued on how to fill in the MedWatch 3500 form may help those reporting adverse events to submit accurate, appropriate information.

Data Analysis: Generating Signals

Data mining is defined as the analysis of observational data sets to find unsuspected relationships and to summarize the data in novel ways that are both understandable and useful to the data user (Hand et al., 2001). Different forms of data mining can be used when the data sets are large, as in the case of adverse-event reports for medications.

The methods commonly used in pharmacovigilance to identify associations account for the variability typically found with small report counts. Quantitative evaluation can be derived from the relationships between the frequency of use of a substance and events reported, taking into consideration also all other substances' concomitant use and events (Almenoff et al., 2005). When evaluating these data, a typical challenge derives from a lack of data for the "denominator" (i.e., number of users for each dietary supplement) and low "numerator" data (i.e., number of adverse events reported for a particular dietary supplement). Data on dietary supplement sales and use (e.g., from commercial vendors or surveys) are valuable when estimating the percentage of the population that uses a dietary supplement. Signals detected by measuring disproportionality of drug-event combinations compared to known ratios from premarket efficacy trials are only statistical indicators of possible safety issues. Rare events (e.g., birth defects) are easiest to detect, but events that are commonly experienced by the population (e.g., diarrhea) are difficult to associate with the consumption of a specific dietary supplement or dietary supplement ingredient. The topic of data analysis and mining from adverse event reports is complex and has been extensively reviewed by others (Almenoff et al., 2005; Strom, 2005). Unfortunately, for the reasons described above, the quantity and quality of data reported from dietary supplement-related events is often less than desirable, resulting in weak signals for safety concerns. If higher reporting rates accompany the increase in use, awareness, and new legal requirements to report adverse events, then data mining tools might be more useful in the future.

In the case of medications, suggested signals derived from adverse event reports are complemented by other available information on the safety of the substance, such as adverse events described in clinical studies, case reports, or cohort studies (Strom, 2005). Because there is no premarket approval requirement to conduct a safety assessment for dietary supplements, manufacturers might not perform these studies, and safety data on health effects from products or interactions with other supplements or with other bioactive substances are mostly lacking. Still, both the published literature and studies sponsored by the National Center for Complementary and Alternative Medicine of the National Institutes of Health (NIH) can be used to support the attribution of adverse events to use of a particular dietary supplement. It is also encouraging that an increasing number of reports describe events from drug–dietary supplement interactions, although many are from case studies and not clinical trials.

With these serious limitations in the data quality and quantity and with reviews often conducted on a case-by-case basis, the extensive experience and appropriate expertise of the reviewers become critical when identifying signals.

THE MILITARY'S SYSTEM TO MONITOR ADVERSE EVENTS

The monitoring of adverse events related to dietary supplement use as a signal detection system within the military is integral to maintaining the health and optimal performance of military personnel. This monitoring system would be a key component of the framework recommended in Chapter 5 and would serve as a criterion to initiate reviews of research and provide important input to military commanders' policy decisions, as described in Chapter 5. It is especially important that such a system be operational at installations where military personnel face extraordinary physical and mental challenges. The military has a system to monitor adverse events from medications but does not currently have a separate and distinct system to monitor adverse events from dietary supplements. Many of the elements needed to implement such a system are already in place. The U.S. Army Medical Command has the official responsibility to make decisions regarding nutrition for all military services and would most likely address dietary supplement use and surveillance as part of that responsibility. This committee commends the military for their initiative in seeking methods to manage the safe use of dietary supplements by the troops; that is, conducting specific surveys of dietary supplement use as well as implementing educational programs and policies. The committee also acknowledges the value of past cooperation between the military and the FDA in evaluating adverse event reports from military installations at the time of high concern over ephedra use. This section describes and recommends improvements to the military adverse event monitoring system. It also describes ongoing educational efforts in the military.

Military Adverse Event Monitoring System for Medications

Each military service has established a system to collect and evaluate data on adverse events related to medication usage. Reports of adverse events are received and evaluated at the local medical treatment facility (MTF). In addition, summary reports are aggregrated and reviewed by the medical headquarters of each service as well as by the Office of the Assistant Secretary of Defense (Health Affairs). In some cases, data are also evaluated at the major command level within each service (e.g., Air Mobility Command, U.S. Army Special Operations Command, or Military Sealift Command).

All adverse events potentially associated with the use of medications by Army personnel are reported using MEDMARX,[2] a subscription-based, adverse drug reaction database. Briefly, health care personnel (physician, nurse, pharmacist, or other) at an MTF report an event to the MTF pharmacy; it would then be entered into a MEDMARX Adverse Drug Reaction (ADR) Data Entry Form (see Appendix E) by the patient safety manager or other designated person at the pharmacy. The ADR form allows MEDMARX subscribers to collect and analyze reports of adverse drug reactions. The ADR module collects information that describes the adverse reaction, the body system involved, the seriousness of the event, and the result of the reaction on level of patient care; the form also includes the Naranjo Probability Assessment Scale to determine the likelihood that use of a specific substance resulted in the adverse reaction. Adverse event reports might also be submitted via the Vaccine Adverse Event Reporting System (of the Centers for Disease Control and Prevention and the FDA) form or MedWatch 3500 form (Appendix E).

The Pharmacy and Therapeutics (P&T) Committee at each MTF—composed of physicians, nurses, pharmacists, and logisticians—is an advisory group on all matters relating to the acquisition and use of medications in an MTF. These include review of policies, review of medication errors, evaluation of clinical data on new drugs and preparations requested for use in the MTF, maintenance of the formulary of authorized medications for the installation, and review of drug adverse event reports. The P&T Committee also proposes policy decisions to the medical commander (see Hoerner in Appendix B), from medication selection to restricting availability or issuing warnings and framing educational activities. It would appear sensible for the P&T Committee in each MTF to oversee the dietary supplement functions related to adverse-event monitoring at the local level.

[2]A national, Internet-accessible database that hospitals and health care systems use to track and trend adverse drug reactions and medication errors. Hospitals and health care systems participate in MEDMARX voluntarily and subscribe to it on an annual basis. It facilitates productive and efficient documentation, reporting, analysis, tracking, trending, and prevention of adverse drug events. It allows subscribing facilities to learn valuable lessons from the experiences of other users. Subscribers can access data from a national database of more than 1.1 million adverse drug event records. The data within MEDMARX follow standardized definitions.

Military Policies on Reporting of Adverse Events and Use of Dietary Supplements

Regulations

A review of the military policies currently in place for dietary supplements revealed that they are limited. It has been the policy of the Army Surgeon General to follow the FDA's guidance and regulations concerning such products. For example, in 2005, when the FDA announced a crackdown on products containing androstenedione (commonly known as "andro"), its possession without a prescription became a Class II felony. Possession of the substance by a service member was therefore subject to action under the Uniform Code of Military Justice.

In its Nuclear Weapons Personnel Reliability Program Regulation (DoD, 1995), the Department of Defense (DoD) establishes requirements and procedures for the implementation of the program to ensure that only the most reliable people perform duties associated with nuclear weapons. Although there is mention of prohibition of the use of alcohol and certain drugs under this program for safety reasons, there is no mention of restricting the use of dietary supplements. Likewise, there is no reference to the use of dietary supplements or reporting of adverse events included in medical requirements for Army aviation personnel (DoA, 2007).

In 2000, the Army's Office of the Surgeon General implemented policy specific to dietary supplements with a memorandum directing health care providers to document in the patient's medical record adverse events believed to be associated with dietary supplements. Health care providers should also notify the local MTF P&T Committees of any such adverse event (DoA, 2000). The memorandum also directed health care providers to report adverse events to the FDA using the MedWatch 3500 form. In addition, per the 2007 Heat Injury Prevention Policy Memorandum from the Army's Office of the Surgeon General, all cases of heat exhaustion and heatstroke reported to the Army Medical Surveillance Activity through the Reportable Medical Events System should include any history of dietary supplement use within the previous 2 weeks (USARIEM, 2007). In contrast, while heat injuries are reportable events for all services, neither the Navy nor the Air Force requires dietary supplement use to be reported (personal communication, Asha Riegodedios, Navy Environment Health Center, October 26, 2007).

There are other entities whose personnel undertake tasks with high risks and demands (e.g., Coast Guard personnel or airline pilots), and their policies to restrict the accessibility and use of dietary supplements are presented here. Recognizing the potential risks associated with dietary supplements, the U.S. Coast Guard, a branch of the Department of Homeland Security, has recently implemented regulations to manage the use of dietary supplements. They include not only specifications of the kinds of dietary supplements that may be used by all active duty members and aviators (U.S. Coast Guard, 2003), but also provisions for the submission of all reports of patient adverse reactions associated with dietary supplement use (U.S. Coast Guard, 2007). According to Coast Guard regulations, clinics shall submit all pertinent patient adverse reactions or product quality problems to the Commandant and the Maintenance and Logistics Command, using the MedWatch 3500 form. Coast Guard pharmacies are not allowed to dispense any product not approved by the FDA (i.e., any herbal supplement or other dietary supplement), with the exception of vitamins having an established Recommended Dietary Allowance. The Federal Aviation Administration, responsible for the safety of civil aviation, does not have any regulations or policy guidance concerning the use of vitamins or dietary supplements per se, except for a restriction on the use of melatonin (i.e., its use is prohibited within 12 hours of flight duty). The Air Line Pilots Association advises pilots to avoid dietary supplements that are banned by the FDA or purchased overseas (personal communication, Bill Edmunds, Air Line Pilots Association, January 25, 2008).

Education

Efforts to educate service members on the safety of specific dietary supplements include brochures and websites (Evans U.S. Army Community Hospital, 2006; Hooah 4 Health, 2007; NEHC, 2004; USACHPPM, 2000, 2003). The Navy and Marine Corps Public Health Center website provides, as part of their ShipShape weight management program, information on dietary supplements and links to the NIH Office of Dietary Supplements (ODS) website (Navy and Marine Corps Public Health Center, 2007). The ODS website offers information on dietary supplements for both the general public and scientists. The Air Force provides online information through the Human Performance Training Team website on its Air Force Knowledge Now portal. The Army offers information on dietary supplements on the Army Knowledge Online portal as part of its Ultimate Warrior Hooah Bodies and Weigh to Stay sites.

However, there is currently no centralized educational program that is effectively and consistently applied across military services and that considers specific military needs. One promising educational tool currently under development is a joint, online community of health care providers and active duty military personnel (see Jaghab in Appendix B; USACHPPM, 2007). This interactive website provides information about general nutrition, weight maintenance, and behavior management, and could be used as a centralized educational system to provide information about dietary supplements.

The importance of educating health care providers about dietary supplements was indicated by results from a 2002 survey of Army Medical Department health care providers conducted by the DoD Nutrition Committee in partnership with the U.S. Army Center for Health Promotion and Preventive Medicine, in which health care providers asked to be provided with professional development regarding dietary supplements (Corum, 2004). The Aerospace Medicine program for physicians training to become flight surgeons includes specific information on dietary supplements and active ingredients of safety concern in their online preparation materials for the Aerospace Medicine Primary course. However, it does not mention how to report adverse events involving dietary supplements, nor does the curriculum include any additional formal training on dietary supplements during the residency phase (Air Force Medical Service, 2007).

Physical trainers in military fitness centers or assigned to organizational units are also key sources of information on nutrition and health. Moreover, the more casual environment and camaraderie experienced at fitness centers may encourage openness about sharing and requesting information about nutrition needs for optimal performance, health concerns, and even adverse events experienced.

Adverse Event Data Collection Process and Analysis: Challenges and Opportunities Unique to the Military

In addition to the complications highlighted above that are commonly encountered in monitoring adverse events within the general population, the military faces unique challenges related to the activities of service members and the locations, culture, and settings in which they operate. Challenges and opportunities discussed below relate to the collection of data and analysis by using the electronic health records system.

Data Collection Process

Low reporting rate in the military Factors contributing to a low reporting rate in the general civilian population are also encountered by the military: inconsistent definitions of the term *adverse event*, a voluntary monitoring system, poor communication with health care providers (e.g., reluctance to report dietary supplement use and adverse events as well as lack of discussions about dietary supplement use during medical visits), little consumer awareness of their potential harmful effects, belief that the federal government regulates dietary supplements in the same manner as medications, and a perception that dietary supplements are inherently safe.

Other factors also affect the reporting level in the military. For example, there is no separate system to report adverse events associated with dietary supplements. The extent to which military health care providers are following the few existing military policies on dietary supplement use is also not known. Despite policies and educational efforts mentioned in the section above, recent surveys of military personnel presented to this committee indicate that a low percentage of respondents (33 percent of men and 53 percent of women among those confirming use of dietary supplements during the previous 12 months) discuss the use of dietary supplements with their health care providers (see Marriott et al. in Appendix B). Likewise, a 2002 survey conducted by the DoD Nutrition Committee in partnership with the U.S. Army Center for Health Promotion and Preventive Medicine found that only about 60 percent of primary health care providers ask their patients about dietary supplement use (Corum, 2004). Data suggest that the military reporting rate may be lower than that in the civilian population, as shown in a survey about reporting smallpox vaccine adverse events, even when adjusting for differences in representation of age and gender of subjects (McMahon et al., 2007). McMahon et al. speculated that factors contributing to this finding could be related to differences in behavior (i.e., civilian population having a lower threshold for reporting adverse events), accessibility to forms, or differences in policy implementation.

Contributing to the problem of low reporting rate is the fact that those responsible for providing education about healthy and safe behaviors, such as military commanders or medical personnel, are themselves inadequately informed about the benefits and risks of consuming dietary supplements (Corum, 2004). Physical trainers at fitness centers and assigned to organizational units might also lack such information. As a result, service members are not educated about dietary supplements at the fitness center or the treatment facility. The lack of knowledge in both patient and health care provider (or physical trainer) about dietary supplements of specific interest to the military would contribute to the infrequency of reporting adverse events associated with dietary supplement use.

An already low rate of reporting within the U.S. civilian population might be further diminished within the military by the fact that commanders have access to service members' protected health information. For example, medical officers are allowed to share patients' medical information with the commanding officer without requiring specific consent, provided that service members are adequately warned that medical record information is not confidential (DoD, 2003). This practice may restrain the willingness of service members to talk freely with military health care providers about their dietary supplement use. Other factors that may contribute to a low reporting rate might be related to unique political and cultural characteristics of military service, including mobility of the troops.

Quality of data collected The causes for low data quality or gaps in data that were identified in the FDA monitoring system are also relevant to the military system: lack of familiarity with medical reporting procedures, absence of a formalized process to probe for additional information, and challenges in obtaining data on dose consumed and dietary supplement product ingredients as well as effects from simultaneous consumption of other dietary supplements or medications. In addition, adverse event data may be submitted through various methods (e.g., FDA MedWatch forms, MEDMARX form, or the Army Reportable Medical Events System); this lack of integration allows for both duplication and absence of event reports.

Electronic Health Record Limitations and Opportunities

The military has unique opportunities not only because health care for most service members is provided within a single DoD system, but also because the military is taking pioneering steps toward the development of an electronic health records system. Despite its potential to be a state-of-the-art system, the current electronic medical record-keeping system (Armed Forces Health Longitudinal Technology Application) does not include dietary supplements as part of the patient's medication profile. Their use can be missed if the health care provider is not trained to inquire about it. Only some dietary supplements (i.e., vitamins and minerals) are included in the medication formulary of an MTF; their use can then be entered into the patient's record, which allows for the possibility of establishing relationships between reported adverse events and the use of these dietary supplements.

The switch from a paper-based system to an electronic system of documenting health-related data is in progress and will result in a longitudinal, centralized health care records system that is accessible anywhere, from the battlefield to large hospitals. This system will serve as a central, integrated clinical data repository where each patient has a single record; it will allow for aggregate analysis of data, drug interaction alerts, and patient allergy notifications (Charles et al., 2004). Such a modern computerized system will improve the ability to detect and attribute adverse events. For instance, such a system might be used to create computer-generated signals as a tool for identifying (and possibly preventing) likely specific adverse events or high-risk interactions of dietary supplements with medications or other dietary supplements, as an additional strategy to detect adverse events (Gardner and Evans, 2004). For example, a physician entering a prescription medication might be alerted to the specific risks of product interaction if the patient is using a given dietary supplement. A number of vendors have developed programs that are capable of generating alerts for medication interactions, but for most dietary supplements, the knowledge base for a similar system is not yet available. Clearly, it would be advantageous, albeit time-consuming, for the military to establish place-, unit-, or mission-specific alert rules in a manner that results exclusively in alerts that are pertinent (i.e., false alerts are minimized). In summary, if a module including dietary supplements were developed and incorporated in the patient's medication profile, this improved electronic system would permit not only the analysis of an individual adverse event, but also the analysis of dietary supplement use and adverse event trends among users in military subpopulations. Strategies to automate alerting mechanisms to prompt evaluation and reporting of adverse effects might help compensate for the problem of low reporting rates.

PROPOSED ADVERSE EVENT SURVEILLANCE SYSTEM FOR DIETARY SUPPLEMENTS FOR THE MILITARY

The Dietary Supplement and Nonprescription Drug Consumer Protection Act of 2007 mandates that dietary supplement manufacturing companies report life-threatening events to the FDA. Non-life-threatening adverse events are to be recorded by the manufacturer, and records retained for 6 years in case the FDA needs to inspect the information. This act defines the term *adverse event* very broadly as any health-related event associated with the use of a dietary supplement that is adverse.

The term *adverse event* might identify a different effect in the context of the military. That is, the success of a military operation depends on each member's optimal performance, and thus effects that might not be perceived as a serious problem in the general population (e.g., dehydration) might constitute a significant problem in the military context, depending on the unit and task. It is therefore critical that specific adverse effects that might pose harm to military performance be reported so that leadership can take appropriate actions. With this in mind, the committee has chosen to use the FDA's definitions of adverse events and serious adverse events. For the military, the distinction between them is based on the extent of decrement to either the performance or the survivability of service members, taking into consideration their tasks (both physical and mental), the environmental surroundings (e.g., high altitude, extreme temperatures), and risks (e.g., bleeding, dehydration, infection, stress). A list of conditions to help categorize adverse events as of high, moderate, low, and minimal concern is shown in Box 5-1.

The committee's reviews of selected dietary supplements show that some supplements in popular use might present health and performance problems if misused, particularly for those subpopulations facing demanding tasks. For example, *Ginkgo biloba* and garlic have anticoagulant effects that in a combat situation might result in extended bleeding, jeopardizing health and mission success. Other supplements should not be taken while performing tasks that require alertness because of their potential for sedative effects (e.g., valerian or melatonin). The use of ephedrine-like substances is also of concern because of potential harmful cardiac effects. In addition, sales data provided to the committee indicate high use of some multi-ingredient dietary supplements; the effects of ingredient interactions are mostly unknown and present concerns. Based on the heightened risks, frequency of use among military service members, the lack of consistent policies, and the absence of a military process to report adverse events, a separate system for use by the military to monitor and evaluate adverse effects from dietary supplements is warranted. This section describes the committee's recommendations to establish such a system.

Ideally, a successful surveillance system will be economical, simple to use, and easily accessible, and yield data that are accurately representative of the population (Woolf, 2006). The data should be collected efficiently and in a consistent, unbiased manner. Vital to the effectiveness of the system is a database that allows for integrated and expeditious data analysis so that dissemination of findings to key public health officials and commanders is timely. It is also critical that encouragement to report adverse events be provided by broadening educational programs and outreach activities addressing various aspects of dietary supplement use, particularly the importance of reporting adverse events.

The lower cost of a voluntary system would make it more appropriate than an active system for use within the military population, provided that rates of response are substantially increased by educational programs and outreach activities. Active surveillance should be conducted occasionally as a tool to detect or investigate signals of concern from dietary supplements at installations whose military personnel face highly demanding tasks (e.g., Rangers or Special Forces). An active system entails a regular, periodic collection of case reports from health care providers or other personnel at those military installations. To support the data, questions about adverse effects should be included in surveys of dietary supplement use administered at these sentinel installations (see Chapter 2).

The committee also emphasizes that there is much to be gained from collaboration with other groups. The regulatory environment has not always been able to keep up with the market growth of dietary supplements. There is no single system in place for surveillance of adverse events associated with dietary supplements; nongovernmental organizations, government agencies, and manufacturers have implemented new systems or adapted systems that were already in operation for other products. Any military system of surveillance should complement its data with data from other governmental agencies and industry. Clearly, there are many limitations that would impede comparisons with databases maintained by other organizations (e.g., Consumer Product Safety Commission, the FDA, the American Association of Poison Control Centers), manufacturers, and trade associations (e.g., the American Chemistry Council, Consumer Specialty Products Association) (see description of their limitations in Kingston in Appendix B). While it is not feasible to directly integrate or equate data from these various sources, it is advisable to make in-depth comparisons, taking into consideration differences and limitations of data collection. A key committee recommendation is the formation of a partnership in which various parties with common interests work together in building knowledge by sharing collected data. Appendix B includes a description of postmarket surveillance efforts by both the private and public sectors. Also described is the surveillance system for products regulated by the U.S. Environmental Protection Agency, a system that engages the manufacturer as the primary point of contact for reporting adverse events. This industry role entails a significant training component or outsourcing of the surveillance system and design of a database and collection system.

The following section describes the committee's recommendations in three different areas: (1) the collection and analysis of adverse event surveillance data, (2) sharing of adverse event surveillance data, and (3) training and outreach. To increase the reporting rate of adverse events, various strategies have been recommended: (1) the education of commanders, service members, and military health care personnel; (2) dual mechanisms for reporting adverse events, that is, one directly from service members and one from health care personnel; (3) a centralized reporting system; and (4) the establishment of a forum or coalition with other groups to share data from the general population on adverse events.

Recommendations present actions to take and identify the military organization logically responsible for implementing them. The committee did not attempt to include all the military organizations that might be involved with educational, decision-making, research, or other activities, but rather provided a broad organizational picture of the responsibilities.

Recommendations for the Collection and Analysis of Adverse Event Data

The recommendations in this section are related to the following questions: What is the process by which the military should monitor adverse events resulting from the use of dietary supplements? How would commanders get information in a timely fashion? How can reporting rates and data quality be improved?

A critical analysis of the 2002 survey by the U.S. Army Center for Health Promotion and Preventive Medicine recommends various educational tools, but also urges that reports of adverse events associated with dietary supplements be reported through the Army Reportable Medical

Events System. Regardless of the form used to report adverse events (e.g., MEDMARX, MedWatch 3500 form, Army Reportable Medical Events System's ADR, or other), the analysis and decision-making activities would be realized more efficiently by using a centralized process in which data are reported through an integrated electronic health record system as described earlier in this chapter. The following are recommendations to expand the current system to include reporting of adverse events from dietary supplements. Since collaboration will be critical to the success of an adverse-event monitoring system, other organizations may also play a contributory role in collecting or sharing information.

> **Recommendation 7: The military should use a centralized monitoring system for reporting dietary supplement adverse events (and data on use), in which data are recorded through the integrated electronic health record system already being implemented in the military.**

Improvement of the Electronic Health Records System

The military should ensure that future electronic health records adequately capture dietary supplement use and adverse event data. (As the military continues to move toward a single electronic health record for each service member, provisions will be needed to ensure entry of data on dietary supplement use and adverse events when service members receive health care from providers not located in the MTFs.) Implementation of a centralized system will have to address difficulties such as the need for additional staff time and training efforts to collect, identify, and code dietary supplements being used. In particular, the electronic system should do the following:

- Prompt the health care provider to ask the patient about dietary supplement use, safety, and benefits and to submit adverse event reports. It would also be appropriate to add a standard assessment question(s) as part of the routine office check-in, including inquiry about the patient's reasons for taking any supplements reported used.
- Create standardized reports that can be aggregated for analysis (e.g., at the MTF, or based on common mission requirements, deployment status, and branch of service). Reports would include data on frequency of use and adverse events.
- Generate automated alerts in response to significant change in usage or reports of adverse events attributed to a dietary supplement of particular interest, which would help with adverse event attribution and identification of trends. This feature could be customized for use at various

levels (e.g., at the MTF, or based on common mission requirements, deployment status, or branch of service).

- Generate automated alerts for individual patients when there is a risk of dietary supplement interaction with a medication or other treatment.

Recommendation 8: The military should designate a committee or military entity to be responsible for the oversight and coordination of dietary supplement-related activities, such as overseeing the adverse-event surveillance system and parallel educational components.

Based on the heightened risks, the frequency of use among military service members, the lack of consistent policies, the suspected associations between adverse events in the field and the use of dietary supplements, the absence of a military system to report these adverse events, and the potential consequences of the unguided use of dietary supplements for an individual's health or mission success, a military entity or committee (hereafter referred to as the designated oversight committee) should be designated to oversee, coordinate, and provide guidance related to the use of dietary supplements by military personnel. The alternative, continuing without a designated group, would perpetuate the suboptimization of the existing resources and data and continue to put military members at risk owing to a lack of science-based guidance, education, and policy. The committee recognizes that establishing a new entity might not be feasible, and the tasks of an existing military committee or entity could be expanded to include responsibilities related to dietary supplements. In addition to a key role in designing an adverse event reporting system for dietary supplements, this oversight committee should have access to military and nonmilitary information and data, and provide advice on surveillance, educational programs, adverse event reporting, and research activities (see a description of these tasks below). The actual operational and data collection activities would rest with other existing military organizations, such as U.S. Army Research Institute of Environmental Medicine (research), the Center for Health Promotion and Preventive Medicine (educational materials), or DoD's Health Affairs Office (surveillance).

This designated oversight committee should include the expertise of nutritionists, dietitians, epidemiologists, toxicologists, pharmacists, experts on adverse event reporting, physiologists, health promotion staff, health educators, physicians and health care providers, and military leadership.

One possibility to consider would be to include oversight for these activities in the formal charter of the DoD Dietary Supplement and Other Self-Care Products Committee under the authority of the Office of the Assistant Secretary of Defense (Health Affairs) (see Box 6-1), which addresses nutrition issues including those relating to dietary supplements.

BOX 6-1
Dietary Supplement and Other Self-Care Products Committee

The Dietary Supplement and Other Self-Care Products Committee (DSOPC) has requested an official charter from DoD Health Affairs. According to their draft charter, the DSOPC shall use peer-reviewed and militarily relevant research, evidence-based data, and the consensus of subject-matter experts to develop recommendations that support DoD activities, policies, and instructions relating to dietary supplements and other self-care products used to enhance health and human performance. Specifically, the DSOPC should do the following:

- Establish Memorandums of Understanding with the FDA (1) to identify, in collaboration with the FDA, adverse events and their association, when possible, with particular dietary supplements and other self-care products used by the U.S. population; (2) to monitor and evaluate records of adverse outcomes for military beneficiaries.
- Recommend methodologies for assessing prevalence of use of dietary supplements and other performance-enhancing/self-care products across and within DoD active duty populations and their family members.
- Review trends on the use of dietary supplements and other performance-enhancing/self-care products.
- Assemble and document servicewide activities relating to dietary supplement use, education, and research.
- Review servicewide educational approaches for military health care providers (physicians, nurses, dietitians, etc.) and for the active duty population regarding the benefits and hazards of dietary supplement and other self-care product use.
- Provide recommendations for and prioritize an operationally relevant research agenda on dietary supplements for health and human performance as well as other self-care products.
- Develop evidence-based recommendations, in collaboration with other agencies, for servicewide policies that provide guidance on the use of dietary supplements and other self-care products for health and human performance for active duty personnel.
- Make recommendations to the Office of the Assistant Secretary of Defense for Health Affairs regarding appropriate resourcing and resource sharing for DSOPC initiatives among the services.
- Recommend methodology for development of a DoD system-wide communication process for reporting and dissemination of all adverse events, current research initiatives, educational programs, and implementation instructions relating to dietary supplements and other self-care products.
- Serve as a consultant on the role of dietary supplements and other self-care products in human performance and health and medical conditions for unified and specified commands upon request.

SOURCE: Personal communication, Patricia Deuster, Uniformed Services University of the Health Sciences, June 22, 2007.

This committee should review on an annual basis reported adverse events as well as surveys of supplement use by military personnel and, as indicated, recommend to the military leadership immediate action and/or conducting a review of published science-based safety reviews by the review panel. The following are specific responsibilities of the designated oversight committee.

Develop adverse event submissions systems The committee recommends the development of two reporting mechanisms, one for use by the health care provider and one for use directly by the service member. The health care provider would enter dietary supplement use information in the patient's record and submit appropriate adverse event forms to the MTF P&T Committee. In addition, service members should be able to report adverse events without having to arrange a medical appointment. Adverse event report data should be submitted through a toll-free telephone number or interactive website that allows for follow-up by medical personnel. These data should be provided to the MTF P&T Committee in a timely manner to be evaluated along with other adverse events reported from health care providers.

The designated oversight committee will clearly define the systems intended to submit the adverse event reports, including the forms to be used (e.g., MedWatch, MEDMARX ADR) by health care providers and directly by service members; the committee will also designate a system to categorize adverse events by level of severity.

Participate in forum or coalition The designated oversight committee should participate in a forum or coalition of military (i.e., the DoD and the corresponding support structures within each military service) and non-military groups for the exchange of data and information related to dietary supplements, including data on adverse event reports (see below).

Develop and implement reporting mechanisms For an adverse event reporting approach to be of value, it is critical to have an efficient system to provide timely information about adverse events to those who need it (e.g., MTF P&T Committees, commanders, fitness centers and unit trainers, health care providers). After adverse event report summaries are written (see below), the flow of information to share adverse event data and summaries by the various military groups should be defined (e.g., frequency of reporting and recipients of information). The designated oversight committee should establish a system of information flow that is effective (i.e., information is delivered to decision makers and educators) and timely (see Figure 6-1).

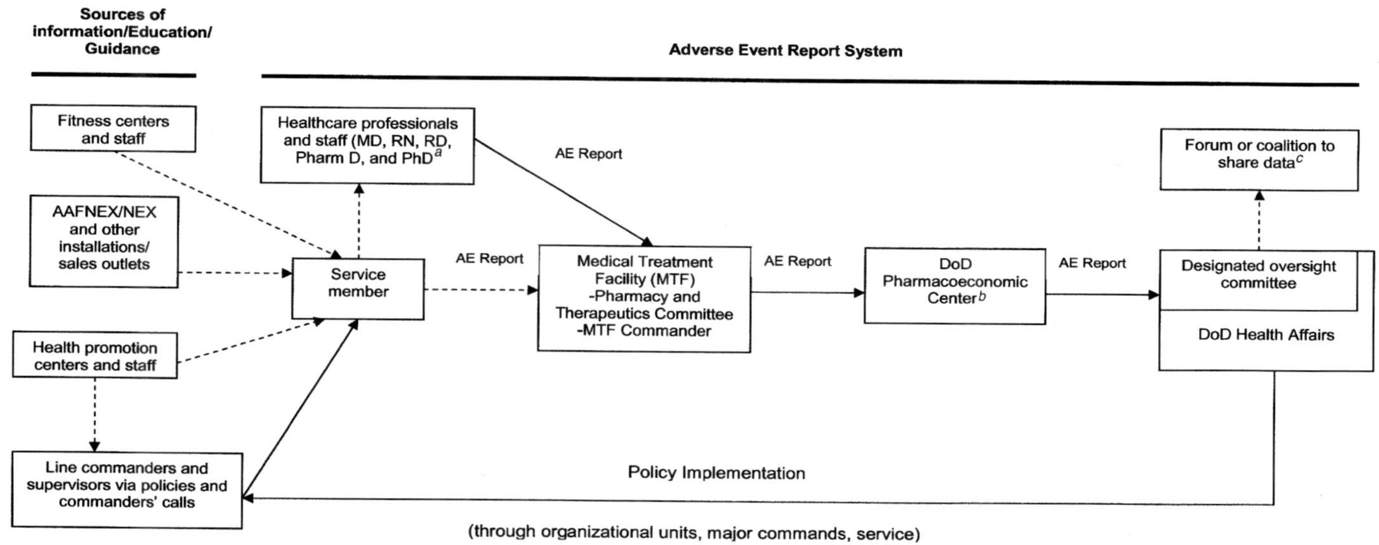

FIGURE 6-1 Proposed information flow for the recommended adverse-event monitoring system.
——▶ Formal Chain of Command.
- - - -▶ Input, coordination, and collaboration.

[a]MD (Doctor of Medicine); RN (Registered Nurse); RD (Registered Dietitian); PharmD. (Doctor of Pharmacy); PA (Physician Assistant).

[b]Representatives from each military service, pharmacists, epidemiologists, clinicians, nutritionists, pharmacoepidemiologists.

[c]Designated oversight committee members, registered dietitians from each military service, USARIEM, pharmacist from the DoD Pharmacoeconomic Center and services, medical representative from each service, FDA's Center for Food Safety and Applied Nutrition, Federal Trade Commission, NIH's Office of Dietary Supplements, AAFEX/NEX (Army and Air Force Exchange Service/Navy Exchange Service), and other sales outlets located on military installations; industry trade association; Health and Wellness and Health Promotion Centers from the services, fitness centers or units trainers from the services.

Collect relevant data The designated oversight committee should identify relevant databases and efforts related to surveillance of adverse events associated with the use of dietary supplements by military and nonmilitary groups. The following information should be collected:

- Data on adverse events—This task is related to the designated oversight committee's participation in a partnership with other military and nonmilitary groups (see below for a list of the type of data and information to be collected).
- Information on dietary supplement product ingredients to create a database in collaboration with the FDA, the NIH's Office of Dietary Supplements, the U.S. Department of Agriculture, and the U.S. Pharmacopeia—In the future, such a database would be useful to estimate dosage and ingredients consumed and, in turn, to analyze adverse event data.
- Data on dietary supplement use and associated benefits and risks, including those from interactions with medications, other dietary supplements, or foods—of particular interest are data on risks and benefits when subjects are in environments similar to those experienced by military personnel. These data should be obtained from the expert panel conducting reviews of dietary supplements under the oversight of USARIEM (see Chapter 5).

Recommend policy The designated oversight committee should provide guidance to the DoD on military policies and regulations on the safety (and efficacy) of dietary supplement usage, such as strategies, educational programs, and materials highlighting benefits and risks of dietary supplement use for military members, as well as for health care professionals (see below).

> **Recommendation 9: The responsibility of the local Medical Treatment Facilities' Pharmacy and Therapeutics Committees should be extended to reviewing and summarizing the adverse event reports as submitted by health care providers or service members, and preparing and providing summaries via a process recommended by the designated oversight committee.**

Extension of the responsibility of the MTF's P&T Committees The military should assign specific responsibility for the oversight and coordination of the monitoring system and parallel education components at the local level. Because the local MTF P&T Committees already review adverse reactions to drugs, the committee concludes that it would be feasible to expand their responsibilities to review adverse reactions to dietary supplements at the local level. Modifications of the pertinent regulations (e.g., AFI 44-102,

Medical Care Management, Paragraph 10.9) to include review and analysis of dietary supplement adverse events at the local level will ensure that local actions are initiated when appropriate. It may also be appropriate to identify the need for organizational units (e.g., Aerospace Medicine and U.S. Army Center for Health Promotion and Preventive Medicine) at the installation level to address dietary supplement usage and safety, as these organizational units have the responsibility to "optimize and enhance human performance" (e.g., AFI 40-101, *Health Promotion Program*; AFPD 48-1, *Aerospace Medical Program*; AFI 48-101, *Aerospace Medical Program*; AFI 40-104, *Nutrition Education*; AR 40-3, *Medical, Dental, and Veterinary Care*; and NAVMED P-117, *Manual of the Medical Department*).

Review of adverse events associated with dietary supplement use The committee supports the 2000 memorandum from the Army's Office of the Surgeon General (DoA, 2000) stating that adverse events believed to be associated with dietary supplements should be documented by health care providers in the patient's medical record. The committee also supports the local MTF P&T Committees' notification of any such adverse event by health care providers. The MTF P&T Committees should develop summaries of these adverse event reports highlighting dietary supplements of concern and associated adverse events, and particularly emphasizing those concerns related to military performance and environments of specific military groups (e.g., Special Forces, Rangers).

Enhance the expertise of adverse event reviewers Adverse event reviewers should include experts on epidemiology and adverse event surveillance, data mining and statistical techniques, nutrition, toxicology, diagnosis of diseases or conditions, physiology, and botany and pharmacognosy. Reviewers should be familiar with the demands and conditions unique to military operations and experienced in identifying serious or unexpected adverse effects, especially when relevant to military performance.

Submit reports on adverse events through the military system To ensure that data are available in a timely manner to military commanders and then released to the FDA as the military deems appropriate, summaries of the adverse event reports should be submitted by the MTF's P&T Committees through a designated system. The frequency and specific process to submit these summaries should be established by the designated oversight committee.

Recommendation to Share Adverse Event Data and Other Information Related to Dietary Supplements

Recommendation 10: The committee recommends that a coalition or forum be established for the exchange of data and information related to dietary supplements, such as data from surveillance of dietary supplement use and adverse events.

The committee found that only by establishing a joint forum or coalition will there be assurance that key data about reported adverse events would be shared by the FDA, military institutions, PCCs, and others. Although it is not appropriate to make direct comparisons of the data because of differences in data collection approaches, it is advisable to make in-depth examinations that take into consideration these differences and other data limitations. Members of this forum will also share other valuable information regarding new products in the market, increases in popularity of products, and latest research updates (see a list of suggested data and information to share below). With effective communication, there is much to be gained from such collaboration.

The members of this forum or coalition would update or add new data to a database established for this purpose. They could also meet periodically to present data and information updates. Members of the designated committee to oversee dietary supplement activities would participate in this coalition and have access to the database. Participants of the forum should include, among others, experts in toxicology and safety evaluation of natural products.

Representatives from the following groups could be invited to become part of this partnership:

- Designated oversight committee (recommended by this committee to come under the purview of the DoD)
- Registered dietitians from the U.S. Air Force, U.S. Army, and U.S. Navy (DoD Nutrition Committee)
- USARIEM
- Pharmacists from the DoD Pharmacoeconomic Center, U.S. Air Force, U.S. Army, and U.S. Navy
- Medical representatives from the U.S. Air Force, U.S. Army, and U.S. Navy
- FDA's Center for Food Safety and Applied Nutrition
- Federal Trade Commission (FTC)
- NIH Office of Dietary Supplements
- Army and Air Force Exchange Service/Navy Exchange Service (AAFES/NEX)

- Other sales outlets located on military installations
- Industry trade associations
- Health and Wellness and Health Promotion Centers from the U.S. Air Force, U.S. Army, and U.S. Navy
- Fitness centers or unit trainers from the U.S. Air Force, U.S. Army, and U.S. Navy
- Other representatives

To support the goal of the partnership, the collaboration might include sharing information and fostering discussion on the following topics:

- Sales outlet reports from AAFES/NEX, Defense Commissary Agency, and/or other sources at military installations to compare sales of dietary supplements from year to year and identify new products introduced to the market
- Reports from industry trade associations on changes in products and sales trends
- Summary of adverse events from specific military installations to identify regional differences, active surveillance data on adverse events at sentinel installations, and overall trends
- Summary of FDA adverse event reports as available, including relevant data from the PCCs; in addition, data on health claims of efficacy for dietary supplements would also be shared as appropriate
- Summary of FTC evaluation of dietary supplement products
- Summary of clinical trials registered by the NIH Center for Alternative Medicine evaluating dietary supplements
- Reports about dietary supplement use from in-depth surveys on sentinel installations—sentinel sites would be selected based on the mission of forces stationed at the installation (e.g., Rangers, Army Special Forces, Air Force Special Operations Command, B-1B long-range bomber crew, Navy Seals) as well as the capacity to conduct such a survey (i.e., provision of electronic health records, health care personnel to manage the additional data collection) (see Chapter 2)
- Reports from USARIEM on performance-enhancing supplements selected for review as well as a summary of research findings and protocols
- Summary of medication and dietary supplement education and materials (e.g., on safety, efficacy, interaction with medications) provided by pharmacy, health-promotion, dietetics, nursing, and medical staff to meet the requirements of the Joint Commission on the Accreditation of Healthcare Organizations (JCAHO, 2007)
- Review of efforts by each service to provide education on dietary

supplements to their personnel (e.g., usage of websites and attendance of meetings about dietary supplements)

- Results from DoD's Survey of Health Related Behaviors that summarize trends in use and the characteristics of dietary supplement users

Recommendations to Expand Education: Training and Outreach

Recommendation 11: Military service members and commanders should be educated to recognize both the potential adverse effects and benefits from using specific dietary supplements and the importance (and the process) of reporting an adverse event.

Recommendation 12: Health care personnel should be trained in evaluating dietary supplement use, informing and obtaining information from their patients, and appropriately reporting adverse events.

The committee recommends expansion of all educational programs and outreach activities to increase awareness about the use of dietary supplements. These educational elements are key to the support of an effective, centralized adverse event monitoring system. If the evaluation of these educational activities shows that they are ineffective at improving the quality or rate of adverse event reporting from dietary supplement use, the military could explore additional strategies. For instance, in addition to continuing educational efforts, the DoD could subcontract a dietary supplement information and safety hotline service for military personnel to communicate, anonymously, with a health care specialist. This hotline service would serve two purposes, education of the service member and data collection of adverse events.

The following are recommendations for educational activities:

Develop educational materials on dietary supplements and balanced nutrition, tailored to military members The proposed designated oversight committee should oversee the development of educational materials to be disseminated through a variety of methods (e.g., posters, websites, or point-of-sale brochures). Such educational materials on dietary supplements will describe potential benefits, mechanisms of action, and how to report adverse effects. These materials should focus on the military's special performance requirements and the need to protect each individual's body and health; messages should connect the need to protect health with the importance of reporting adverse events. These messages should also emphasize that while some symptoms (e.g., diarrhea) are not particularly problematic while in garrison, they may be of concern during deployment when mission readiness becomes critical. When available or displayed at point of sale, these materials will remind and encourage the service member to contact the user's primary physician or emergency room in the event that adverse effects are experienced, even if they do not require medical intervention.

Actively pursue outreach activities Service members and their commanders must be educated so that they recognize both the potential adverse effects and the benefits from the use of a given dietary supplement, and the importance of reporting any adverse events to health care providers. This may be achieved through the following approaches:

- Include information about dietary supplements in routine commanders' calls and communication regarding force protection/performance enhancement and health promotion, to reinforce the concept that some dietary supplements should be used with care and the importance for force protection of reporting adverse effects. Military commanders will be made aware of issues surrounding dietary supplement use as part of their formal education and routinely rely on their medical staff for input. There will also be direct communication with the designated oversight committee or via summary tables and monographs, produced by the review panel, or other educational materials that are provided both to medical staff and commanders.
- Consider modifying current contracts for sale of dietary supplements to include requirements to allow placement of outreach and educational materials about dietary supplements at point of sale on military installations (e.g., AAFES/NEX outlets and fitness centers).

Provide appropriate training and continuing education for health care personnel Health care personnel (e.g., emergency room staff, flight surgeons, medics, dietitians, pharmacists, and health promotion personnel) should improve their abilities to evaluate dietary supplement use, to inform military members, and to appropriately report adverse events. Education should be included in existing programs (e.g., Uniformed Services University of Health Sciences, internships and residencies, aerospace medicine training, independent duty medical technician training, and mandatory continuing education at medical staff meetings).

Education and training should emphasize the following objectives:

- Enhance health care personnel's awareness of and ability to pose relevant questions and provide information to patients about the use of dietary supplements. Identify and direct their patients to credible sources of information (e.g., NIH Office of Dietary Supplements).
- Provide guidelines on how to effectively report adverse events. Training should address the following topics: (1) identification of adverse

events of interest to the military (see Box 5-1), (2) the forms and process used to report adverse events, (3) effective collection of the data necessary to evaluate an adverse event (e.g., include listing of different names by which the dietary supplement is known; prompt patient on whether the product information was confirmed from product label or website, whether product was taken in accordance with instructions on the product label, and to identify any other medications, dietary supplements, or foods consumed; verify contact information for follow-up), and (4) actions likely to be considered based on adverse event monitoring reports.

REFERENCES

Air Force Medical Service. 2007. *AMP aerospace medicine primary course. Self-imposed stressors.* http://63.166.150.212/amp/Mod02/SCO10/asset1.htm (accessed November 8, 2007).

Almenoff, J., J. M. Tonning, A. L. Gould, A. Szarfman, M. Hauben, R. Ouellet-Hellstrom, R. Ball, K. Hornbuckle, L. Walsh, C. Yee, S. T. Sacks, N. Yuen, V. Patadia, M. Blum, M. Johnston, C. Gerrits, H. Seifert, and K. LaCroix. 2005. Perspectives on the use of data mining in pharmacovigilance. *Drug Saf* 28(11):981-1007.

Ashar, B. H., R. G. Miller, C. P. Pichard, R. Levine, and S. M. Wright. 2008. Patient's understanding of the regulation of dietary supplements. *J Community Health* 33(1):22-30.

Charles, M. J., B. J. Harmon, and P. S. Jordan. 2004. Improving patient safety with the military electronic health record. *Adv Patient Saf* 3:23-34.

Corum, S. J. C. 2004. Dietary supplement use in the military: Do Army health care providers know enough? *AMEDD* PB 8-04-1/2/3:36-38.

DoA (Department of the Army). 2000. *Memorandum: OTSG policy on medical screening for dietary supplement use.* http://chppm-www.apgea.army.mil/doem/pgm34/HIPP/PolicyScreeningDietarySupplementUse.pdf (accessed March 11, 2008).

DoA. 2007. *Army regulation 40–501: Standards of medical fitness.* http://www.apd.army.mil/pdffiles/r40_501.pdf (accessed October 25, 2007).

DoD (Department of Defense). 1995. *Nuclear Weapons Personnel Reliability Program (PRP).* http://www.fas.org/nuke/guide/usa/doctrine/dod/dodd-5210_42.htm (accessed September 6, 2007).

DoD. 2003. *DoD health information privacy regulation.* http://www.dtic.mil/whs/directives/corres/pdf/602518r.pdf (accessed October 25, 2007).

Evans U.S. Army Community Hospital. 2006. *Safety awareness bulletin for dietary supplements.* http://evans.amedd.army.mil/ncd/dietarysupplementalert.htm (accessed October 24, 2007).

FDA (U.S. Food and Drug Administration). 2007. *From test tube to patient: The FDA's drug review process: Ensuring drugs are safe and effective.* http://www.fda.gov/fdac/special/testtubetopatient/drugreview.html (accessed September 4, 2007).

Figueiras, A., F. Tato, J. Fontainas, and J. J. Gestal-Otero. 1999. Influence of physicians' attitudes on reporting adverse drug events: A case-control study. *Med Care* 37(8):809-814.

Gardner, R. M., and R. S. Evans. 2004. Using computer technology to detect, measure, and prevent adverse drug events. *J Am Med Inform Assoc* 11(6):535-536.

Haller, C. A., T. Kearney, S. Bent, R. Ko, N. L. Benowitz, and K. Olson. In Press. Dietary supplement adverse events: Report of a one-year poison control center surveillance project. *J Med Toxicol.*

Hand, D. J., H. Manilla, and P. Smyth. 2001. *Principles of data mining*. Cambridge, MA: MIT Press.

Hooah 4 Health. 2007. *Herbs for health*. http://www.hooah4health.com/body/nutrition/herbs.htm (accessed March 20, 2007).

IOM (Institute of Medicine). 2005. *Dietary supplements: A framework for evaluating safety*. Washington, DC: The National Academies Press.

IOM. 2007. *The future of drug safety: Promoting and protecting the health of the public*. Washington, DC: The National Academies Press.

JCAHO (Joint Commission on the Accreditation of Healthcare Organizations). 2007. *Comprehensive accreditation manual for hospitals: The official handbook*. Chicago: Joint Commission Resources.

LSRO (Life Sciences Research Office). 2004. *Recommendations for adverse event monitoring programs for dietary supplements*. Bethesda, MD: Life Science Research.

McMahon, A. W., C. Zinderman, R. Ball, G. Gupta, and M. M. Braun. 2007. Comparison of military and civilian reporting rates for smallpox vaccine adverse events. *Pharmacoepidemiol Drug Saf* 16(6):597-604.

Navy and Marine Corps Public Health Center. 2007. *Weight management (SHIPSHAPE)*. http://www-nehc.med.navy.mil/hp/shipshape/ShipShape_Nutrition/About_Nutrition.htm (accessed December 4, 2007).

NEHC (Navy Environmental Health Center). 2004. *NEHC nutri-facts dietary supplements*. http://www-nehc.med.navy.mil/downloads/hp/NutrFact_Dietary%20Supplements.pdf (accessed October 24, 2007).

OIG (Office of Inspector General). 2001. *Adverse event reporting for dietary supplements: An inadequate safety valve*. Department of Health and Human Services OEI-01-00-00180.

Strom, B. L. 2005. *Pharmacoepidemiology*, 4th ed. Chichester, England: John Wiley & Sons.

USACHPPM (U.S. Army Center for Health Promotion and Preventive Medicine). 2000. *Module 5: Dietary supplements: A basic guide*. http://chppm-www.apgea.army.mil/dhpw/Wellness/PPNC/PM_MOD5.pdf (accessed October 24, 2007).

USACHPPM. 2003. *The warfighter's guide to dietary supplements: What you really need to know*. http://chppm-www.apgea.army.mil/documents/TG/TECHGUID/TG295.pdf (accessed October 24, 2007).

USACHPPM. 2007. *U.S. Army Center for Health Promotion and Preventive Medicine*. http://chppm-www.apgea.army.mil/ (accessed October 29, 2007).

USARIEM (U.S. Army Research Institute of Environmental Medicine). 2007. *Memorandum: Heat injury prevention policy*. http://www.usariem.army.mil/DOWNLOAD/HeatInjuryPrevention2007.pdf (accessed October 25, 2007).

U.S. Coast Guard. 2003. *Coast Guard aviation medicine manual*. http://www.uscg.mil/directives/cim/6000-6999/CIM_6410_3.pdf (accessed November 6, 2007).

U.S. Coast Guard. 2007. Chapter 10: Pharmacy operations and drug control. In *Coast Guard medical manual*. http://www.uscg.mil/hq/cg1/cg112/docs/mm/ch2/mmch10.pdf (accessed November 6, 2007).

Woolf, A. D. 2006. Safety evaluation and adverse events monitoring by poison control centers: A framework for herbs and dietary supplements. *Clin Toxicol (Phila)* 44(5):617-622.

7

Research Needs

The committee was requested to select a limited number of dietary supplements to review and then determine whether further examination and integrative evaluation or research on each is warranted. There are numerous research questions about the safety and efficacy of the selected dietary supplements. A first step in developing a research agenda, however, is to set priorities to deliver answers to the questions most critical to the military with the most efficient use of resources. In a complex institution like the military, whose subpopulations within the various services might have different tasks, the coordination of efforts to prioritize research needs is key to the success of this endeavor. Consequently, the committee did not attempt to provide an exhaustive listing of research needs for any dietary supplement; instead, the committee presents an approach for the military to use to prioritize research needs. For example, research might focus on supplements with anticoagulant effects as a potential critical concern, regardless of the potential benefit for which they are marketed. Box 7-1 lists examples of research needs for the supplements reviewed in this report.

Future studies on dietary supplement use in the military should be approached from an etiological or mechanistic perspective, focusing on areas of particular concern or potential benefit for health, performance, and survivability (e.g., fitness level, hydration; gastrointestinal tract, hepatic, and cardiovascular function; and cognitive and neurobehavioral function). In agreement with the committee's recommendation that both risks and benefits be considered in management decisions about dietary supplements, studies that focus on answering questions about potential safety concerns and putative benefits may need to be prioritized separately according to the

BOX 7-1
Examples of Potential Research Questions on the Dietary Supplements Selected for Committee Evaluation

Of the supplements selected for review, the committee found no compelling reason for the military to make research on the following dietary supplements a high priority at this time: chromium, dehydroepiandrosterone, garlic, ephedra, ginseng, melatonin, valerian, and *Ginkgo biloba*. For the remaining dietary supplements reviewed by the committee, further investigation into the following specific questions may be warranted:

- What is the range of consumption of caffeine in the military population? What are the sources and amounts of total intake? To what extent are patterns of consumption approaching the limits for operationally effective doses of caffeine?
- What are the beneficial or adverse effects of long-term use of tyrosine? Of creatine?
- Are there tolerance or withdrawal effects from using creatine, caffeine, or other dietary supplements?
- Given that β-Hydroxy-β-methylbutyrate (HMB) appears to improve muscle function or mass in physically untrained subjects or those in a catabolic state, what are the effects of HMB in new recruits or those with hypocaloric intake?
- What are the effects of varying the protein content (amount and composition of amino acids) in sports bars or drinks and the timing of their consumption on recovery from strenuous activity (e.g., on reduction of immune suppression after exercise, hydration, or reduction of muscle soreness)?
- Are there any dietary supplements (e.g., quercetin) that help reduce post-stress health effects such as respiratory infections?

special needs of military subpopulations. The military has unusual access to its members' medical records, and its population is in better general health and includes fewer individuals at risk for certain diseases and drug interactions, all of which should facilitate the identification of potential concerns and possible benefits associated with the use of dietary supplements by service members.

KEY CONSIDERATIONS FOR CONDUCTING MILITARY NUTRITION RESEARCH

Study Designs

In conducting research of interest to the military, it is critical that the efficacy and safety of dietary supplements be tested with representative subjects engaged in training that is similar to combat and in specific military conditions (e.g., in situations of sleep deprivation, extreme environments, moderate physical activity of long duration). Study designs should continue to include human models that mimic some of the physical stresses and environments that accompany military missions and training programs. For example, a human model could consist of individuals exercising on a predefined, outdoor running and obstacle course or a specific physical activity in an environmentally controlled laboratory setting.

The selection of study subjects should take into consideration physiological differences (e.g., blood pressure, body mass index) that reflect demographic factors (i.e., gender, age, or ethnicities) of the military population that might result in differential effects of dietary supplements. Research populations should represent the current targeted population participating in garrison training, serving in combat, or both.

Animal Models

Although the military can conduct studies of the effects of dietary supplements on subjects undergoing the physical stresses of training or conditions simulating combat, using human models for the simulation of severe mental and emotional stress presents practical and ethical limitations. Likewise, some procedures (e.g., multiple liver biopsies) would be difficult to justify on humans. The military should therefore continue the development of animal model systems that mimic the stresses of garrison training and combat to allow screening for the physiological effects of dietary supplements under extreme conditions. Screening with well-designed and ethical animal studies could be followed with more focused and better-designed human studies. These models would not only provide preliminary information about the effects of dietary supplements but could also be applied to obtaining preliminary information about the effects of other interventions in preventing and treating diseases and injuries under conditions of garrison training and combat. To maximize and coordinate efforts in this area, collaboration with civilian researchers is of vital importance. The following paragraphs describe key elements of an animal model research program.

Animal–Human Transposition

This committee recommends that the military support and conduct experiments to understand animal–human transpositions. It is increasingly apparent that it is not possible to directly extrapolate data obtained in animal studies to humans (IOM, 2006; NRC, 2005, 2007). Not only are there differences in biological regulation between species, but the premises for most safety studies might also be inappropriate. For example, feeding test animals with multiples of expected exposure levels to increase the sensitivity of a test may yield inaccurate results as substances may act metabolically quite differently at low levels than they do at high levels. The development of animal models allowing animal–human transposition will require better understanding of fundamental biology. For example, better understanding of the molecular and genetic regulatory bases of physiological responses to extreme environments will permit more credible qualitative and quantitative comparisons of animal and human outcomes, and hence more precise predictions of adverse effects in humans.

Methods to Quantify Stress

There are many stressors experienced by deployed service members and the corresponding stress responses can be perceived in the short or long term. Stress frequently results from military situations that include thermoregulatory challenges, physical exertion, inadequate sleep and rest, and psychological stressors such as confronting unknown, high-risk situations and the threat of death. Because of the multidimensional nature of stress, its measurement will continue to be difficult. The military should support or conduct studies on improving the methods to quantify stress.

APPROACHES TO IDENTIFYING AND SELECTING RESEARCH NEEDS

Coordinating Efforts Among Military Services

To identify dietary supplement research topics of interest to the military, a clear coordinating process needs to be implemented between all services. Ideally, this process will include input from all the services and will evaluate the potential topics as well as the feasibility and implementation of the research methods.

The highest-priority research should be performed or sponsored by the military and should occur in conjunction with monitoring the results of research conducted in the civilian population for potential military implications. As with other aspects of dietary supplement management, recommending research to be conducted or sponsored by the military should be a task for the designated oversight committee (see Chapter 6). Specific criteria for priorities or concerns might be set by the individual services and submitted to the Dietary Supplement Oversight Committee.

Identification of Research Needs for Specific Dietary Supplements

This committee recommends that gaps in data or information be identified based on the following elements of the recommended approach to manage dietary supplement use: (1) the results of the surveillance system evaluating the use of dietary supplements within the military (Chapter 2);

(2) gaps identified in the reviews conducted for specific dietary supplements, especially those issues relevant to military performance and survivability (Chapter 5); and (3) the occurrence of adverse events of military importance associated with the use of specific dietary supplements (Chapter 6). As the committee evaluated dietary supplements (Chapters 3 and 4) using the framework, it identified examples of potential research questions for the selected dietary supplements (Box 7-1).

Safety

Following the framework illustrated in Figure 5-1, the military should develop a list of adverse effects of particular concern for service members (e.g., interference with blood clotting). One potential response for the military would be to generate requests for proposals for methods to evaluate safety in these areas or to identify any particular classes of compounds that could be expected to cause such safety concerns.

Benefit

There is a long history of use of botanicals (e.g., Chinese traditional medicines) with putative beneficial effects that could be the subject of research by the military. The committee recommends that the military narrow its research questions to those traditional botanicals that are believed to affect physical and mental functions; one approach to focus their searches might be consultation with expert ethnobotanists and pharmacognocists.

In addition, the military should consider conducting research to develop a framework approach to determine the efficacy of dietary supplements. Such an approach should consist of a mechanism to determine the level of benefit to service members under specific environmental conditions and for specific military tasks; it should include elements such as recommendations for appropriate research designs, for conducting literature reviews, and for identifying research gaps.

Concomitantly, the military could take a similar approach as that suggested for safety, that is, to make requests for proposals that address methods for evaluation of efficacy, any particular class of compound that might be expected to confer these benefits, or both.

POTENTIAL RESEARCH AREAS OF INTEREST

Research on Adverse Effects from Supplements Relevant to the Military

As mentioned above, the military should determine the adverse effects of dietary supplements in the context of specific military environments and tasks. Broad research areas that would shed light on the safety of dietary supplements are described below. As with benefits, for all areas of research described, it is necessary to determine the dosage and duration of use of the dietary supplement leading to adverse effects and to consider the impact of unique military environments on these effects.

Frequency and Severity of Adverse Events

Before prioritizing research on adverse effects or taking management action, it is important to determine the frequency and severity of adverse events of interest to the military; one way to acquire this information is the use of well-designed surveys (Chapter 2). Another approach recommended by the committee is the implementation of an adverse-event monitoring system for the military (Chapter 6).

Identification of Ingredients Associated with Adverse Events

The concomitant analytical evaluation of the identity and integrity of the supplement products associated with reported adverse events is a key element in managing the use of dietary supplements. One potential strategy to conduct these analyses would be to contract with appropriate research facilities that are equipped for and experienced in chemical analysis of natural products.

Interactions with Other Compounds

When designing surveys and studies and interpreting their results, researchers should be mindful of the large number of dietary supplements available, which are often consumed in combination and whose composition is often changed or is unknown. Intake of multiple supplements could lead to interactions having either synergistic or antagonistic effects. Likewise, dietary supplements could interact with other food components or medications. Speculation on the impact of the interactions is possible based on mechanisms of action or other factors, but there is minimal research in this area.

Tolerance and Withdrawal Effects

Research should assess the development of tolerance and/or withdrawal effects following chronic use of those dietary supplements frequently consumed by the military (e.g., caffeine, creatine, tyrosine).

Multi-Ingredient Dietary Supplement Products

Multi-ingredient dietary supplements, which are frequently reformulated and for which safety data are limited, will continue to be available and used by military service members. It is critical to identify concerns (or potential benefits) associated with these products. Use of the framework developed by the committee is recommended to identify concerns associated with the use of multi-ingredient dietary supplements; the same criteria for initiating a review (i.e., frequency of use and adverse event reporting) should be followed. A high prevalence (or significant increase) of use indicated by the surveillance system, adverse event reports suggesting a potential for concern, or a known hazardous component in a multi-ingredient dietary supplement constitute signals calling for review and possibly management action. If literature reviews fail to reveal any safety data, then the military should consider conducting safety evaluation studies of the product or significant ingredients and potential effects of ingredient interactions (see above). The development of methodologies to evaluate multi-ingredient products, including potential interactions, is an area of reasearch that should be supported by the military.

Research on Beneficial Effects from Supplements Relevant to the Military

When prioritizing research on potentially beneficial dietary supplements, the military might consider the general topics described below. For all topics, determining the dosage and length of exposure necessary to observe benefits and the impact of the military's tasks and extreme operational environments on those effects are crucial research questions. (The reader is referred to the World Health Organization monographs, a series of four volumes published by the Traditional Medicines Programme in Geneva, Switzerland; the German E monographs; or the United States Pharmacopeia monographs.) In all cases, these putative benefits of dietary supplements need to be proven scientifically and compared to those provided by alternative compounds (drugs) currently used as the standard of care.

Mitigation of the Adverse Effects of Stressors on Service Member Performance

One important category of research is determining which dietary supplements would be useful in alleviating physiological fatigue resulting from sleep deprivation, shift work, and transmeridian travel. An existing example of military interest in these types of supplements is the addition of caffeinated chewing gum to some military rations. Aside from research assessing the effects of caffeine on fatigue, few studies have been conducted to evaluate the actions of other naturally occuring stimulants, despite their worldwide use.

Another category of research that might be addressed is the use of dietary supplements to moderate physiological responses to extreme environments, such as hypoxia and altitude sickness. Indigenous peoples in the Himalayan and Andes Mountains tolerate high altitude and cold with a hardiness for which no genetic link has been scientifically proven (Wu and Kayser, 2006). These groups use various herbs and other nutrients to maintain their strength and prevent altitude sickness, and these may be of interest to the military.

Other stressors regularly encountered by military personnel that might be mitigated by dietary supplements are dehydration, radiation from explosive sources, physiological and psychological stress, and exhaustion.

Prevention or Treatment of Injuries

In addition to promoting recovery from the previously mentioned stressors, dietary supplements might also facilitate wound healing, a process frequently encountered in a military setting. Many plants have been used worldwide for wound healing and related concerns (e.g., sunburn relief). Some in vitro and in vivo data suggest the beneficial effects of these plants; however, there are few experimental studies on their value in human populations.

Surveys on Dietary Supplement Use

Analysis of surveys to determine the pattern and extent of dietary supplement use is a critical element of a dietary supplement research agenda. This need has been amply discussed in Chapter 2. Briefly, the committee recommends continuing the collection of usage data by expanding the Department of Defense Health Related Behaviors Survey; it also recommends that more comprehensive surveys be conducted at select military sites where service members are likely to face higher risks due to the intensity of their training or exposure to extreme environments. As described in Chapter 5, adequate surveillance systems will help alert the military to potential concerns.

Validation of the Recommended Approach to Manage Dietary Supplements

Validation of the approach laid out by this committee is strongly recommended, especially for these elements of the approach: the surveillance system; the adverse event report monitoring system; and the framework for safety, including the recommendation to integrate consideration of risks and benefits as the basis for taking action. The efficacy of this overall approach will best be determined by an annual status report and a five-year review of results from the surveillance, the adverse-event report monitoring system, and the effectiveness of command recommendations to allow or restrict the use of specific supplements. The designated oversight committee should decide on a timeline and specific criteria to validate this approach as well as to review the results.

Research on Education Methods

Research should be conducted to identify the effectiveness of various methods of communication and outreach to educate service members, commanders, health care personnel, and physical training and fitness centers staff on the use of dietary supplements. Information should be obtained on the awareness of use and knowledge about supplements among military personnel, commanders, and military physicians.

REFERENCES

IOM (Institute of Medicine). 2006. *Dietary reference intakes research synthesis: Workshop summary.* Washington, DC: The National Academies Press.

NRC (National Research Council). 2005. *Application of toxicogenomics to cross-species extrapolation: A report of a workshop.* Washington, DC: The National Academies Press.

NRC. 2007. *Toxicity testing in the 21st century: A vision and a strategy.* Washington, DC: The National Academies Press.

Wu, T., and B. Kayser. 2006. High altitude adaptation in Tibetans. *High Alt Med Biol* 7(3):193-208.

Appendix A

Workshop Agenda

Dietary Supplement Use by Military Personnel

Food and Nutrition Board, Institute of Medicine
The National Academies,
2101 Constitution Avenue, NW, Washington, DC
Lecture Room
February 12–13, 2007

February 12, 2007

1:00 **Welcome and Introductory Remarks**
M.R.C. Greenwood, Committee Chair

SESSION 1: INTRODUCTION

Moderator: John Erdman, Committee on Military Nutrition Research

1:15 **Perspectives on Committee's Task and Workshop Goals: Prospective Uses**
Andrew Young, U.S. Army Research Institute of Environmental Medicine

1:35 **Physiological Demands and Nutritional Needs of Military Personnel**
Scott Montain, U.S. Army Research Institute of Environmental Medicine

1:50 **Efficacy of Dietary Supplements: Physical and Cognitive Performance**
Harris Lieberman, U.S. Army Research Institute of Environmental Medicine

2:20 **Discussion**

3:00 **Break**

3:15 **Health Policy Development and Implementation for Military Personnel**
Lynn Pahland, Office of the Assistant Secretary of Defense (Health Affairs)

3:45 **Monitoring Dietary Supplements of Military Medical Facilities**
Paul Hoerner, Lt Col USAF, BSC, Department of Defense Patient Safety Center

4:15 **Design of Surveys on Dietary Supplement Use: Factors to Consider**
David Kaufman, Boston University

4:45 **Discussion**

5:30 **Adjourn**

February 13, 2007

SESSION 2: SURVEYS ON USE OF DIETARY SUPPLEMENTS

Moderator: Wayne Askew, Committee on Military Nutrition Research

8:00 **Dietary Supplement Use in the United States Adult Population: An Analysis of the National Databases**
Paula Gardiner, Harvard Medical School

8:30 **Insights into Dietary Supplement Usage by U.S. Active Military Personnel**
Steve French, National Marketing Institute

9:00 **Beyond the DFAC (Dinning Facilities Administration Center): What Supplements Soldiers Are Taking and Why**
Sonya Corum, Lt Col, U.S. Army Training and Doctrine Command

9:30 **2006 Air Force Dietary Supplement Use Survey Information About Usage**
Charity J. Thomasos, Lt Col MIL USAF, Eglin Hospital, Eglin Air Force Base, FL

10:00 **Break**

10:30 **Dietary Supplement Use in the Last 12 Months as Reported by Active Duty Military Personnel**
Bernadette Marriot, Abt Associates, Inc.

11:00 **Army Health Care Providers' Knowledge of Dietary Supplement Usage**
Danny Jaghab, Lt Col, U.S. Army Center for Health Promotion and Preventive Medicine

11:30 **Dietary Supplement Use in U.S. Army Personnel**
Harris Lieberman, U.S. Army Research Institute of Environmental Medicine

12:00 **Summary**
Cheryl Anderson, Johns Hopkins University

12:15 **Open Discussion**

12:45 **Lunch**

SESSION 3: FRAMEWORK FOR EVALUATING SAFETY

Moderator: Johanna Dwyer, Committee on Military Nutrition Research

1:45 **What Do We Know About Safety and Adverse Effects of Dietary Supplements Commonly Used for Physical Performance and for Weight Loss?**
Mary Hardy, University of California, Los Angeles

2:15 **Dietary Supplements: An IOM Framework for Evaluating Safety**
Elizabeth Jeffery, University of Illinois

2:45 **Approaches for Postmarketing Adverse Effect Surveillance of Drugs and Biologicals**
Gerald J. Dal Pan, Office of Surveillance and Epidemiology, FDA

3:15 **Break**

3:30 **Current Approaches for Postmarketing Adverse Effect Surveillance of Foods and Dietary Supplements**
Bill Frankos, Division of Dietary Supplements Program, FDA

4:00 **Corporate Approaches to Safety and Postmarketing Adverse Effect Surveillance of Dietary Supplements**
Rick Kingston, SafetyCall International

4:30 Summary
Sanford Miller, University of Maryland

4:45 Discussion

5:30 Adjourn

Appendix B

Workshop Papers

The contents of Appendix B are provided on the CD in the back of the book.

Appendix C

Findings from Recent Surveys on Dietary Supplement Use by Military Personnel and the General Population

TABLE C-1 Findings from Recent Surveys on Dietary Supplement Use by Military Personnel and the General Population[a]

Reference	Demographics	Group	Questions
MILITARY PERSONNEL			
Corum, 2007	2003–2005 Mean age: 25.4 years (n=5,206) Response rate not known	Soldiers (ranks: E1–E9)	Health Promotion and Prevention Initiative, dietary supplements questionnaire "Estimate how often you use each of the following individual vitamin and mineral supplements (pills, tablets, gel caps, etc). For each supplement listed below: Step 1: Select ONE bubble in the yellow section that best describes how frequently you use a supplement. Step 2: Select ONE or MORE check boxes in the blue section to select the reasons you use that supplement."

Findings: Usage	Other Findings	Authors' Conclusions and Study Limitations
Vitamins/minerals: Multivitamin: 33.8% Vitamin C: 24.4% Calcium: 19.3% Iron: 14.4% Potassium: 12.1% Vitamin A: 12.5% Vitamin B_6: 11.5% **Ergogenic aids:** Sports drinks: 42.8% Sports bars: 17.3% Protein: 13.7% Ephedra-free: 10.1% **Herbal supplements:** Caffeine: 17.5% Ginseng: 6.7% Garlic: 5% Ginkgo: 3.9% Echinacea: 3.6%	**Motivation** Vitamins/minerals: Health Prevent illness Ergogenic aids: Performance enhancement Strength Herbal supplements: Prevent fatigue **Sources of information:** (n=2,241) Friends: 36% Magazines: 31.7% Internet: 22.1% Sales associates: 10.4% Doctors: <10% TV/radio/newspaper: <5% **Supplement purchase:** (n=2,241) Commissary/PX: 35.6% Nutrition/health food store on post: 25.3% Nutrition/health food store off post: 25.3% Mail order/Internet: 13.2% **Adverse effects:** (n=951) Abdominal pain, breathing difficulty, chest pain, dehydration, diarrhea, dizziness, heart attack, heat stroke, loss of consciousness, muscle cramping, nausea/vomiting, numbness in extremities, palpitations, tremors	**Conclusions:** • 16% listed dehydration as an adverse effect (concern) • Women and men tend to use different dietary supplements (DS) • Many of the DS used were associated with palpitations or anxiety, which could be due to caffeine • Perception that if something is sold in the base, it means it is safe **Limitations:** • Surveys not designed to relate adverse effects or benefits to any particular DS • Response rate not known • Results might be skewed because it was completed voluntarily • They do not have dietary pattern surveys of respondents • Adverse effects are *not* usually reported to health care providers

continued

TABLE C-1 Continued

Reference	Demographics	Group	Questions
French, 2007	2005 Men and women 18 y and older (n=376) Response rate: 60%	Nationally representative group of U.S. adults "currently serving in the military, national guard, or reserve"	The Natural Marketing Institute ESP (E-screener panel) Questionnaire Index Supplement use in past 3 mo

Findings: Usage	Other Findings	Authors' Conclusions and Study Limitations
Supplement use: Any: 69% Multivitamin only: 23% Two or more supplements: 46% **Categories:** Protein powders: 14% Weight loss: 9% Herbal: 8% Sports nutrition: 8% Fiber: 4% Children's: 3% Homeopathic: 2% Condition specific: 2% **Specific:** Multivitamins: 57% Calcium: 13% Vitamin E: 9% Vitamin B: 8% Glucosamine/Chondroitin: 7% Creatine: 6% Fish oil: 5% Omega-3: 4% Flaxseed oil: 4% Amino acids: 4% Vitamin D: 3% Conjugated linoleic acid (CLA): 3% Lycopene: 2% Arginine: 1%	**Supplement purchase** (by age, military only): **18–29 years:** GNC: 28% Internet: 19% Nutrition/health food store: 8% Natural food market: 6% Mail order/catalog: 4% **30–44 years:** GNC: 19% Internet: 17% Natural food market: 12% Nutrition/health food store: 7% Mail order/catalog: 5% **45 years and older:** Internet: 23% GNC: 13% Nutrition/health food store: 13% Mail order/catalog: 10% Natural food market: 8%	**Conclusions:** • Supplement use increases with age (over age 45 y more likely), higher income, and higher education in military • Military more likely to use multivitamins only, significantly more sports-related supplement products • Study also gives information on overall use by gender • Study provides brand names of sports nutrition and muscle-building supplements used

continued

TABLE C-1 Continued

Reference	Demographics	Group	Questions
French, 2007	2005 Men and women 18 y and older Response rate: 60%	Nationally representative group of U.S. adults (nonmilitary)	The Natural Marketing Institute ESP (E-screener panel) Questionnaire Index Supplement use in past 3 mo

Findings: Usage	Other Findings	Authors' Conclusions and Study Limitations
Supplement use: Any: 73% Multivitamin (only): 18% 2 or more supplements: 55% **Categories:** Protein powders: 4% Weight loss: 7% Herbal: 12% Sports nutrition: 2% Fiber: 8% Children's: 3% Homeopathic: 4% Condition specific: 3% **Specific:** Multivitamins: 58% Calcium: 26% Vitamin E: 20% Vitamin B: 14% Glucosamine/chondroitin: 11% Creatine: 1% Fish oil: 9% Omega-3: 7% Flaxseed oil: 6% Amino acids: 2% Vitamin D: 8% CLA: 1% Lycopene: 2% Arginine: 1%		**Conclusions:** • See above for general comments (French, 2007) • Supplement use increases with age • Nonmilitary significantly higher in DS use for specific supplements *except* for creatine, CLA, amino acids

continued

TABLE C-1 Continued

Reference	Demographics	Group	Questions
GENERAL POPULATION			
Gardiner, 2007	2002 18–30 y (n=6,666) Response rate: 73.4%	National Health Interview Survey (NHIS) In-person interviews	NHIS "Have you ever used a multivitamin or vitamin?" "During the past 12 months, did you use natural herbs for your own health or treatment?"

Findings: Usage	Other Findings	Authors' Conclusions and Study Limitations
Supplement use Vitamin (ever): 63% Nonvitamin mineral: 17% **Of the 17%:** Echinacea: 47% Ginseng: 36% Gingko: 23% Garlic: 16% St. John's wort: 15% Peppermint: 15% Ginger: 11% Chamomile: 9% Kava: 9% Glucosamine: 4% Ephedra: 7% Prevalence of supplement use by physical activity level (any/nonvitamin): Sedentary: 34%/9% Moderate: 22%/19% High: 43%/23% Prescription medication users also taking nonvitamin/mineral supplement: 22%		**Conclusions:** • Nonvitamin and mineral supplement users were more likely to have high education, high physical activity, poor self-perceived health status; and be prescription medication users **Limitations:** • DS use is underrepresented because only those that responded positively to the question: "have you ever used a natural herb?" were further surveyed about use of specific DS; "natural herb" may be misleading • Only 35 herbs listed in survey; thousands are sold • Herbs have unique common names based on region or cultural background

continued

TABLE C-1 Continued

Reference	Demographics	Group	Questions
Gardiner, 2007	1999–2002 18–30 y (n=3,231) Response rates: 1999–2000: 82%, 2001–2002: 84%	National Health and Nutrition Examination Survey (NHANES) In-person interviews	NHANES "Have you used or taken any vitamins, minerals, or other dietary supplement in the past month?" If Yes, asked to provide dose, frequency, and duration of use and to show supplement container. If container was not available, asked for exact name.

Findings: Usage	Other Findings	Authors' Conclusions and Study Limitations
Supplement use: Any DS: 37% Nonvitamin/mineral: 7% **Of the 37%:** Multivitamin (any): 23% Vitamin C: 7% Vitamin E: 2% Vitamin B: 1.4% Iron: 2.1% Calcium: 2.6% **Of the 7%:** Sport: 2% Weight loss: 3% Herbs: 4% Prevalence of DS use by physical activity level (any DS/nonvitamin): Sedentary: 30%/5% Moderate: 38%/5% High: 41%/9% Prevalence of DS use among prescription medication users (any DS/nonvitamin): 45%/7%		**Conclusion:** Supplement users more likely to be ages 23–30 y female, non-Hispanic white, have high self-perceived health status, and have high physical activity level **Limitations:** • DS use likely underrepresented because survey does not include teas, loose herbs, etc., or DS without a bottle or label • Did not record reason for use or health condition associated with use • Did not ask about sports drinks, teas, or fortified foods

continued

TABLE C-1 Continued

Reference	Demographics	Group	Questions
Jaghab, 2007	(n=1,200) **Participation rate:** 15%	Army physicians (n=573) Ancillary (n=614) Located in: Iraq >40% Afghanistan >20% Other >9%	Electronic survey on Army Medical Department (AMEDD) Knowledge Management website

<table>
<tr><th>Findings: Usage</th><th>Other Findings</th><th>Authors' Conclusions and Study Limitations</th></tr>
<tr><td>Top 10 supplements reported to physicians/ ancillary:
Creatine: 32.5%/27%
Protein: 16.2%/26.2%
Multivitamin and minerals: 13.4%/20.2%
None: 11.9%/10.4%
Weight loss: 10.5%/19.1%
Metabolism boosters: 8.6%/8.8%
Ephedra: 7.7%/5.2%
Bodybuilders: 6.6%/7.7%
Glucosamine and chondroitin: 3.5%/3.7%
Nitrous oxide: 2.8%/5.7%
Caffeine: 2.8% (to physicians)
Herbal preparations: 3.7% (to ancillary)</td><td>Top 5 reasons took supplements reported to physicians/ancillary:
Performance enhancer: 52.5%/48.5%
Gain weight: 24.3%/22.1%
Lose weight: 23.9%/27%
Increase muscle mass/ conditioning/strength: 6.1%/6.5%
Cognitive enhancer/stay awake: 3.7% (to physicians only)
Supplement diet/health maintenance: 3.6% (to ancillary only)

Supplement purchase:
PX: 52%/59.3%
Online: 35.4%/39.9%
GNC: 22%/15%
Given or sent: 13.1%/14.2%
Unknown: 11.7%/4.9%
Local markets: 2.8%/1.8%</td><td>Educational suggestions:
• Which supplements work and don't work
• Better nutrition in general
• General risks of taking supplements
• Weight-loss supplement education

Study also provides top 5 brands of supplements used

Concerns about side effects (from physicians and ancillary):
• Interaction of supplements with medications or other supplements
• Dehydration
• Side effects (general)
• Renal/kidney functions
• Heat injury/heat stress
• Supplements are not regulated by the FDA
• Safety of taking supplements
• Cardiac issues
• Overuse of supplements
• DS users don't understand the risks and complications of the supplements
• Long-term effects</td></tr>
</table>

continued

TABLE C-1 Continued

Reference	Demographics	Group	Questions
Kaufman, 2007	2005 Men and women, all ages Adults (n=2,684) Children (<18 y) (n=581) (if under 14 y, parents answer) **Participation rate:** 57%	National survey Telephone interviews, random digit dialing	Slone survey "We are interested in all medicines which you have taken in the past 7 days. These include prescriptions from your doctor or clinic, nonprescription medicines, vitamins, herbs, or alternative medicines." Asked to retrieve bottle and provide information on container.

Findings: Usage	Other Findings	Authors' Conclusions and Study Limitations
Supplement use (most commonly used): Vitamins (any): 40% Multivitamins: 26% Herbal/natural (any): 23% Lutein: 9.4% Lycopene: 7.8% Glucosamine: 4.0% Garlic: 2.6% Chondroitin: 2.5% *Ginkgo biloba*: 1.6% Co-enzyme Q: 1.5% **Other:** Prescription medication users who take one or more herbals: 30%		Slone data used as an example of survey design age group not the same as military

continued

TABLE C-1 Continued

Reference	Demographics	Group	Questions
Lieberman et al., 2007	(ongoing) Men and women (n=484) Average age: 29 y Response rate: 80%	General Army	

Findings: Usage	Other Findings	Authors' Conclusions and Study Limitations
Supplement use at least once per week: Males: 55% Females: 70% **Top 10 supplements:** **Men:** Multivitamins: 30% Sports drink: 20% Vitamin C: 13% Protein powder: 13% Vitamin E: 6% Calcium: 6% Vitamin D: 5% Vitamin A: 5% Creatine: 5% Sport bar: 5% **Women:** Multivitamins: 28% Sports drink: 28% Calcium: 15% Folate: 13% Vitamin C: 13% Iron: 10% Vitamin B_6: 10% Vitamin D: 8% Vitamin E: 8% Protein powder: 8% **Number of different supplements used per week:** **Men:** 1–2: 30% 3–4: 12% 5+: 14% **Women:** 1–2: 35% 3–4: 18% 5+: 18%	**Top 5 reasons for supplement use:** **Men:** Health Performance Muscle strength Other Energy **Women:** Health Other Energy Performance/weight loss/not sure Endurance/strength	**Conclusions:** • All Army populations surveyed consume high levels of DS • Different Army populations have different patterns of use • Editorial comment: Scientific justification for this level of supplement use is lacking Study also provides information on supplement use by age, education, occupation; supplement knowledge; and money spent on supplements per wk

continued

TABLE C-1 Continued

Reference	Demographics	Group	Questions
Lieberman et al., 2007	April 1999 men (n=768) Average age: 23.6 y Response rate not known	U.S. Army Rangers	
Lieberman et al., 2007	July 2000 Men (n=152) Average age: 31.3 y Response rate not known	Special Forces	

Findings: Usage	Other Findings	Authors' Conclusions and Study Limitations
Supplement use at least once per week: 81% **Top 10 supplements:** Sports drink: 41% Multivitamins: 23% Creatine: 19% Protein/amino acids: 18% Antioxidants: 14% Herbs (ginseng, garlic, etc.): 9% Carbohydrate beverage: 7% Androstenedione: 7% Sports bar: 6% Sports gel: 3% **Number of different supplements used per week:** 1–2: 45% 3–4: 19% 5+: 15%	**Top 5 reasons for supplement use:** Energy Health Muscle strength Other Physician	General comments (see above)
Supplement use at least once per week: 65% **Top 10 supplements:** Sports drink: 36% Multivitamins: 32% Protein powder: 16% Creatine: 16% Sports bar: 15% Vitamin C: 11% Meal replacement beverage: 9% Vitamin E: 7% Antioxidants: 6% Androstenedione: 6% **Number of different supplements used per week:** 1–2: 41% 3–4: 14% 5+: 7%	**Top 5 reasons for supplement use:** Health Performance Energy Other Physician	General comments (see above)

continued

TABLE C-1 Continued

Reference	Demographics	Group	Questions
Lieberman et al., 2007	1999–2001 Men and women (n=315) Average age: 44 y Response rate not known	Army War College (mid to upper management)	

Findings: Usage	Other Findings	Authors' Conclusions and Study Limitations
Supplement use at least once per week: Men: 71% Women: 81% **Top 10 supplements** **Men:** Multivitamins: 39% Vitamin E: 22% Vitamin C: 17% Sports drink: 10% Antioxidants: 7% B-complex: 6% Garlic: 6% Beta-carotene: 5% *Ginkgo biloba*: 5% Calcium: 5% **Women:** Multivitamins: 52% Calcium: 32% Vitamin E: 32% Vitamin C: 29% Antioxidants: 23% Beta-carotene: 16% Magnesium: 13% Folate: 13% B-complex: 13% Vitamin B_6: 10% **Number of different supplements used per week** **Men:** 1–2: 29% 3–4: 14% 5+: 12% **Women:** 1–2: 36% 3–4: 6% 5+: 23%	**Top 5 reasons for supplement use** **Men:** Health Other Performance/energy Poor diet Physician **Women:** Health Performance/energy Other Poor diet Physician	General comments (see above)

continued

TABLE C-1 Continued

Reference	Demographics	Group	Questions
Marriott, 2007	April–August 2005 (n=16,146) Response rate overall: 51.8%	Active duty military (worldwide) All four branches and pay grades Army (n=3,636) Navy (n=4,626) Marine (n=3,356) Air Force (n=4,627)	DoD Survey of Health Related Behaviors Among Military Personnel plus added questions on diet, DS, CAM

Findings: Usage	Other Findings	Authors' Conclusions and Study Limitations
Supplement use (last 12 months): Any: 60.3% Multivitamin: 45% Individual vitamin/mineral: 26.9% Antioxidants: 20.8% Bodybuilding: 20.5% Herbal: 11.7% Weight loss: 18% Joint health: 8.5% Performance: 8.4% Other types: 9.1% **Frequency of use:** Once a month: 8.3% Once a week: 7.6% Every other day: 7.7% Once a day: 30.7% 2 times or more a day: 12.8% **Reporting use to military personnel:** To doctor: 36.6% To nurse/physician assistant: 21.7% Indicated on health record: 12.8% Women: 62.5% Men: 45.2% Reporting increases with age **Reporting to doctor by military branch:** Air Force: 49.5% Navy: 32.6% Army: 31.5% Marine: 25.3%	**Reasons for use:** Supplement diet Improve health Improve mental health Improve cognitive function Improve physical performance Increase muscle mass Lose weight Specific health problems **Information sources:** Personal contacts: 47.9% Print media: 29.1% Friends/family: 24.8% Multimedia nonprint: 23% Health professionals: 17.3% Sales store associates: 5.7%	**Conclusions:** • Nutrient supplements provided through military health care • Diet: <10% eat three or more servings of fruit and vegetables per day • Women in the Navy highest reported fruit (10.7%) and vegetable (12.9%) of three or more servings per day • Military dining services may represent an opportunity for increased communication about healthy diet and dietary supplement use Study also includes information on: Bodybuilding supplements, performance-enhancing supplements, and weight-loss supplements by pay grade, gender, age, education, BMI, activity, smoking, drinking, and supplement use overall by gender, military branch Author suggestions: analysis of specific information on exact supplements used with estimates of nutrient intake from food and supplements

continued

TABLE C-1 Continued

Reference	Demographics	Group	Questions
Thomasos, 2007	2006 (spring/summer) (n=10,985)	Air Force enlisted and officers	Adapted from the U.S. Army Center for Health Promotion and Preventive Medicine Dietary Supplement Questionnaire "Have you ever used any type of dietary supplement?"

NOTE: BMI=body mass index; CAM=complementary and alternative medicine; DS=dietary supplement; PA=physical activity.

Findings: Usage	Other Findings	Authors' Conclusions and Study Limitations
Supplement use: Currently using: 38% Past use only: 31% Never used: 31% **Most common supplements used** (5 or more times/wk): Multivitamin Multimineral Creatine Glutamine Vitamin C Caffeine Calcium Protein powders Fish oils Hydroxycut Chondroitin NO_2	**Primary reasons for use** (from most to least commonly reported): Promote health, weight loss, strength, lean muscle mass, stamina, fatigue reduction, cognition/alertness, memory, other **Most common supplement used:** (1) Senior enlisted: for weight loss (2) Junior enlisted/officers: for strength and lean body mass gains **Sources of information** (most to least commonly reported): Magazines, friends/family, books/journals, internet sites, health care providers, tv/radio/newspaper, store salesperson **Supplement purchase:** Commissary/PX: >40% Other on-base stores: ~25% Off-base stores: ~24% Internet/mail order: <10% **Adverse effects** (most to least commonly reported): Palpitations, anxiety, dehydration, nausea/vomiting, chest pain, dizziness/confusion, abdominal pain, tremors, diarrhea, muscle pain, numbness/tingling, breathing problems, heart attack, blood in urine, heat injury, visual disturbances, fainting	**Conclusions:** • Most U.S. Air Force members using DS • >60% DS bought on base • Most spend between \$11–\$50/mo • Most members do not report having adverse effects on this survey • Adverse effects are *not* usually reported to health care providers • Education on DS is needed **Additional information:** • Supplements were categorized into "like types" • Study also provides information on supplement use by: Occupation Grade (O1–O6 and E1–E9)

TABLE C-2 Surveys on Use of Dietary Supplements by Military Personnel

Reference	Demographics	Group	Questions	Findings: Usage
Arsenault and Kennedy, 1999	n=2,215 males, Average age: 25 (18–47 y) Response rate: 99%	Men entering U.S. Army Special Forces and Ranger training schools	Use of vitamins, minerals, pro-performance or other supplements	**Supplement use:** Past and/or present: 85% **Current use:** Any kind: 64% Ergogenics: 29% Multivitamin: 37% Vitamin C: 20% Creatine: 18% Ginseng: 9% **Daily use:** Any kind: 35% Ergogenics: 14%
Bovill et al., 2000[a]	n=152 male Average age: 31 y Response rate not known	U.S. Army Special Forces	Surveys asked about nutrition, supplement use, demographics, and health habits	**Supplement use:** 86% occasionally **Frequency:** Sports drinks: 66% Sports bars: 43% Multivitamins: 42% Vitamin C: 22% Protein powder: 22%

Findings: Motivation	Other Findings	Authors Conclusions and Study Limitations
Use for: General health, performance enhancement, interest in preventing infectious diseases, physical performance, and wound healing	• Use is higher than in general population of young men (39% use them occasionally) • Supplement use associated with higher scores for Army physical fitness tests, daily exercise, weight lifting, and nonsmokers • Not associated with age, ethnicity, BMI, chewing tobacco, or alcohol use	**Conclusions:** • Military population is at risk for potential adverse effects of inadequate use of DS, including abrupt cessation when deployed in operations or entering training • Presence of DS on military bases and discontent with food might result in higher use of DS **Recommendations:** • Further studies of benefits and risks are necessary • Routine one-size-fits-all advice should not be given • OK to treat deficiencies but questions about performance effects • Military health care professionals should be well informed about risks and benefits
General health: 63% Performance: 20%	• Supplement use associated with frequency of strength training • Not associated with age or habitual exercise • Information on nutrition from: Magazines/newspapers/books: 76% Friends: 54% Radio/TV: 34% Physicians/nurses: 33% Internet: 30%	

continued

TABLE C-2 Continued

Reference	Demographics	Group	Questions	Findings: Usage
Bovill et al., 2003	n=157 male (119 Special Forces, 38 non-Special Forces) Response rate: 89%	U.S. Army Special Forces and support soldiers (non-Special Forces)		**Supplement use:** Current: 87% **Specific use:** Similar to above (Bovill et al., 2000)

Findings: Motivation	Other Findings	Authors Conclusions and Study Limitations
A majority (64%) of soldiers incorrectly believed that protein is used for energy for short-term athletic events, 58% believed that vitamins provide energy	• Supplements used by more Special Forces (90%) than non-Special Forces (76%) • Supplement use associated with more frequent exercise and greater nutrition knowledge • Not associated with age, weight, ethnicity • Information on nutrition similar to above (Bovill et al., 2000)	**Conclusions:** Possible trend in increased use of supplements in military

continued

TABLE C-2 Continued

Reference	Demographics	Group	Questions	Findings: Usage
Brasfield, 2004	n=874 750 men 124 women Average age: 24.9 y (17–49 y) Response rate: 64%	Enlisted U.S. Army, active duty Representative sample of soldiers	Use of supplements and motivation	**Supplement use:** 60.9% **Frequency:** Multivitamin: 56% Vitamin C: 28% Creatine: 23% Ephedra: 21% Ginseng: 21% Calcium: 20% Vitamin E: 15% Vitamin A: 13% Iron: 13% Garlic: 12% **DS users consumed:** Three or more DS: 53% Two DS: 22% One DS: 25%
Deuster et al., 2003	n=38 Average age: 25 y (18–40 y) Response rate: 100%	U.S. Army Rangers	Nutrient, alcohol, DS intake, and physical activity level	**Daily supplement use:** 81.5% **Most common:** CHO/electrolyte fluids Protein powder: 24% Creatine: 13% Ephedrine: 13% Also reported use of ginseng, glutamine, vitamins/minerals

Findings: Motivation	Other Findings	Authors Conclusions and Study Limitations
General health, performance enhancement, prevent illness	**Source of information** (in order of frequency): Other (friends, family, etc.) Magazines Store salesperson Internet Doctors Books TV More females than males consumed a DS; however, more men consumed creatine, ginseng, and garlic No association with aerobic exercise frequency **Adverse events:** 18% Palpitations: 46% Dizziness/confusion: 30% Tremors: 26% Abdominal pain: 24% Numbness/tingling extremities: 16% Loss of consciousness: 4%	**Conclusions:** High number of adverse effects that might be attributed to DS use **Recommendations:** • Use of some DS should be discontinued prior to undergoing surgery • Health care screening • Routine assessment • Education • Further surveys recommended **Limitations:** • Self-reporting might result in misunderstanding and misreporting • Generalizations to general population are not possible • Categorization of DS Stores on military bases specifically to sell DS, in 2004, 92 stores worldwide on military installations
		Conclusions: Use of supplements is not necessary based on the dietary intakes of protein by the Rangers

continued

TABLE C-2 Continued

Reference	Demographics	Group	Questions	Findings: Usage
Johnson et al., In press	n=294 Average age: 23 y (survey was conducted in 1999) Response rate: 40%	U.S. Army Rangers	Use of supplements; potential factors associated: age, participation in competitive or recreational athletics, weight training; sources of nutritional information	**Supplement use:** 56% **Frequency:** Whole protein: 62% Creatine: 46% Thermogenics: 44% Anabolic steroids: <2%
McGraw et al., 2000	n=367 Average age: 22 y Response rate not known	U.S. Army Rangers	Use of supplements and associated factors	**Supplement use:** 36% **Frequency:** Creatine: 19% Multivitamin/ multimineral: 16% Protein/Amino acids: 14% Vitamin C: 7% Sport bars: 6%
McPherson and Schwenka, 2004	n=291 Average age: 39 y (18–83 y) Response rate: 73%	U.S. soldiers, retirees, spouses in military hospital	Use of complementary and alternative medicine (CAM)	Massage and supplements were most commonly used **CAM use:** Active duty: 72% Retiree: 85% Family: 89% **Supplement use:** Herbal supplements: 36% Nutritional food supplements: 36%

Findings: Motivation	Other Findings	Authors Conclusions and Study Limitations
	• No difference in age of user compared to nonuser • Supplement use associated with recreational activities, weight training • Source of information: Other soldiers: 59% Fitness magazines: 46% Internet: 18% Nutritionist: 8% Unit surgeon: 6%	**Conclusions:** • Soldiers consume ergogenics at the same rate as other athletic populations • Supplement use is inversely correlated to nutritional knowledge **Recommendation:** Further education of unit surgeons **Limitation:** Self-exclusion of soldiers with higher usage might result in low response and apparently lower supplement use level
	• Supplement use lower than general male population (42%), elite athletes (59%), or U.S. Army Special Operations candidates (64%) • Supplement use associated with frequency of strength training • Not associated with smoking or aerobic training.	
Pain, stress, anxiety, depression, weight loss	81–98% thought the treatment was effective	**Conclusions:** • Health providers need to become educated in CAM therapies • Further studies needed **Limitation:** Geographical area might have biased the results, Western region (increased CAM, more providers)

continued

TABLE C-2 Continued

Reference	Demographics	Group	Questions	Findings: Usage
Schneider et al., 1998	n=91 Response rate not known	Naval Sea, Air, Land (SEAL) personnel		**Supplement use:** 78% Using more than one supplement concurrently: 4–9 DS: 32% 3 DS: 34% 2 DS: 18% 1 DS: 16%
Sheppard et al., 2000	n=229 (133 military) Response rate: 40%	U.S. civilian and military health clubs	Use of creatine and other supplements	**Creatine use:** 12.2 g/d for 40 wk **Military supplement use:** Vitamin: 65% Mineral: 47% Protein: 45% Creatine: 29% Herbal: 21% Androstenedione: 13% Hydroxy-β-methyl-butyrate (HMB): 10% Anabolic/androgenic steroids: 3%

[a]Some of the findings from Bovill et al. (2000) and Bovill et al. (2003) are virtually the same and might come from the same study.

Findings: Motivation	Other Findings	Authors Conclusions and Study Limitations
Increase muscle mass, strength, and power; provide energy; improve general health		**Notes:** Navy, concurrent supplements
	• Supplement use associated with resistance training goal of strength • Creatine use associated with male gender, goal of strength training, lower frequency and duration of aerobic training, use of protein, andro/DHEA, and HMB • Information on creatine from: Popular media: 69% Physicians: 14% Dieticians: 10%	**Conclusions:** • Concerns: creatine use with other anabolic supplements • Popular magazines as main source of information • Education and access to information of users is critical • 45% of current creatine users reported adverse effects: gastrointestinal, muscle cramping/spasms, dehydration

REFERENCES

Arsenault, J., and J. Kennedy. 1999. Dietary supplement use in U.S. Army Special Operations candidates. *Mil Med* 164(7):495-501.

Bovill, M. E., S. M. McGraw, W. J. Tharion, and H. R. Lieberman. 2000. Supplement use and nutrition knowledge in a Special Forces unit. *FASEB Journal* 15(5):A999.

Bovill, M. E., W. J. Tharion, and H. R. Lieberman. 2003. Nutrition knowledge and supplement use among elite U.S. army soldiers. *Mil Med* 168(12):997-1000.

Brasfield, K. 2004. Dietary supplement intake in the active duty enlisted population. *US Army Med Dept J* (Oct-Dec):44-56.

Corum, S. J. C. 2007. *Dietary supplements questionnaire.* Paper presented at the Institute of Medicine Workshop on Dietary Supplement Use by Military Personnel, Washington, DC, February 13. Institute of Medicine Committee on Dietary Supplement Use by Military Personnel.

Deuster, P. A., A. Sridhar, W. J. Becker, R. Coll, K. K. O'Brien, and G. Bathalon. 2003. Health assessment of U.S. Army Rangers. *Mil Med* 168(1):57-62.

French, S. 2007. *Insights into dietary supplement usage by U.S. active military personnel.* Paper presented at the Institute of Medicine Workshop on Dietary Supplement Use by Military Personnel, Washington, DC, February 13. Institute of Medicine Committee on Dietary Supplement Use by Military Personnel.

Gardiner, P. 2007. *Prevalence of dietary supplements in the U.S. young adult population.* Paper presented at the Institute of Medicine Workshop on Dietary Supplement Use by Military Personnel, Washington, DC, February 13. Institute of Medicine Committee on Dietary Supplement Use by Military Personnel.

Jaghab, D. 2007. *Survey of Army health care providers concerning dietary supplements.* Paper presented at the Institute of Medicine Workshop on Dietary Supplement Use by Military Personnel, Washington, DC, February 13. Institute of Medicine Committee on Dietary Supplement Use by Military Personnel.

Johnson, A. E., C. A. Haley, and J. A. Ward. In Press. *Hazards of dietary supplement use.*

Kaufman, D. W. 2007. *Design and conduct of surveys on dietary supplement use.* Paper presented at the Institute of Medicine Workshop on Dietary Supplement Use by Military Personnel, Washington, DC, February 12. Institute of Medicine Committee on Dietary Supplement Use by Military Personnel.

Lieberman, H. R., T. Stavinoha, S. McGraw, and L. Sigrist. 2007. *Use of dietary supplements in U.S. Army populations.* Paper presented at the Institute of Medicine Workshop on Dietary Supplement Use by Military Personnel, Washington, DC, February 13. Institute of Medicine Committee on Dietary Supplement Use by Military Personnel.

Marriott, B. M. 2007. *Dietary supplement use by active duty military personnel: A world wide sample.* Paper presented at the Institute of Medicine Workshop on Dietary Supplement Use by Military Personnel, Washington, DC, February 13. Institute of Medicine Committee on Dietary Supplement Use by Military Personnel.

McGraw, S. M., W. J. Tharion, and H. R. Lieberman. 2000. Use of nutritional supplements by U.S. Army Rangers. *FASEB J* 14(4):A742.

McPherson, F., and M. A. Schwenka. 2004. Use of complementary and alternative therapies among active duty soldiers, military retirees, and family members at a military hospital. *Mil Med* 169(5):354-357.

Schneider, K., L. Hervig, W. Y. Ensign, Jr., W. K. Prusaczyk, and H. W. Goforth, Jr. 1998. Use of supplements by U.S. Navy SEALS. *Med Sci Sports Exerc* 30:S60.

Sheppard, H. L., S. M. Raichada, K. M. Kouri, L. Stenson Bar Maor, and J. D. Branch. 2000. Use of creatine and other supplements by members of civilian and military health clubs: A cross-sectional survey. *Int J Sport Nutr Exerc Metab* 10(3):245-259.

Thomasos, C. 2007. *Assessment of Air Force dietary supplement usage by major commands.* Paper presented at the Institute of Medicine Workshop on Dietary Supplement Use by Military Personnel, Washington, DC, February 13. Institute of Medicine Committee on Dietary Supplement Use by Military Personnel.

Appendix D

Case Studies

THE CASE OF DEHYDROEPIANDROSTERONE: DECISIONS FOR ACTION

Dehydroepiandrosterone (DHEA) was selected for a review of safety and efficacy because, as the committee compiled data about the use of dietary supplements by military personnel, anabolic supplements or body-building supplements were highlighted as one of the categories of dietary supplements that were most popular. DHEA is a steroid compound that is also popular in the civilian population because of its alleged effect in increasing muscle mass and enhancing physical performance. It is no surprise then that, performance enhancement being one of the main reasons military personnel cite for taking dietary supplements, DHEA has become popular among military members. DHEA was among the top 10 dietary supplements used at least once a week by Rangers (7 percent) and Special Forces (6 percent) in surveys conducted in 1999 and 2000, respectively (Lieberman et al., 2007). In another survey comparing civilian and military use of dietary supplements among members of health clubs, as many as 13 percent of military personnel were using DHEA (Sheppard et al., 2000). When asked by health care providers about "bodybuilder supplement use," 6.6 percent of military members reported using them (Jaghab, 2007); DHEA may have been among them. In addition, the most recent U.S. Department of Defense (DoD) Survey of Health Related Behaviors Among Military Personnel (Marriott, 2007) found that as many as 20.5 percent of military personnel used bodybuilder supplements within the last 12 months. As a variety of sources suggested a high level of use, the committee initiated a review of DHEA safety and efficacy. The committee searched for literature reviews (Figures 4-1 and 4-2) conducted over the previous 10 years as well as more recent original studies not included in reviews. In addition, a search was conducted for articles specifically designed to signal safety or performance effects of critical importance to the military.

Surprisingly, the popular view that DHEA increases muscle mass and therefore might improve performance appears to be based largely on the findings of a 1998 paper that had significant methodological limitations (Morales et al., 1998). The various reviews of the literature addressing efficacy indicate that there is little substantiation for such a performance claim. There is a gender-specific effect on blood testosterone that perhaps merits further research to determine effects of DHEA on lean tissue and bone density gain in women during resistance training. Some reviews found that the use of DHEA by women increases testosterone concentration. Other reviews evaluated suspected benefits on cognition, mood, and bone strength from consuming DHEA. A search for original articles on studies that include situations or conditions of particular relevance for the military yielded no result. Based on Table 4-2 and the findings from literature reviews, the committee agrees that there is a low level of benefit to be gained by military personnel from using DHEA. Reviews highlighted adverse androgenizing effects experienced by women, and other minor effects such as facial acne or increased sebum production; there was no adverse effect identified that would decrease the readiness of military personnel. There was some theoretical increased risk of cardiovascular disease in women due to the reduction in high-density lipoprotein noted in some studies.

Although some drugs are known to either increase or decrease blood DHEA, there were no reports that supplementary DHEA affected the action of most drugs. Other prescription steroid hormones (e.g., testosterone analogs, estrogen) may be exceptions; it is possible that DHEA consumption could affect the metabolism of those drugs.

One long-term theoretical but critical adverse effect uncovered during the safety reviews is the potential association of DHEA levels in blood with a higher risk of breast cancer seen in various epidemiological studies. The potential for hepatic neoplasia was also suggested by results from a review of animal studies. This potential adverse effect is serious enough that, although a cause and effect could not be established from those studies, a high level of concern was determined for DHEA (Box 4-1).

The military should decide on the course of action based on the high level of concern and low benefit derived from its use. A course of action might be to do the following:

- Follow up with the research community to determine whether the equivocal animal data related to neoplasia are translated to humans and to monitor future research on either safety or benefits to determine if it needs to be reclassified in the future, which would likely lead to different management actions. Research on DHEA should be monitored to determine if it should be reclassified as future research unfolds.

- Develop an outreach strategy to educate military members about the high risks and low benefits of using DHEA by
  - including DHEA in a list of dietary supplements to avoid. Recommend the use of alternative products (e.g., creatine, beta-hydroxy-beta-methylbutyrate [HMB]) or strategies (modification of resistance training regime, increase of energy intake) that might provide similar desired effects;
  - informing military health care providers, fitness trainers and therapists, registered dietitians, nutritionists, commanders, and other educators about the risks and benefits of using DHEA and recommend alternative products or foods; and
  - monitoring use and potential adverse effects among military personnel.

THE CASE OF EPHEDRA: DECISIONS FOR ACTION

Ephedra (*Ephedra sinica* Stapf and other ephedrine-containing *Ephedra* species) was selected for a review of safety by the committee for various reasons. First, due to the severe adverse effects reported, the sale of ephedra in dietary supplements has been banned in the United States since 2004 (Rados, 2004); it is therefore the first and only dietary supplement that has been banned since the Dietary Supplement Health and Education Act was implemented (the ephedra alkaloids ephedrine and pseudoephedrine, however, are allowed to be sold as over-the-counter medications in the United States). A study by Deuster et al. (2003) reported that 13 percent of the U.S. Army Rangers surveyed used ephedrine. Similarly, a high percentage (21 percent) of ephedra users were calculated from a self-reporting questionnaire distributed among U.S. Army active duty personnel (Brasfield, 2004). These surveys, however, were conducted prior to the ephedra ban in the United States; the impact of the ban on the use of ephedra and its alkaloids is not known. A survey focusing on supplement use that was distributed among Army health care providers revealed that 5.2 and 7.7 percent of soldiers reported use of ephedra to their physicians or other health care personnel, respectively (Jaghab, 2007). Although these numbers might not be representative of the military population, they do raise safety concerns about the use of ephedra. The odds of adverse events from misuse of over-the-counter medications containing ephedra alkaloids might be small but continue to be of concern. Also, botanicals that are chemically similar to ephedra and might mimic its effects are still available in the market.

Although initially the military had considered ephedra among the dietary supplements likely to be efficacious and of interest, defense applications for use of ephedra were never developed by The Technical Cooperation Program (TTCP) panel[1] because of safety concerns (Lieberman et al., 2007). These safety concerns and its use among military personnel prompted a safety evaluation of ephedra.

The committee initiated a safety review by applying Figures 5-1 and 5-2 (see Chapter 5). An initial search for reviews of ephedra was carried out in appropriate databases such as PubMed, Napralert, Toxline, SciFinder, UIC, and Company Digital Libraries. Among the terms used in the search were *ephedra* and Latin binomials, *healthy*, *performance*, *ergogenic*, *memory*, *interactions*, *adverse*, *toxicity*, and *infection*. The review only focused on perceived benefits such as increased weight loss and performance enhancement as relevant benefits for military personnel. A few studies demonstrate a statistically significant weight loss using ephedra versus placebo. Most studies, however, showed a weight loss of only 0.6–0.8 kg per month using ephedra, or 1.0 kg with ephedra-caffeine combinations. The committee concluded that these effects are not clinically relevant. Moreover, there are no clinical studies with long-term data. Likewise, clinical studies with ephedra alkaloids have not been shown to result in significant improvements in performance for the specific modalities tested. However, combinations of ephedrine HCl (synthetic ephedrine) and caffeine seem to enhance various measurements of performance.

During clinical trials it was noted that the risk of adverse events increased two- to fourfold and that the adverse effect profile of ephedra was primarily related to serious cardiovascular effects, from palpitations to tachycardias and strokes. Although most adverse effects are relevant to the general population, some of them, such as psychosis, vision impairment, dehydration, or muscle failure, would specifically present heightened risks for military personnel. Interaction with sympathomimetic drugs as well as the occurrence of palpitations should be of concern. Some of the adverse events (e.g., psychosis, increased heart rate and blood pressure, myocardial infarction, arrhythmias) were also seen in studies when ephedra and caffeine were provided in combination.

The committee concluded that the use of ephedra (and related alkaloids) presents a high level of concern. With only moderate potential for benefits and the high level of concern, this committee supports the current ban on ephedra use. Military leadership might decide to take the following actions on ephedra and its alkaloids, particularly directed toward popula-

[1]The TTCP panel is an international panel of military scientists whose mission is to conduct research, share information, and write papers on performance-enhancing treatments for potential operational use.

tions that might use performance enhancers, such as Rangers or Special Operations forces:

- Develop an outreach strategy to educate soldiers about the high risks and low benefits of using ephedra and its alkaloids by

  – including ephedra and its alkaloids in outreach materials listing dietary supplements to avoid. Recommend the use of alternative products (e.g., creatine, HMB) or strategies (modification of resistance training regime, increase of energy intake) that might provide similar desired effects;

  – informing military health care providers, fitness trainers and therapists, registered dietitians, nutritionists, commanders, and other educators about the risks and benefits of using ephedra and its alkaloids and recommend alternative products or foods; and

  – monitoring use and potential associated adverse effects among military personnel.

THE CASE OF MELATONIN: DECISIONS FOR ACTION

The committee's interest in melatonin originated from its potential value for use by military personnel as a sleep enhancer and for reentrainment following rapid deployment across time zones (Lieberman et al., 2007). Although melatonin was not reported as being used in any of the military surveys reviewed, melatonin is being used at a high rate as a dietary supplement in the general population. This committee anticipates that in the future, military personnel might be taking melatonin to achieve circadian reentrainment or to improve sleep; therefore, the committee selected melatonin as being of interest to the military and supports a review of safety and efficacy before decisions about its value for military personnel are made.

Melatonin is a hormone secreted in the brain by the pineal gland and also reportedly found in a number of plants. It has widespread effects in the body, many of them poorly understood. Endogenous secretion of melatonin is believed to help maintain internal circadian synchrony among organ systems throughout the body. Exogenous melatonin is available over the counter in the United States. Literature searches conducted by the committee focused on ingestion of melatonin for inducing diurnal sleep in healthy adults, for improving nocturnal sleep in persons with insomnia, and for circadian reentrainment (e.g., for jet lag or night-shift work). The searches were conducted in Thomson ISI and PubMed. There are numerous published clinical studies and experiments. This committee reviewed the findings from three recent reviews (Arendt and Skene, 2005; Morin et al., 2007; Wagner et al., 1998) and three meta-analyses (Brzezinski et al., 2004; Buscemi et al., 2005, 2006). The committee concluded that there is moderate potential for benefits (very modest evidence of improvement of sleep, but moderate to good evidence of circadian reentrainment under controlled conditions).

Mild adverse effects that might affect military performance have been identified, such as drowsiness, core body heat loss, and gastrointestinal distress (e.g., nausea); serious adverse effects were not found. Putative synergistic effects of exogenous melatonin with sedative hypnotics were not found. Given the moderate concern and moderate potential for benefits of exogenous melatonin, the military leadership could initiate the following activities:

- Follow up with the scientific community conducting research on the effects of melatonin for sleep and circadian reentrainment during operations in environments inconducive to sleep, to determine if melatonin has advantages over sedative-hypnotics that have carryover effects on performance.
- Develop an outreach strategy to educate military members, military health care providers, fitness trainers and therapists, registered dietitians, nutritionists, and commanders about the potential interaction of melatonin with sedative-hypnotic medications and the potential for increased heat loss.

REFERENCES

Arendt, J., and D. J. Skene. 2005. Melatonin as a chronobiotic. *Sleep Med Rev* 9(1):25-39.

Brasfield, K. 2004. Dietary supplement intake in the active duty enlisted population. *US Army Med Dept J* (Oct-Dec):44-56.

Brzezinski, A., M. G. Vangel, R. J. Wurtman, G. Norrie, I. Zhdanova, A. Ben-Shushan, and I. Ford. 2005. Effects of exogenous melatonin on sleep: A meta-analysis. *Sleep Med Rev* 9(1):41-50.

Buscemi, N., B. Vandermeer, N. Hooton, R. Pandya, L. Tjosvold, L. Hartling, G. Baker, T. P. Klassen, and S. Vohra. 2005. The efficacy and safety of exogenous melatonin for primary sleep disorders—A meta-analysis. *J Gen Intern Med* 20(12):1151-1158.

Buscemi, N., B. Vandermeer, N. Hooton, R. Pandya, L. Tjosvold, L. Hartling, S. Vohra, T. P. Klassen, and G. Baker. 2006. Efficacy and safety of exogenous melatonin for secondary sleep disorders and sleep disorders accompanying sleep-restriction: Meta-analysis. *Br Med J* 332(7538):385-393.

Deuster, P. A., A. Sridhar, W. J. Becker, R. Coll, K. K. O'Brien, and G. Bathalon. 2003. Health assessment of U.S. Army Rangers. *Mil Med* 168(1):57-62.

Jaghab, D. 2007. *Survey of Army health care providers concerning dietary supplements*. Institute of Medicine Committee on Dietary Supplement Use by Military Personnel meeting, Washington, DC, February 13.

Lieberman, H. R., T. Stavinoha, S. McGraw, and L. Sigrist. 2007. *Use of dietary supplements in U.S. Army populations*. Institute of Medicine Committee on Dietary Supplement Use by Military Personnel meeting, Washington, DC, February 13.

Marriott, B. M. 2007. *Dietary supplement use by active duty military personnel: A worldwide sample.* Institute of Medicine Committee on Dietary Supplement Use by Military Personnel meeting, Washington, DC, February 13.

Morales, A. J., R. H. Haubrich, J. Y. Hwang, H. Asakura, and S. S. Yen. 1998. The effect of six months treatment with a 100 mg daily dose of dehydroepiandrosterone (DHEA) on circulating sex steroids, body composition and muscle strength in age-advanced men and women. *Clin Endocrinol (Oxf)* 49(4):421-432.

Morin, A. K., C. I. Jarvis, and A. M. Lynch. 2007. Therapeutic options for sleep-maintenance and sleep-onset insomnia. *Pharmacotherapy* 27(1):89-110.

Rados, C. 2004. Ephedra ban: No shortage of reasons. *FDA Consum* 38(2):6-7.

Sheppard, H. L., S. M. Raichada, K. M. Kouri, L. Stenson Bar Maor, and J. D. Branch. 2000. Use of creatine and other supplements by members of civilian and military health clubs: A cross-sectional survey. *Int J Sport Nutr Exerc Metab* 10(3):245-259.

Wagner, J., M. L. Wagner, and W. A. Hening. 1998. Beyond benzodiazepines: Alternative pharmacologic agents for the treatment of insomnia. *Ann Pharmacother* 32(6):680-686.

Appendix E

Adverse Event Reporting Forms

MEDMARX[SM] Adverse Drug Reaction Data Entry Form

***Required Information**

***Date of reaction:**____________________(mm/dd/yyyy) ***Source of reaction:** ☐ Inpatient ☐ Outpatient

***Description of reaction:**

____

____

____

____

____

***Body system(s) involved:**

☐ Allergy & Immune System	☐ Cardiac/Heart	☐ Gastrointestinal/Digestive System	☐ Renal & Urinary System
☐ Blood/Bone Marrow/Lymphatic System	☐ Circulation/Vascular & Coagulation	☐ Liver/Hepatobiliary & Pancreas	☐ Reproduction & Pregnancy
☐ Body as a Whole, General/Constitutional	☐ Ears/Auditory, Nose & Throat	☐ Mental Health & Behavior	☐ Respiratory/Pulmonary, & Thoracic
☐ Bones/Joints, Muscles & Connective Tissue	☐ Endocrine System (Hormones)	☐ Metabolism & Nutrition	☐ Skin/Subcutaneous Tissues, Hair & Nails
☐ Brain, Neurologic, & Nervous System	☐ Eyes/Ocular & Vision	☐ Mouth & Teeth	

***Reaction summary terms:**

☐ Abnormal, Diagnostic test	☐ Dry skin	☐ Irregular menses	☐ Rash
☐ Abnormal, Laboratory value	☐ Dysphagia (difficulty swallowing)	☐ Ischemia	☐ Red-man syndrome
☐ Acidosis	☐ Dyspnea (shortness of breath)	☐ Keratitis	☐ Renal failure
☐ Adult respiratory distress syndrome (ARDS)	☐ Edema	☐ Lethargy	☐ Respiratory arrest
☐ Alkalosis	☐ Erectile dysfunction	☐ Leukopenias	☐ Respiratory distress/depression
☐ Allergic reaction/hypersensitivity	☐ Extrapyramidal/movement disorder	☐ Libido alteration	☐ Rhabdomyolysis
☐ Anemias	☐ Fatigue	☐ Liver dysfunction/failure	☐ Rhinitis
☐ Angina	☐ Feminization of male	☐ Loss of consciousness/syncope	☐ Rigors/chills
☐ Anorexia	☐ Fever	☐ Malignancy	☐ Salivary gland changes
☐ Apnea	☐ Fistula	☐ Masculinization of female	☐ Seizure
☐ Arthritis	☐ Flatulence	☐ Melena	☐ Serum sickness
☐ Ascites	☐ Flushing	☐ Memory impairment	☐ Somnolence/depressed consciousness level
☐ Ataxia	☐ Gastritis	☐ Mucositis/stomatitis	☐ Speech impairment
☐ Autoimmune disorder	☐ Glaucoma	☐ Multi-organ failure	☐ Stevens-Johnson syndrome
☐ Bruising	☐ Glucose metabolism disorder	☐ Muscle weakness	☐ Sweating
☐ Cardiac arrhythmia	☐ Gynecomastia	☐ Nail changes	☐ Syndrome inappropriate antidiuretic hormone
☐ Cardiac conduction abnormality	☐ Hair loss/alopecia	☐ Nausea	☐ Syndrome, Other
☐ Cardiac failure	☐ Headache	☐ Neuropathy	☐ Taste alteration
☐ Cardiac infarction	☐ Hearing changes	☐ Nystagmus	☐ Thombocytopenia
☐ Cardiac ischemia	☐ Heartburn/dyspepsia	☐ Obstruction	☐ Thrombosis/embolism
☐ Cardiac rate abnormal	☐ Hematemesis	☐ Otitis	☐ Thyroid dysfunction
☐ Cardiomyopathy	☐ Hematuria	☐ Pain	☐ Tremor
☐ Cataract	☐ Hemolysis	☐ Palpitations	☐ Tumor lysis syndrome
☐ Cerebral ischemia	☐ Hemoptysis	☐ Pancreatitis	☐ Ulcer
☐ Coagulopathy	☐ Hemorrhage	☐ Pericardial effusion	☐ Urinary electrolyte wasting
☐ Colitis	☐ Hiccups	☐ Petechiae/purpura	☐ Urinary frequency/urgency
☐ Confusion	☐ Hives	☐ Pharyngitis	☐ Urinary retention
☐ Conjunctivitis	☐ Hot flashes/flushes	☐ Phlebitis	☐ Urine color change
☐ Constipation	☐ Hypertension	☐ Photosensitivity	☐ Vaginal dryness
☐ Cough	☐ Hypotension	☐ Pigmentation changes	☐ Vaginitis
☐ Cushing's syndrome/appearance	☐ Hypoxia	☐ Pleural effusion	☐ Vascular leak syndrome
☐ Dehydration	☐ Ileus	☐ Pneumonitis/pneumonia	☐ Vasculitis
☐ Depression/mood alteration	☐ Incontinence	☐ Pneumothorax	☐ Vision Changes
☐ Diarrhea	☐ Infection	☐ Proctitis	☐ Voice changes
☐ Dizziness	☐ Infertility/sterility	☐ Pruritus/itching	☐ Vomiting
☐ Dry eye syndrome	☐ Injection site reaction/extravasation	☐ Psychosis	☐ Watery eye
☐ Dry mouth/salivary gland	☐ Insomnia	☐ Pulmonary fibrosis	☐ Weight change

***Suspected medication (generic name):**__________________________ ***Patient age:**_________(days, weeks, months, years) Circle one

***Seriousness Criteria**

- ☐ Intervention to prevent incapacity
- ☐ Is life-threatening
- ☐ Other medically important condition
- ☐ Results in death
- ☐ Is a congenital anomaly or birth defect
- ☐ Not serious (none of the above apply)
- ☐ Requires initial/prolonged hospitalization
- ☐ Results in persistent/significant incapacity

***Patient location:**

- ☐ Admitting Department
- ☐ Cardiac Catheterization Laboratory
- ☐ Cardiovascular / Pulmonary Services
- ☐ Clinic, Outpatient
- ☐ Dialysis Unit
- ☐ Emergency Department
- ☐ Emergency Transport Vehicle
- ☐ Endoscopy / GI Lab
- ☐ Hospice
- ☐ Hospital, another
- ☐ Intensive Care Unit, Coronary
- ☐ Intensive Care Unit, General
- ☐ Intensive Care Unit, Medical
- ☐ Intensive Care Unit, Neonatal
- ☐ Intensive Care Unit, Pediatric
- ☐ Intensive Care Unit, Surgical
- ☐ Labor / Delivery
- ☐ Long-Term Care Facility
- ☐ Maternity
- ☐ Nursery
- ☐ Nursing (Patient Care) Unit
- ☐ Obstetrical Recovery Room
- ☐ Occupational Therapy
- ☐ Operating Room
- ☐ Oncology Department
- ☐ Outpatient Surgery Department
- ☐ Patient home / Residence
- ☐ Pediatrics
- ☐ Pharmacy, Inpatient
- ☐ Pharmacy, Outpatient
- ☐ Physical Therapy
- ☐ Post-anesthesia Care Unit
- ☐ Pre-Op holding
- ☐ Psychiatric, Inpatient
- ☐ Psychiatric, Outpatient
- ☐ Radiology
- ☐ Rehabilitation Care Unit
- ☐ Transplant Unit

***Outcome of reaction:**

- ☐ Fatal
- ☐ Not recovered/not resolved
- ☐ Recovered/resolved
- ☐ Recovered/resolved with sequelae
- ☐ Recovering/resolving
- ☐ Unknown

***Result of reaction on patient level of care:**

- ☐ A level of care not determined
- ☐ Airway established / patient ventilated
- ☐ Antidote administered
- ☐ Cardiac defibrillation performed
- ☐ CPR administered
- ☐ Dialysis
- ☐ Drug therapy initiated / changed
- ☐ Hospitalization, initial
- ☐ Hospitalization, prolonged 1-5 days
- ☐ Hospitalization, prolonged 6-10 days
- ☐ Hospitalization, prolonged >10 days
- ☐ Laboratory tests performed
- ☐ Narcotic antagonist administered
- ☐ None
- ☐ Observation initiated / increased
- ☐ Oxygen administered
- ☐ Surgery performed
- ☐ Transferred to higher level of care
- ☐ Vital signs / monitoring initiated / increased
- ☐ X-ray / MRI / other diagnostic test performed

***Preventability assessment:**

- ☐ Considered preventable, Other
- ☐ Documented drug interaction involved
- ☐ Dose/route/frequency inappropriate
- ☐ Drug inappropriate for clinical condition
- ☐ History of allergy/previous reaction
- ☐ Not considered preventable
- ☐ Poor compliance involved
- ☐ Required monitoring/tests not performed
- ☐ Unknown/Unable to assess

***Action(s) taken:**

- ☐ Documented ADR-other
- ☐ Documented ADR-patient chart
- ☐ Documented ADR-prescription entry system
- ☐ Formulary changed
- ☐ Informed patient/caregiver
- ☐ Informed patient's physician
- ☐ Other Medication(s) Dose changed/withdrawn
- ☐ Policy/Procedure changed
- ☐ Policy/Procedure instituted
- ☐ Provided Supportive/Palliative Care
- ☐ Submitted FDA MedWatch Form
- ☐ Suspected Medication(s) Discontinued
- ☐ Suspected Medication(s) Dose Increased
- ☐ Suspected Medication(s) Dose Reduced
- ☐ Suspected Medication(s) Dose Unchanged
- ☐ Unknown

***Naranjo Scale**
Probability/Causality Assessment

Question	Yes	No	Do Not Know
1. Are there previous conclusive reports on this reaction?			
2. Did the adverse event appear after the suspected drug was administered?			
3. Did the adverse reaction improve when drug was discontinued or a specific antagonist was administered?			
4. Did the adverse reaction appear when the drug was readministered?			
5. Are there alternative causes (other than the drug) that could on their own have caused the reaction?			
6. Did the reaction appear when a placebo was given?			
7. Was the drug detected in the blood (or other fluids) in concentrations known to be toxic?			
8. Was the reaction more severe when the dose was increased, or less severe when the dose was decreased?			
9. Did the patient have a similar reaction to the same or similar drugs in any previous exposure?			
10. Was the adverse event confirmed by any objective evidence?			

Brand Name:____________
Dosage form:____________
Batch Lot number:____________
Strength/Concentration:____________
Dosage Interval:____________
Medication Start Date:____________

Manufacturer:____________
Intended route of administration:____________
Investigational drug name:____________
Indication:____________
Dosage Information Detail:____________
Medication End Date:____________

Therapeutic Classification:____________
Labeler:____________
Compounded ingredients:____________
Dosage:____________
Reaction Latency:____________

Detection Method:

- ☐ Patient-Objective Evidence
- ☐ Triggers-Medication Orders/Lab Values
- ☐ Patient-Subjective Complaint
- ☐ Spontaneous report
- ☐ Chart Review
- ☐ Other
- ☐ ICD-9 Code Review

Patient Sex: ☐ Male ☐ Female ☐ Unavailable

Patient weight:____________ **Location detail:**____________ **Duration of reaction:**____________

Pertinent medication history; medical history, including relevant pre-existing conditions; concomitant drug therapy, with dates:

____

Results of relevant tests/procedures to the reaction:

____

Reporter level of staff:

☐ Anesthesiologist	☐ Dentist and related specialties	☐ Dialysis Technician	☐ Dietary Personnel
☐ Emergency Medical Services	☐ Laboratory Personnel	☐ Management Personnel	☐ Nuclear Medicine Technician
☐ Nurse Anesthetist	☐ Nurse Practitioner/Advanced Practice Nurse	☐ Nurse, Graduate	☐ Nurse, Licensed Practical/Vocational
☐ Nurse, Registered	☐ Nurse, Travel	☐ Nursing Assistant/Aide	☐ Nursing Personnel, non-specific
☐ Optometrist	☐ Patient/Family Member/Caregiver	☐ Pharmacist	☐ Pharmacy Personnel, non-specific
☐ Pharmacy Technician	☐ Phlebotomist	☐ Physical Therapist	☐ Physician
☐ Physician Assistant	☐ Physician, Intern	☐ Physician, Resident	☐ Psych Tech/Mental Health Technician
☐ Radiology Technician	☐ Respiratory Therapist	☐ Student	☐ Unit Secretary/Clerk
☐ Unlicensed Assistive Personnel			

Action taken and recommendations to avoid future reactions:

____

Internal control:____________ **Serum Creatinine:**____________ **milligrams per deciliter**

Physician Service detail:____________ **Patient detail:**____________ **Reporter detail:**____________

This document is part of a quality improvement process
CONFIDENTIAL-Not to be included as part of the patient medical record

Patient Name:____________
Medical Record #:____________
Signature of Unit Manager:____________

U.S. Department of Health and Human Services

MEDWATCH

The FDA Safety Information and Adverse Event Reporting Program

For VOLUNTARY reporting of adverse events, product problems and product use errors

Page ____ of ____

Form Approved: OMB No. 0910-0291, Expires: 10/31/08
See OMB statement on reverse.

FDA USE ONLY

Triage unit sequence #

PLEASE TYPE OR USE BLACK INK

A. PATIENT INFORMATION

1. **Patient Identifier** — In confidence
2. **Age at Time of Event, or Date of Birth:**
3. **Sex** ☐ Female ☐ Male
4. **Weight** ______ lb or ______ kg

B. ADVERSE EVENT, PRODUCT PROBLEM OR ERROR

Check all that apply:

1. ☐ **Adverse Event** ☐ **Product Problem** *(e.g., defects/malfunctions)*
☐ **Product Use Error** ☐ **Problem with Different Manufacturer of Same Medicine**

2. **Outcomes Attributed to Adverse Event** *(Check all that apply)*
☐ Death: ______ *(mm/dd/yyyy)* ☐ Disability or Permanent Damage
☐ Life-threatening ☐ Congenital Anomaly/Birth Defect
☐ Hospitalization - initial or prolonged ☐ Other Serious (Important Medical Events)
☐ Required Intervention to Prevent Permanent Impairment/Damage (Devices)

3. **Date of Event** *(mm/dd/yyyy)*
4. **Date of this Report** *(mm/dd/yyyy)*
5. **Describe Event, Problem or Product Use Error**
6. **Relevant Tests/Laboratory Data, Including Dates**
7. **Other Relevant History, Including Preexisting Medical Conditions** *(e.g., allergies, race, pregnancy, smoking and alcohol use, liver/kidney problems, etc.)*

C. PRODUCT AVAILABILITY

Product Available for Evaluation? *(Do not send product to FDA)*

☐ Yes ☐ No ☐ Returned to Manufacturer on: ______ *(mm/dd/yyyy)*

D. SUSPECT PRODUCT(S)

1. **Name, Strength, Manufacturer** *(from product label)*
#1
#2

2. **Dose or Amount** | **Frequency** | **Route**
#1
#2

3. **Dates of Use** *(If unknown, give duration) from/to (or best estimate)*
#1
#2

4. **Diagnosis or Reason for Use** *(Indication)*
#1
#2

5. **Event Abated After Use Stopped or Dose Reduced?**
#1 ☐ Yes ☐ No ☐ Doesn't Apply
#2 ☐ Yes ☐ No ☐ Doesn't Apply

6. **Lot #**
#1
#2

7. **Expiration Date**
#1
#2

8. **Event Reappeared After Reintroduction?**
#1 ☐ Yes ☐ No ☐ Doesn't Apply
#2 ☐ Yes ☐ No ☐ Doesn't Apply

9. **NDC # or Unique ID**

E. SUSPECT MEDICAL DEVICE

1. **Brand Name**
2. **Common Device Name**
3. **Manufacturer Name, City and State**
4. **Model #** | **Lot #**
Catalog # | **Expiration Date** *(mm/dd/yyyy)*
Serial # | **Other #**
5. **Operator of Device**
☐ Health Professional
☐ Lay User/Patient
☐ Other:
6. **If Implanted, Give Date** *(mm/dd/yyyy)*
7. **If Explanted, Give Date** *(mm/dd/yyyy)*
8. **Is this a Single-use Device that was Reprocessed and Reused on a Patient?**
☐ Yes ☐ No
9. **If Yes to Item No. 8, Enter Name and Address of Reprocessor**

F. OTHER (CONCOMITANT) MEDICAL PRODUCTS

Product names and therapy dates *(exclude treatment of event)*

G. REPORTER *(See confidentiality section on back)*

1. **Name and Address**

Phone # | **E-mail**

2. **Health Professional?** ☐ Yes ☐ No
3. **Occupation**
4. **Also Reported to:**
☐ Manufacturer
☐ User Facility
☐ Distributor/Importer
5. **If you do NOT want your identity disclosed to the manufacturer, place an "X" in this box:** ☐

FORM FDA 3500 (10/05) **Submission of a report does not constitute an admission that medical personnel or the product caused or contributed to the event.**

ADVICE ABOUT VOLUNTARY REPORTING

Detailed instructions available at: http://www.fda.gov/medwatch/report/consumer/instruct.htm

Report adverse events, product problems or product use errors with:

- Medications *(drugs or biologics)*
- Medical devices *(including in-vitro diagnostics)*
- Combination products *(medication & medical devices)*
- Human cells, tissues, and cellular and tissue-based products
- Special nutritional products *(dietary supplements, medical foods, infant formulas)*
- Cosmetics

Report product problems - quality, performance or safety concerns such as:

- Suspected counterfeit product
- Suspected contamination
- Questionable stability
- Defective components
- Poor packaging or labeling
- Therapeutic failures (product didn't work)

-Fold Here-

Report SERIOUS adverse events. An event is serious when the patient outcome is:

- Death
- Life-threatening
- Hospitalization - initial or prolonged
- Disability or permanent damage
- Congenital anomaly/birth defect
- Required intervention to prevent permanent impairment or damage
- Other serious (important medical events)

Report even if:

- You're not certain the product caused the event
- You don't have all the details

How to report:

- Just fill in the sections that apply to your report
- Use section D for all products except medical devices
- Attach additional pages if needed
- Use a separate form for each patient
- Report either to FDA or the manufacturer *(or both)*

Other methods of reporting:

- 1-800-FDA-0178 -- To FAX report
- 1-800-FDA-1088 -- To report by phone
- www.fda.gov/medwatch/report.htm -- To report online

If your report involves a serious adverse event with a device and it occurred in a facility outside a doctor's office, that facility may be legally required to report to FDA and/or the manufacturer. Please notify the person in that facility who would handle such reporting.

-Fold Here-

If your report involves a serious adverse event with a vaccine call 1-800-822-7967 to report.

Confidentiality: The patient's identity is held in strict confidence by FDA and protected to the fullest extent of the law. FDA will not disclose the reporter's identity in response to a request from the public, pursuant to the Freedom of Information Act. The reporter's identity, including the identity of a self-reporter, may be shared with the manufacturer unless requested otherwise.

The public reporting burden for this collection of information has been estimated to average 36 minutes per response, including the time for reviewing instructions, searching existing data sources, gathering and maintaining the data needed, and completing and reviewing the collection of information. Send comments regarding this burden estimate or any other aspect of this collection of information, including suggestions for reducing this burden to:

Department of Health and Human Services
Food and Drug Administration - MedWatch
10903 New Hampshire Avenue
Building 22, Mail Stop 4447
Silver Spring, MD 20993-0002

Please DO NOT RETURN this form to this address.

OMB statement:
"An agency may not conduct or sponsor, and a person is not required to respond to, a collection of information unless it displays a currently valid OMB control number."

U.S. DEPARTMENT OF HEALTH AND HUMAN SERVICES
Food and Drug Administration

FORM FDA 3500 (10/05) (Back) **Please Use Address Provided Below -- Fold in Thirds, Tape and Mail**

DEPARTMENT OF HEALTH & HUMAN SERVICES

Public Health Service
Food and Drug Administration
Rockville, MD 20857

Official Business
Penalty for Private Use $300

NO POSTAGE NECESSARY IF MAILED IN THE UNITED STATES OR APO/FPO

BUSINESS REPLY MAIL

FIRST CLASS MAIL PERMIT NO. 946 ROCKVILLE MD

MEDWATCH

The FDA Safety Information and Adverse Event Reporting Program
Food and Drug Administration
5600 Fishers Lane
Rockville, MD 20852-9787

Form Approved: OMB No. 0910-0291, Expires: 10/31/08
See OMB statement on reverse.

U.S. Department of Health and Human Services
Food and Drug Administration

MEDWATCH

FORM FDA 3500A (10/05)

For use by user-facilities, importers, distributors and manufacturers for MANDATORY reporting

Page ____ of ____

Mfr Report #

UF/Importer Report #

FDA Use Only

A. PATIENT INFORMATION

1. **Patient Identifier** — In confidence
2. **Age at Time of Event:** ____ or **Date of Birth:**
3. **Sex** ☐ Female ☐ Male
4. **Weight** ____ lbs or ____ kgs

B. ADVERSE EVENT OR PRODUCT PROBLEM

1. ☐ **Adverse Event** and/or ☐ **Product Problem** *(e.g., defects/malfunctions)*
2. **Outcomes Attributed to Adverse Event** *(Check all that apply)*
   - ☐ Death: ____ *(mm/dd/yyyy)*
   - ☐ Disability or Permanent Damage
   - ☐ Life-threatening
   - ☐ Congenital Anomaly/Birth Defect
   - ☐ Hospitalization - initial or prolonged
   - ☐ Other Serious (Important Medical Events)
   - ☐ Required Intervention to Prevent Permanent Impairment/Damage (Devices)
3. **Date of Event** *(mm/dd/yyyy)*
4. **Date of This Report** *(mm/dd/yyyy)*
5. **Describe Event or Problem**
6. **Relevant Tests/Laboratory Data, Including Dates**
7. **Other Relevant History, Including Preexisting Medical Conditions** *(e.g., allergies, race, pregnancy, smoking and alcohol use, hepatic/renal dysfunction, etc.)*

PLEASE TYPE OR USE BLACK INK

Submission of a report does not constitute an admission that medical personnel, user facility, importer, distributor, manufacturer or product caused or contributed to the event.

C. SUSPECT PRODUCT(S)

1. **Name** *(Give labeled strength & mfr/labeler)*
   #1
   #2
2. **Dose, Frequency & Route Used**
   #1
   #2
3. **Therapy Dates** *(If unknown, give duration) from/to (or best estimate)*
   #1
   #2
4. **Diagnosis for Use** *(Indication)*
   #1
   #2
5. **Event Abated After Use Stopped or Dose Reduced?**
   #1 ☐ Yes ☐ No ☐ Doesn't Apply
   #2 ☐ Yes ☐ No ☐ Doesn't Apply
6. **Lot #**
   #1
   #2
7. **Exp. Date**
   #1
   #2
8. **Event Reappeared After Reintroduction?**
   #1 ☐ Yes ☐ No ☐ Doesn't Apply
   #2 ☐ Yes ☐ No ☐ Doesn't Apply
9. **NDC# or Unique ID**
10. **Concomitant Medical Products and Therapy Dates** *(Exclude treatment of event)*

D. SUSPECT MEDICAL DEVICE

1. **Brand Name**
2. **Common Device Name**
3. **Manufacturer Name, City and State**
4. **Model #** / **Lot #** / **Catalog #** / **Expiration Date** *(mm/dd/yyyy)* / **Serial #** / **Other #**
5. **Operator of Device**
   ☐ Health Professional
   ☐ Lay User/Patient
   ☐ Other: ____
6. **If Implanted, Give Date** *(mm/dd/yyyy)*
7. **If Explanted, Give Date** *(mm/dd/yyyy)*
8. **Is this a Single-use Device that was Reprocessed and Reused on a Patient?**
   ☐ Yes ☐ No
9. **If Yes to Item No. 8, Enter Name and Address of Reprocessor**
10. **Device Available for Evaluation?** *(Do not send to FDA)*
    ☐ Yes ☐ No ☐ Returned to Manufacturer on: ____ *(mm/dd/yyyy)*
11. **Concomitant Medical Products and Therapy Dates** *(Exclude treatment of event)*

E. INITIAL REPORTER

1. **Name and Address** / **Phone #**
2. **Health Professional?** ☐ Yes ☐ No
3. **Occupation**
4. **Initial Reporter Also Sent Report to FDA**
   ☐ Yes ☐ No ☐ Unk.

MEDWATCH

FORM FDA 3500A (10/05) *(continued)* **Page ____ of ____**

FDA USE ONLY

F. FOR USE BY USER FACILITY/IMPORTER *(Devices Only)*

1. **Check One**
   ☐ User Facility ☐ Importer
2. **UF/Importer Report Number**
3. **User Facility or Importer Name/Address**
4. **Contact Person**
5. **Phone Number**
6. **Date User Facility or Importer Became Aware of Event** *(mm/dd/yyyy)*
7. **Type of Report**
   ☐ Initial
   ☐ Follow-up # ________
8. **Date of This Report** *(mm/dd/yyyy)*
9. **Approximate Age of Device**
10. **Event Problem Codes** *(Refer to coding manual)*
    Patient Code ☐ - ☐ - ☐
    Device Code ☐ - ☐ - ☐
11. **Report Sent to FDA?**
    ☐ Yes ________ *(mm/dd/yyyy)*
    ☐ No
12. **Location Where Event Occurred**
    ☐ Hospital
    ☐ Home
    ☐ Nursing Home
    ☐ Outpatient Treatment Facility
    ☐ Outpatient Diagnostic Facility
    ☐ Ambulatory Surgical Facility
    ☐ Other: ________ *(Specify)*
13. **Report Sent to Manufacturer?**
    ☐ Yes ________ *(mm/dd/yyyy)*
    ☐ No
14. **Manufacturer Name/Address**

G. ALL MANUFACTURERS

1. **Contact Office - Name/Address** ***(and Manufacturing Site for Devices)***
2. **Phone Number**
3. **Report Source** *(Check all that apply)*
   ☐ Foreign
   ☐ Study
   ☐ Literature
   ☐ Consumer
   ☐ Health Professional
   ☐ User Facility
   ☐ Company Representative
   ☐ Distributor
   ☐ Other:
4. **Date Received by Manufacturer** *(mm/dd/yyyy)*
5. (A)NDA # ________
   IND # ________
   STN # ________
   PMA/ 510(k) # ________
   Combination Product ☐ Yes
   Pre-1938 ☐ Yes
   OTC Product ☐ Yes
6. **If IND, Give Protocol #**
7. **Type of Report** *(Check all that apply)*
   ☐ 5-day ☐ 30-day
   ☐ 7-day ☐ Periodic
   ☐ 10-day ☐ Initial
   ☐ 15-day ☐ Follow-up # ____
8. **Adverse Event Term(s)**
9. **Manufacturer Report Number**

H. DEVICE MANUFACTURERS ONLY

1. **Type of Reportable Event**
   ☐ Death
   ☐ Serious Injury
   ☐ Malfunction
   ☐ Other: ________
2. **If Follow-up, What Type?**
   ☐ Correction
   ☐ Additional Information
   ☐ Response to FDA Request
   ☐ Device Evaluation
3. **Device Evaluated by Manufacturer?**
   ☐ Not Returned to Manufacturer
   ☐ Yes ☐ Evaluation Summary Attached
   ☐ No *(Attach page to explain why not)* or provide code:
4. **Device Manufacture Date** *(mm/yyyy)*
5. **Labeled for Single Use?**
   ☐ Yes ☐ No
6. **Evaluation Codes** *(Refer to coding manual)*
   Method ☐ - ☐ - ☐ - ☐
   Results ☐ - ☐ - ☐ - ☐
   Conclusions ☐ - ☐ - ☐ - ☐
7. **If Remedial Action Initiated, Check Type**
   ☐ Recall ☐ Notification
   ☐ Repair ☐ Inspection
   ☐ Replace ☐ Patient Monitoring
   ☐ Relabeling ☐ Modification/ Adjustment
   ☐ Other: ________
8. **Usage of Device**
   ☐ Initial Use of Device
   ☐ Reuse
   ☐ Unknown
9. **If action reported to FDA under 21 USC 360i(f), list correction/ removal reporting number:**

10. ☐ **Additional Manufacturer Narrative** and / or 11. ☐ **Corrected Data**

The public reporting burden for this collection of information has been estimated to average 66 minutes per response, including the time for reviewing instructions, searching existing data sources, gathering and maintaining the data needed, and completing and reviewing the collection of information. Send comments regarding this burden estimate or any other aspect of this collection of information, including suggestions for reducing this burden to:

Department of Health and Human Services
Food and Drug Administration - MedWatch
10903 New Hampshire Avenue
Building 22, Mail Stop 4447
Silver Spring, MD 20993-0002

Please DO NOT RETURN this form to this address.

OMB Statement:
"An agency may not conduct or sponsor, and a person is not required to respond to, a collection of information unless it displays a currently valid OMB control number."

Appendix F

Biographical Sketches of Workshop Speakers

LT. COL. Sonya Corum, M.B.A., is currently serving as Director of the Experimentation and Analysis Element at the U.S. Army Training Center, Fort Jackson, South Carolina. She graduated with a B.S. in Food and Nutrition from Appalachian State University in Boone, North Carolina, in 1988. Her first assignment after completing the Dietetic Internship at Brooke Army Medical Center was at Ireland Army Community Hospital, Fort Knox, Kentucky, as the Chief, Clinical Dietetics. Since that time, Lieutenant Colonel Corum has held a number of positions in medical treatment facilities including Chief, Production and Service at William Beaumont Army Medical Center, and Chief, Nutrition Care at Fort Campbell. She also deployed with the 86th Combat Support Hospital in support of Hurricane Mitch relief. She has served as the Executive Fellow to the Chief, Medical Specialist Corps. Lieutenant Colonel Corum was the Nutrition Staff Officer at the U.S. Army Center for Health Promotion and Preventive Medicine (USA-CHPPM) where she spearheaded the Army's Dietary Supplement Education Campaign. She also deployed with the 31st Combat Support Hospital in support of Operation Iraqi Freedom. Lieutenant Colonel Corum received an M.B.A. from the University of Texas, El Paso, and is a Command and General Staff College graduate.

Gerald J. Dal Pan, M.D., M.H.S., is the Director of the Office of Surveillance and Epidemiology in the U.S. Food and Drug Administration's Center for Drug Evaluation and Research (FDA/CDER). Prior to that, he was the Director of the Division of Surveillance, Research, and Communication Support in CDER's Office of Drug Safety, a position he had held since

December 2003. He received his medical degree from Columbia University, and his master's degree in clinical epidemiology from Johns Hopkins University. He trained in internal medicine at the Hospital of the University of Pennsylvania, and in neurology at the Johns Hopkins Hospital. He is board certified in internal medicine and neurology. Dr. Dal Pan was an instructor in the Neurology Department at Johns Hopkins University. He next worked for Guilford Pharmaceuticals in Baltimore, and then for HHI Clinical Research and Statistical Services in Hunt Valley, Maryland. He joined the FDA in July 2000 as a medical officer in the Division of Anesthetic, Critical Care, and Addiction Drug Products.

Vasilios Frankos, Ph.D., serves as the Director, Division of Dietary Supplement Programs (DDSP) and the lead scientist for dietary supplements for the FDA and is responsible for the full implementation of the Dietary Supplement Health and Education Act of 1994. He directs and coordinates policy and administrative activities within the division. He advises on policy and management issues on dietary supplement programs, new dietary ingredient safety assessments, good manufacturing practice, and adverse reaction monitoring, and related activities pertaining to dietary supplements. Before becoming the Director of DDSP, Dr. Frankos also served as Special Assistant for Dietary Supplement Science Review providing toxicological and pharmacological evaluation of data used to assess the risks posed by dietary supplement products, Staff Science Advisor in the Office of the Commissioner, and as a Senior Toxicologist in the Center for Food Safety and Applied Nutrition. Dr. Frankos received his M.S. in molecular biology from the University of Maryland and his Ph.D. in pharmacology and toxicology from the University of Maryland Pharmacy School. He has over 30 years' experience in the toxicological and pharmacological evaluation of data used to assess the safety of FDA-regulated products. In addition to his FDA activities, he spent 18 years as a principal in the consulting firm ENVIRON International Corp.

Steve French, M.B.A., is the Managing Partner of the Natural Marketing Institute, with over 25 years of strategic marketing, business development, market research, and management experience. Complementing a B.S. and M.B.A. in marketing, Mr. French has accumulated extensive insight and knowledge into health, wellness, environmentalism, and social responsibility. He has unparalleled experience across a wide range of corporate business functions and has pioneered a range of consumer research databases. Mr. French is a frequent speaker at many industry events and conferences, and is regularly utilized by television, radio, magazine, newspaper, Internet, and other media sources. He is also an author of numerous published articles and written research reports used across many industries.

Paula Gardiner, M.D., M.P.H., is an Assistant Professor in the Department of Family Medicine at Boston University Medical School. She is a former Research Fellow at the Division for Research and Education in Complementary and Integrative Medical Therapies, Osher Institute, Harvard Medical School. Her research focuses on use of dietary supplements by adults and adolescents in the U.S. population. Additionally, her research has focused on the safety issues surrounding dietary supplements, such as prescription medication and dietary supplement interactions and adverse event reporting. As a member of the United States Pharmacopeia's Dietary Supplements Expert Committee, she has focused on improving adverse event reporting in the United States.

Mary Hardy, M.D., serves as the Codirector of the Integrative Medicine Health and Wellness Program at the Venice Family Clinic, the largest free clinic in the United States. Her clinical practice now involves educating cancer patients in integrative therapies at the Ted Mann Family Integrative Oncology Program at the University of California, Los Angeles. Her current research interests include reviewing the evidence for the safety and efficacy of natural therapies, especially botanicals. Dr. Hardy is board certified in internal medicine and a specialist in botanical and integrative medicine and has actively combined complementary and alternative therapies with traditional Western medicine for many years. A graduate of Louisiana State University School of Medicine in New Orleans, Dr. Hardy completed her internal medicine residency at the Tufts New England Medical Center before studying medical ethics at Harvard Divinity School and Loma Linda University. She completed advanced training in botanical medicine at the Institute for Medical Herbalism and has studied with practitioners in Peru, Kenya, South Africa, and China. She is the complementary and alternative medicine expert for a number of research projects conducted by the Southern California Evidence-Based Practice Center of the RAND Corporation. In addition, she has expanded her interest in botanical research by serving for two and a half years as the Associate Director of the Botanical Research Center of the University of California, Los Angeles, funded by the National Institutes of Health (NIH). Dr. Hardy also serves on the scientific advisory board of the American Botanical Council and the editorial boards of *Alternative Medicine Alert*, *Alternative Therapies in Women's Health*, *Evidence-Based Complementary and Alternative Medicine*, *FACT* as well as *Phytomedicine*. Dr. Hardy is recognized as an authority on integrative medicine and natural products by organizations such as the NIH Office of Dietary Supplements, the California Medical Board, the American Medical Association, the American Pharmaceutical Association, CBS, NBC, Discovery Channel, and the *Los Angeles Times*. She is a founding member of the Advisory Council for the newly established Naturopathic Medicine Board of California and has recently been appointed to the External Advisory Council for the Natural Product Directorate of the Canadian government. The multidisciplinary clinic she founded at Cedars-Sinai Medical Center in the department of Medicine in 1998 allowed her to explore the practical and philosophical issues that both facilitate and impede the development of integrative medicine as a discipline. Contributing to the national development of integrative medicine, she serves as the cochairperson of the Clinical Practice Committee of the Academic Consortium of Integrative Medicine (an organization of the leading medical schools practicing and teaching in this area). Dr. Hardy recently completed a book for Reader's Digest, *Best Remedies*, which focuses on integrative medicine. She is also conducting a review of the quality of research trials in herbal medicine and is finishing a systematic review on the effects of dietary supplements on coagulation for the NIH Office of Dietary Supplements.

LT. COL. Paul J. Hoerner is currently the Deputy Director of the U.S. Department of Defense (DoD) Patient Safety Center (PSC). He directs the daily operations of the PSC, with a budget of $1.5 million, serving more than 576 DoD medical treatment facilities and 9.2 million beneficiaries worldwide. This includes quarterly, annual, and bimonthly publications, safety alerts, and focused analysis for use by DoD, Army, Navy, and Air Force facilities to improve patient safety. Arriving at the PSC in September 2006, he had recently completed a 1-year fellowship at a medial malpractice insurance company. Prior to that assignment, he was the Chief of Pharmacy Operations at David Grant Medical Center. The pharmacy processed over 3,500 outpatient prescriptions and prepared over 1,600 inpatient orders daily. He provided oversight of all aspects of the pharmacy's various elements (clinical, support, inpatient, and outpatient). Colonel Hoerner's career goals are to advance his leadership capabilities and expertise in the fields of pharmacy and patient safety.

LT. COL. Danny B. N. Jaghab has been the Nutrition Staff Officer for the U.S. Army Center for Health Promotion and Preventive Medicine (USACHPPM) at Aberdeen Proving Ground, Maryland, since 2004. His work includes analyzing and assessing current policies and developing and implementing new health promotion and nutrition policies and regulations that better meet the needs of the DoD. He collaborates with federal and national agencies on projects and initiatives as the sole subject-matter expert on nutrition for the U.S. Army. From July 2002 to July 2004, he directed the U.S. Military Dietetic Internship Consortium at the Brooke Army Medical Center in San Antonio, Texas. He was also previously the Chief of the Nutrition Care Division at the DeWitt Army Community Hospital in Fort Belvoir, Virginia. He was a Bronze Star Medal recipient during Operation

Desert Shield/Storm; recipient of the 2004 American Dietetic Association's Media Excellence Award; recipient of the 2004 Department of Defense Patient Safety Award in the category of Technology; and was elected the 2006 Career Guidance Chair, American Dietetic Association's National Organization of Men in Nutrition. He received his B.S. in nutrition and dietetics from Drexel University in Philadelphia, Pennsylvania, and his M.S. in education and counseling from the Long Island University in West Point, New York.

David Kaufman, Sc.D., is Professor of Epidemiology at the Boston University School of Public Health. He obtained his B.A. in 1973 from Bethel College, North Newton, Kansas, and his M.S. in 1979 and Sc.D. in 1983 in Epidemiology from the Harvard School of Public Health. In 1975, he joined the newly created Drug Epidemiology Unit (DEU) (subsequently renamed Slone Epidemiology Unit, and since 2001 the Slone Epidemiology Center) as a Research Associate. Dr. Kaufman was Assistant Director of the Slone Epidemiology Unit from 1986 to 1997, and has been Associate Director since 1998. His early career as an epidemiologist at the DEU was primarily spent in studies of drugs and other factors in relation to cancer, heart disease, and various other conditions. Together with Drs. Slone, Shapiro, and Lynn Rosenberg, he participated in the development of Case-Control Surveillance. In the 1980s, Dr. Kaufman was coinvestigator of the International Agranulocytosis and Aplastic Anemia Study, a pioneering effort in the evaluation of these extremely rare but often drug-induced blood dyscrasias, that was conducted in seven countries with several hundred cases enrolled; he coauthored a book describing the results. He has since directed studies of aplastic anemia in Thailand and the United States and served as an adviser to a study of that disease in Brazil. The Thai study is the largest epidemiological investigation of aplastic anemia that has been conducted, with over 500 cases and 2,200 controls. Dr. Kaufman pursued his interest in rare drug-induced diseases as principal investigator of an international study of Stevens-Johnson syndrome and toxic epidermal necrolysis conducted in four countries in Europe, and a study of anaphylaxis conducted in Spain, Hungary, India, and Sweden. Other major activities have included an international study of analgesics in relation to upper gastrointestinal bleeding, and more recently, the National Analgesic Nephropathy Study, a multicenter study of end-stage renal disease patients in three regions of the United States. Dr. Kaufman worked closely with Allen Mitchell in the development of the Slone Survey, a U.S. population-based survey of medication and dietary supplement use that was initiated in 1998; he is principally responsible for the implementation of that project. Another current study is exploring the relationship of *Oxalobacter formigenes*, an oxalate-metabolizing bacterium found in the colons of about 70 percent of the normal population, and calcium oxalate kidney stones. Dr. Kaufman is also the Principal Investigator of recently launched national patient registries of multiple myeloma and myelodysplastic syndromes (Patient Registries at Slone: Myeloma and MDS).

Rick Kingston, PharmD., is President, Regulatory and Scientific Affairs for SafetyCall International, a multidisciplinary medical practice and poison center focused on corporate postmarket surveillance and product safety for drugs, dietary supplements, and consumer products. He has a 28-year academic career, having attained the rank of full professor in the Department of Experimental and Clinical Pharmacology, and is currently serving as Clinical Professor of Pharmacy in the College of Pharmacy at the University of Minnesota. At the University of Minnesota, he is course director for the didactic course "Therapeutics of Herbs and Other Natural Medicinals" taught in the College of Pharmacy and has previously served as a member of the University's Center for Plants and Human Health and the National Center for Complementary and Alternative Medicine-funded integrative medicine Center for Spirituality and Healing. Previously, Dr. Kingston was cofounder and former Director of the Minnesota Regional Poison Center and its affiliated industry toxicology and product safety surveillance service programs at St. Paul-Ramsey Medical Center in St. Paul, Minnesota. Dr. Kingston completed his B.S. in Pharmacy at the University of New Mexico, his PharmD. in Clinical Pharmacy at the University of Minnesota, and a postdoctoral fellowship in clinical toxicology and pharmacokinetics at St. Paul-Ramsey Medical Center and the University of Minnesota. His 28-year professional experience has been centered in the areas of clinical toxicology and pharmacology, poison control, product postmarket surveillance, and drug and dietary supplement safety. His research and practice interests coincide with SafetyCall International initiatives for corporate clients and include a focus on injury prevention, the epidemiology of toxicology-related incident data, product safety and related regulatory affairs, and specific advances in the clinical management or triage of patients being treated or evaluated for drug, toxin, or consumer product exposures.

Harris R. Lieberman, Ph.D., is a Research Psychologist in the Military Nutrition Division of the U.S. Army Research Institute of Environmental Medicine (USARIEM) in Natick, Massachusetts. He is an internationally recognized expert in the area of nutrition and behavior and has published over 125 original, full-length papers in scientific journals and edited books. Dr. Lieberman received his Ph.D. in Physiological Psychology in 1977 from the University of Florida and then conducted postdoctoral research at the Department of Psychology and Brain Science at the Massachusetts Institute of Technology (MIT). From 1980 to 1990 he was on the staff at MIT, where he examined the effects of food constituents and drugs on human behavior and brain function. In 1990 he joined the civilian research staff of USARIEM where he continued his work in nutrition, behavior, and stress. From 1994 to 2000 he was Chief or Deputy Chief of the Military Nutrition program at USARIEM. His recent research has addressed the effects of various nutritional factors, diets, and environmental stress on cognitive performance and brain function. He holds two patents for novel technologies to assess and enhance cognitive performance. He currently chairs his institute's scientific research committee and serves on the DoD Dietary Supplements Committee and several other national and international committees.

Bernadette M. Marriott, Ph.D., is Principal Associate and Senior Scientist at Abt Associates, and has 38 years of experience in the fields of nutrition, psychology, and comparative medicine, with expertise in diet, nutrition and chronic disease. Dr. Marriott has worked in scientific settings in the federal government, universities, and foundations. Her research has focused on nutrition and related behavioral studies, specifically diet and health research, and food labeling. She currently holds an adjunct full professor position in the Department of Nutritional Sciences, University of North Carolina School of Medicine, and has held previous academic positions of assistant through full professor. Other positions include Vice President for Science Integration, RTI International, Founding Director of the NIH Office of Dietary Supplements, Deputy Director of the Food and Nutrition Board of the Institute of Medicine (IOM), Vice Provost for Research and Dean of Graduate Studies at Northern Arizona University, Vice President for Programs and Communications for the Burroughs Wellcome Fund, and Associate Director of the Caribbean Primate Research Center, University of Puerto Rico. While at the IOM, she oversaw the activities of the Committee on Military Nutrition Research for 8 years and is very familiar with the nutrient requirements of active duty personnel, nutrient composition of ration packages, exercise, and weight management in the military services. At the IOM, she edited, helped write, and/or oversaw the production of 24 reports; of particular relevance to this study are *Food Components to Enhance Performance (DoD)* and *Guiding Principles for Nutrition Labeling and Food Fortification*, for which she was a special consultant and which addresses foods and dietary supplements. Dr. Marriott has extensive experience managing complex programs, building consensus, and working with scientific data. She currently is principal investigator on two NIH-funded projects on adult and child intake, a corporate-funded project on infant feeding, an obesity study supported by the Office of Science and Technology Policy, and was the scientific lead for diet, exercise, weight management, and related health indicators on the *2005 Department of Defense (DoD) Survey of Health Related Behaviors Among Military Personnel* with Bob Bray. Prior to leaving RTI, she was principal investigator on the TRICARE Management Activity-funded *Weight Management Demonstration Project:*

Healthy Eating and Active Living in TRICARE Households (HEALTH). Bernadette Marriott has a B.Sc. in biology/immunology from Bucknell University, a Ph.D. in psychology from King's College, Aberdeen, Scotland, and postgraduate training in trace mineral nutrition, comparative medicine, and advanced statistics. She has published extensively, is on a number of national committees, and is a frequent speaker on diet, dietary supplements, and health.

Scott J. Montain, Ph.D., is a research physiologist working in the Military Nutrition Division at USARIEM, Natick, Massachusetts. Dr. Montain received an M.S. from Ball State University in 1984 and a Ph.D. from the University of Texas at Austin in 1991 before completing postdoctoral training at USARIEM. He is author or coauthor of over 95 peer-reviewed journal articles, book chapters, and reports. Dr. Montain currently serves as Councilor for the Exercise and Environmental Physiology section of the American Physiological Society, and is a Fellow of the American College of Sports Medicine.

LT. COL. Charity Thomasos, M.S., is currently stationed at Eglin Air Force Base, Florida, as the Director of Nutritional Medicine Flight. She earned her B.S. in clinical nutrition/dietetics from West Virginia Wesleyan College, Buckhannon, West Virginia, and her M.S. in human nutrition/biochemistry from the Ohio State University, Columbus. She is a member of the American Dietetic Association and the Nutrition and Complementary Medicine practice group. Lieutenant Colonel Thomasos is the Air Force Dietetics Representative to the DoD Dietary Supplement Committee and a member of the Special Operations Forces subcommittee.

Andrew J. Young, Ph.D., is a research physiologist and Chief of the Military Nutrition Division at USARIEM in Natick, Massachusetts. He obtained a B.S. in biology at Virginia Military Institute and a Ph.D. in physiology at North Carolina State University, then served in the U.S. Army with assignments at USARIEM (1977–1981) and at the Walter Reed Army Institute of Research (1981–1983). After leaving the Army, Dr. Young continued as a civilian scientist at USARIEM. His research has concerned the biological basis for, and strategies to mitigate, performance degradation in people experiencing intense physical exertion, sleep restriction, nutritional deprivation, and exposure to extremes of heat, cold, and high altitude, all of which are characteristics of sustained combat operations. Dr. Young is a member of the American Physiological Society and a Fellow of the American College of Sports Medicine. He is also Editor in Chief of the American College of Sports Medicine's flagship scientific journal, *Medicine and Science in Sports and Exercise*.

Appendix G

Biographical Sketches of Committee Members

M.R.C. Greenwood, Ph.D., is Professor of Nutrition and Internal Medicine, Chair of the graduate group in Nutritional Biology, Director of the Foods for Health Initiative at the University of California, Davis, and Chancellor Emerita, University of California, Santa Cruz. Her previous positions include Chancellor of the University of California, Santa Cruz, from 1996 to 2004 and University of California Provost and Senior Vice President of Academic Affairs. Prior to her Santa Cruz appointments, she was Dean of Graduate Studies and Vice Provost for Academic Outreach and Professor of Biology and Internal Medicine at University of California, Davis. Prior to that, she taught at Vassar College, where she was Chair of the Department of Biology and Director of the Undergraduate Research Summer Institute and was on the adjunct faculty of Columbia University's medical school. From November 1993 to May 1995, while on leave from the University of California, Davis, Greenwood served as Associate Director for Science at the Office of Science and Technology Policy in the Executive Office of the President of the United States. She has been a member of the Institute of Medicine (IOM) of the National Academies (NAS) since 1992. She is currently the Chair of the NAS Policy and Global Affairs Committee. She was a member of the Food and Nutrition Board from 1985 to 1990 and served as chair from 1990 to 1993. She is also a Fellow of the American Academy of Arts and Sciences as well as the American Association for the Advancement of Science, serving as its president in 1998 and chair in 1999. She has been President of the American Society for Clinical Nutrition and NAASO, the Obesity Society. Dr. Greenwood received her A.B., summa cum laude, from Vassar College, and received her Ph.D. from Rockefeller University. Her research areas include obesity, diabetes, and women's health.

Cheryl Anderson, Ph.D., M.P.H., is an Assistant Professor in the Department of Epidemiology at the Johns Hopkins Bloomberg School of Public Health. Previously, she was an Instructor of Epidemiology at the University of Pennsylvania School of Medicine, Center for Clinical Epidemiology and Biostatistics. Dr. Anderson's research centers on diet and the prevention of chronic diseases in minority and underserved populations. Her current research projects address diet and the prevention of cardiovascular disease (CVD) in the context of chronic kidney disease and the optimal macronutrient intake in CVD prevention. Dr. Anderson is a member of the American Heart Association Committee on Nutrition and Physical Activity. She is also a Dannon Institute Nutrition Leadership Institute (NLI) Scholar and the current President of the NLI Alumni Association. She recently served on the National Institutes of Health (NIH) National Institute of Neurologic Disorders and Stroke Writing Group on Primary Prevention of Stroke. She has an A.B. from Brown University, M.P.H. from the University of North Carolina at Chapel Hill, and an M.S. in epidemiology and a Ph.D. in nutritional sciences from the Department of Epidemiology at the University of Washington School of Public Health and Community Medicine.

Bruce R. Bistrian, M.D., Ph.D., is Professor of Medicine at Harvard Medical School and Chief of Clinical Nutrition, Beth Israel Deaconess Medical Center. Formerly he was Codirector of Hyperalimentation Services, New England Deaconess Hospital, and a lecturer in the Department of Nutrition and Food Science, Massachusetts Institute of Technology (MIT). Dr. Bistrian's primary research interests include nutritional assessment, the metabolic effects of acute infections, nutritional support of hospitalized patients, and the pathophysiology of protein-calorie malnutrition. He is a Fellow of the American College of Physicians, and has received an honorary M.A. from Harvard University. Dr. Bistrian is the 2004 recipient of the Goldberger Award of the American Medical Association. Dr. Bistrian has been President of the American Society for Parenteral and Enteral Nutrition, President of the American Society of Clinical Nutrition, and President of the Federation of American Societies of Experimental Biology. He currently serves on the IOM Committee on Military Nutrition Research. Dr. Bistrian has served on the editorial boards of numerous nutrition and medical journals, and is the author or coauthor of over 400 articles for scientific publications. He earned his M.D. from Cornell University, his M.P.H. from Johns Hopkins University, and his Ph.D. in nutritional biochemistry and metabolism from MIT. Dr. Bistrian is board certified in internal medicine and was certified in critical care medicine from 1987 to 2007.

John W. Erdman, Jr., Ph.D., is Professor of Nutrition and Food Science in the Department of Food Science and Human Nutrition and a Professor in the Department of Internal Medicine at the University of Illinois at Urbana-Champaign. His research interests include the effects of food processing on nutrient retention, the metabolic roles of vitamin A and beta-carotene, and the effects of tomatoes and broccoli and their bioactive components on risk of prostate cancer. His research regarding soy protein has extended into studies on the impact of nonnutrient components of foods, such as phytoestrogens, on chronic disease. Dr. Erdman has published over 160 peer-reviewed research papers. He chaired the 1988 Gordon Conference on Carotenoids, and has served as a Burroughs Wellcome Visiting Professor in Basic Medical Sciences at the University of Georgia, and the G. Malcolm Trout Visiting Scholar at Michigan State University. His awards include the Borden Award from the American Society for Nutritional Sciences and the Babcock-Hart Award from the Institute of Food Technologists. Dr. Erdman has served on many editorial boards, and on many program and planning committees for the American Society of Nutritional Sciences, the Institute of Food Technologists, and the NAS. In 1992, he was elected a Fellow of the Institute of Food Technologists, and in 2003 he was elected a Fellow of the American Heart Association. Dr. Erdman was elected to the IOM in 2003. He received his M.S. and Ph.D. in food science from Rutgers University.

William C. Franke, Ph.D., is an Associate Director of the Center for Advanced Food Technology at Rutgers University. He provides technical expertise in the area of product development and food regulations, especially as related to functional foods and nutraceuticals, and develops new opportunities for technology transfer to small and large companies. He also contributes to administration, marketing, and strategic planning. He is a coprincipal investigator for a U.S. Department of Defense contract to develop combat rations to improve the physical and mental performance of soldiers under stress. Previously, he spent 28 years at Lipton/Unilever and served in a number of senior management positions in product development, quality assurance, and regulatory affairs. Most recently, he was Vice President for Scientific and Regulatory Affairs with Unilever United States before he retired. He is a former member of the NAS/IOM Food Forum and served on the IOM expert Committee on Evaluation of the Addition of Ingredients New to Infant Formula. He also served as a member of the board of the Cancer Institute of New Jersey and was recently elected a Fellow of the Institute of Food Technologists. Dr. Franke founded Heart Blend Foods LLC, an R&D company that specializes in the development of heart-healthy foods, in 2005. The company's objective is to license technology and/or bring products to market that improve public health.

Elizabeth Jeffery, Ph.D., is Professor of Nutritional Toxicology and Professor of Nutritional Sciences at the University of Illinois. Dr. Jeffery teaches and performs research in the area of safety and efficacy of functional foods and dietary supplements, with emphasis on biochemical mechanisms of cancer prevention by broccoli and related crucifers. A toxicologist by training, Dr. Jeffery has held elected positions on the Education and Nominating Committees of the Society of Toxicology. She is past President of the Midwest Regional Chapter of the Society of Toxicology and past Chair of the Toxicology specialty section in the American Society for Pharmacology and Experimental Therapeutics. She is past Director of Research Interest Sections and past Chair of the Dietary Bioactive Components Research Interest Section of the American Nutrition Society. She served on the NAS Committee on the Framework for Evaluating the Safety of Dietary Supplements. She has served as an Associate Editor for the *Journal of Toxicology and Applied Pharmacology* and as guest Field Editor for the *Journal of Pharmacology and Experimental Therapeutics*, and is involved in the review of research grant proposals for both the NIH and the U.S. Department of Agriculture (USDA). Dr. Jeffery has a Ph.D. in biochemistry from the University of London, England.

Robin B. Kanarek, Ph.D., is Professor of Psychology at Tufts University in Medford, Massachusetts. Her prior positions include Research Fellow, Division of Endocrinology, University of California, Los Angeles (UCLA) School of Medicine; Research Fellow in Nutrition at Harvard University; and Professor of Nutrition, Chair of the Psychology Department and Dean of the Graduate School of Arts and Sciences at Tufts University. She is a member of the editorial boards of *Physiology and Behavior, Nutritional Neuroscience*, and the *Tufts Diet and Nutrition Newsletter* and is a past Editor in Chief of *Nutrition and Behavior*. Dr. Kanarek has served on ad hoc review committees for the National Science Foundation, the NIH, and USDA nutrition research, as well as the Member Program Committee of the Eastern Psychological Association. She is a fellow of the American College of Nutrition and the North American Society for the Study of Obesity; her other professional memberships include the American Institute of Nutrition, New York Academy of Sciences, Society for the Study of Ingestive Behavior, and Society for Neurosciences. Dr. Kanarek received a B.A. in biology from Antioch College in Yellow Springs, Ohio, and an M.S. and a Ph.D. in psychology from Rutgers University in New Brunswick, New Jersey.

Carl L. Keen, Ph.D., is Chairman of the Department of Nutrition at the University of California, Davis, and a Professor of Nutrition and Internal Medicine. Dr. Keen's research focuses on the influence of diet on embryonic and fetal development, the study of gene–nutrient interactions (emphasizing how subtle changes in cell mineral concentrations influence the expression of select genes), dietary influences on oxidant defense systems and as a consequence the occurrence of cellular oxidative damage, and the influence of dietary flavonoids on vascular health. He has served on numerous government boards including California's Scientific Advisory Board for the Office of Environmental Health Hazard Assessment, numerous Environmental Protection Agency Environmental Health Grant Review Panels, the USDA Human Nutrient Requirements Study Section, and several NIH study sections. He has served on a number of editorial boards and is a member of the American Society for Nutrition, the Teratology Society, the Society for Experimental Biology and Medicine, and the American Association for the Advancement of Science.

Gail B. Mahady, Ph.D., is Associate Professor of Pharmacy Practice and Director of the Clinical Pharmacognosy Laboratory at the University of Illinois at Chicago. Dr. Mahady's research interests include the discovery of novel natural agents for treatment or prevention of infectious disease, specifically plant-based antimicrobial drugs for the prevention and treatment of *Helicobacter pylori* and *Chlamydia* infections in humans; the assessment of clinical safety and efficacy of herbal supplements globally for the symptomatic treatment of menopause, premenstrual syndrome, and chronic urinary tract infections; and the assessment of quality, safety, and efficacy of botanicals for the World Health Organization's (WHO) Traditional Medicines Programme. She is a member of research faculty within the Pan American Health Organization/WHO Collaborating Center for Traditional Medicine at the College of Pharmacy, University of Illinois at Chicago. She is an Elected Member of the United States Pharmacopeia Dietary Supplements Information Expert Panel and a member of the review panel for the National Center for Complementary and Alternative Medicine's Annual Bibliography of Significant Advances in Dietary Supplement Research, among many NIH review panels. Dr. Mahady received her Ph.D. in Pharmacognosy from the University of Illinois at Chicago.

Sanford A. Miller, Ph.D., is a Senior Fellow at the Center for Food and Nutrition Policy at the University of Maryland, College Park. In December 2000, he was named Professor and Dean Emeritus of the Graduate School of Biomedical Sciences at the University of Texas Health Science Center at San Antonio, where he was the Dean of the Graduate School of Biomedical Sciences, and Professor in the Departments of Biochemistry and Medicine from 1987 to 2000. He is the former Director of the Center for Food Safety and Applied Nutrition at the U.S. Food and Drug Administration. Previously, he was a Professor of Nutritional Biochemistry at MIT. Dr. Miller has served on many national and international government and professional society advisory committees, including as Chair of the Joint FAO/WHO

(Food and Agriculture Organization/World Health Organization) Expert Consultation on the Application of Risk Analysis to Food Standards Issues. Dr. Miller's professional honors include the Atwater Memorial Lectureship Award from the USDA Agricultural Research Service, the Babcock-Hart Award from International Life Sciences Institute and the Institute of Food Technologists, the Conrad A. Elvehjem Award of the American Institute of Nutrition, the Esther Peterson Consumer Service Award from the Food Marketing Institute, the Sterling B. Hendricks Award from the USDA, and election as Fellow of the American Society for Nutrition. In June 2000, he was the recipient of the FDA's Distinguished Alumni Award. He has been a member of many NAS committees, including the Food and Nutrition Board's Standing Committee on the Scientific Evaluation of Dietary Reference Intakes, and Subcommittee on Upper Reference Levels of Nutrients and Panel on Macronutrients. He was named a National Associate of NAS in 2002. He is author or coauthor of more than 200 original scientific publications. Dr. Miller received a B.S. in chemistry from the City College of New York, and an M.S. and a Ph.D. in physiology and biochemistry from Rutgers University.

Esther F. Myers, Ph.D., R.D., is Director of Research and Scientific Affairs at the American Dietetic Association (ADA), a position she has held since October 2000, after retiring from the Air Force and serving as Chief Consultant to the Air Force Surgeon General. Dr. Myers currently focuses on research activities needed for the dietetics profession and the association, as well as the ADA strategic leadership initiative on obesity and the ADA Foundation initiative Healthy Weight for Kids. She has been actively involved in the development of ADA's evidence analysis process and in research projects focusing on evaluating the impact of nutrition services in Medicare Demonstration projects and in collaboration with Blue Cross and Blue Shield of North Carolina. She is the ADA staff liaison with the Nutrition Care Process and Standardized Language Committee, which is developing and validating terminology to reflect nutrition care for standardized language systems and electronic health records. Prior to joining ADA, she served as a site visitor for the Commission on Accreditation for Dietetics Education, a peer reviewer for the *Journal of the American Dietetic Association*, and a member of the Health Services Research Task Force overseeing dietetic outcomes research. She was a member of the IOM Committee on Nutrition Services for Medicare Beneficiaries. Dr. Myers received her undergraduate degree from North Dakota State University, her master's degree from the Ohio State University, and her doctorate from Kansas State University.

Janet Walberg Rankin, Ph.D., is a Professor in the Department of Human Nutrition, Foods, and Exercise at Virginia Polytechnic Institute and State

University. She has also served as Chair of its Food, Nutrition, and Health Initiative and acting Department Head as well as Associate Director, and then Interim Director of the University's new Institute for Biomedical and Public Health Sciences. Dr. Rankin's research is related to sports nutrition and interventions for obesity, with specific areas of interest that include the effects of dietary macronutrient mix, energy balance, and dietary supplements on performance, body composition, and immunity. Her current research focuses on dietary manipulations that may affect inflammation and oxidative stress in athletes and obese individuals. Dr. Rankin's affiliation with professional organizations has included membership on the Executive Board and later serving as President of the Southeast Chapter of the American College of Sports Medicine. She is a Fellow of the American College of Sports Medicine, has served as its Vice President, and has been a member or chair on many national committees for this organization. Dr. Rankin received her bachelor's degree in zoology from Duke University and her doctorate in nutrition with a minor in exercise physiology from the University of California, Davis.

Consultant

David F. Dinges, Ph.D., is Professor and Chief of the Division of Sleep and Chronobiology, and Director of the Unit for Experimental Psychiatry in the Department of Psychiatry at the University of Pennsylvania School of Medicine. His research focuses on physiological, neurobehavioral, and psychological effects of sleep loss, disturbances of circadian biology, and stress, and the implications of these unmitigated effects on health and safety. He has performed extensive scientific work on development and validation of behavioral, technological, and pharmacological countermeasures for these effects. His research has been supported by grants from the NIH, the National Aeronautics and Space Administration (NASA), the U.S. Department of Defense, the U.S. Department of Transportation, and the Department of Homeland Security. He currently leads the Neurobehavioral and Psychosocial Factors Team for the NASA-funded National Space Biomedical Research Institute. He is a member of the National Advisory Council for Nursing Research of the NIH. He has been President of the U.S. Sleep Research Society and of the World Federation of Sleep Research and Sleep Medicine Societies, and served on the Board of Directors of the American Academy of Sleep Medicine and the National Sleep Foundation. He is currently Editor in Chief of *SLEEP*. He has received numerous awards, including the 2004 Decade of Behavior Research Award from the American Psychological Association, and the 2007 NASA Distinguished Public Service Medal.

Appendix H

Acronyms and Abbreviations

AAFES	Army and Air Force Exchange Service
ADC	Average daily consumption
ADL	Activities of daily living
AI	Adequate Intake
ALS	Amyotrophic lateral sclerosis
AMDR	Acceptable Macronutrient Distribution Range
AMEDD	Army Medical Department
AMS	Acute mountain sickness
ANS	Autonomic nervous system
APFT	Army Physical Fitness Test
ATP	Adenosine-5′-triphosphate
AUC	Area under the curve
BMD	Bone mineral density
BMI	Body mass index
BP	Blood pressure
CAM	Complementary and Alternative Medicine
CDR	Cognitive drug research
CFF	Critical flicker fusion
CGI	Clinical Global Impression scale
cGMP	Current good manufacturing practice
CHPPM	Center for Health Promotion and Preventive Medicine
CK	Creatine kinase
CNS	Central nervous system

CRT	Choice reaction time
CSFII	Continuing Survey of Food Intakes by Individuals
CVD	Cardiovascular disease
CYP2D6	Cytochrome P450 2D6
DEXA	Dual energy X-ray absorptiometry
DFE	Dietary Folate Equivalents
DHEA	Dehydroepiandrosterone
DHEA-S	the sulfated form of DHEA circulating in the body
DoD	Department of Defense
DRI	Dietary Reference Intake
DS	Dietary supplement
DSHEA	Dietary Supplement Health and Education Act
DSI EC	Dietary supplement information executive committee
DSID	Dietary Supplement Ingredient Database
DSNDCPA	Dietary Supplement and Nonprescription Drug Consumer Protection Act
DSVP	Dietary supplement verification program
EAR	Estimated Average Requirement
ECG	Electrocardiogram
EEG	Electroencephalography
EMG	Electromyography
EOG	Electrooculography
ER	Emergency room
ERGO	Energy rich, glucose optimized
ESP	E-screener panel
FDA	U.S. Food and Drug Administration
FFD&C Act	Federal Food, Drug, and Cosmetic Act
GABA	Gamma-aminobutyric acid
GAS	Ginseng abuse syndrome
GI	Gastrointestinal
GRAS	Generally recognized as safe
HAS	High-altitude sickness
HDL	High-density lipoprotein
HFA	Health and Fitness Assessment
HMB	β-Hydroxy-β-methylbutyrate
HMG-CoA	3-Hydroxy-3-methylglutaryl coenzyme A
HPPI	Health Promotion and Prevention Initiative
HR	Heart rate

IARC	International Agency for Research on Cancer
ICW	Intracellular water
IGF-1	Insulin-like growth factor
IMQ	Index of Memory Quality
INR	International normalized ratio
IOM	Institute of Medicine
LLS	Lake Louise Score
MAJCOM	Major Command (USAF)
MAOD	Maximal accumulated oxygen deficit
MAOI	Monoamine oxidase inhibitor
MAP	Maximal aerobic power
MDRI	Military Dietary Reference Intake
MRCA	Market Research Corporation of America
MRI	Magnetic resonance imaging
MV/MM	Multivitamins/multiminerals supplements
NAS	National Academy of Sciences
ND	Not determined
NE	Niacin Equivalent
NEX	Navy Exchange Service
NF	National Formulary
NFCS	Nationwide Food Consumption Survey
NHANES	National Health and Nutrition Examination Survey
NHIS	National Health Interview Survey
NSORs	Nutritional Standards for Operational Rations
OASD(HA)	Office of the Assistant Secretary of Defense (Health Affairs)
ODS, NIH	Office of Dietary Supplements, National Institutes of Health
OGTT	Oral glucose tolerance test
OIG	Office of the Inspector General
P&T	Pharmacy and Therapeutics
PA	Physical activity
PCC	Poison control center
PGE_2	Prostaglandin E_2
PIF	Proteolysis-inducing factor
PKC	Protein kinase C
PSA	Prostate-specific antigen
PSG	Polysomnography
PUFA	Polyunsaturated fatty acid

RAE	Retinol Activity Equivalent
RDA	Recommended Dietary Allowance
RE	Retinol Equivalent
REE	Resting energy expenditure
RM	Reference material
RMG	Random movement generation test
RVIP	Rapid visual information processing
SBP	Systolic blood pressure
SF	Special Forces
sIgA	Secretory immunoglobulin A
SJS	Stevens-Johnson syndrome
SRT	Selective reminding test
TBW	Total body water
tHcy	Total plasma homocysteine
TNF-α	Tumor necrosis factor-alpha
TTCP	The Technical Corporation Program
UL	Tolerable Upper Intake Level
URTI	Upper respiratory tract infection
USACHPPM	U.S. Army Center for Health Promotion and Preventive Medicine
USAF	U.S. Air Force
USARIEM	U.S. Army Research Institute of Environmental Medicine
USDA	U.S. Department of Agriculture
USP	United States Pharmacopeia
USUHS	Uniformed Services University of the Health Sciences
VCO_2	Rate of elimination of carbon dioxide
V_E	Pulmonary ventilation during exercise
VO_2	Oxygen uptake
WAIS	Wechsler Adult Intelligence Scale
WHO	World Health Organization
WMS	Wechsler Memory Scale
WRAIR	Walter Reed Army Institute of Research

Appendix I

Glossary

Antihyperglycemic	An agent that counteracts high levels of glucose in the blood
Antioxidant	A substance that inhibits the destructive effects of oxidation
Beta-blockers	A class of drugs used for various indications, but particularly for the management of cardiac arrhythmias and cardioprotection after myocardial infarction. They block the action of endogenous catecholamines (epinephrine [adrenaline] and norepinephrine [noradrenaline] in particular) on β-adrenergic receptors, part of the sympathetic nervous system that mediates the fight-or-flight response
Botanicals	A drug, medicinal preparation, or similar substance obtained from a plant or plants
Codex Ebers	A famous Egyptian papyrus recording over 800 medical formulas
CYP2D6	Enzymes involved in the metabolism of xenobiotics in the body

Dietary supplement	A product (other than tobacco) that is intended to supplement the diet; contains one or more dietary ingredients (including vitamins, minerals, herbs or other botanicals, amino acids, and other substances) or their constituents; is intended to be taken by mouth as a pill, capsule, tablet, or liquid; and is labeled in the front panel as being a dietary supplement
Drug	The term *drug* means (A) articles recognized in the official United States Pharmacopeia, official *Homeopathic Pharmacopeia of the United States*, or official *National Formulary*, or any supplement to any of them; and (B) articles intended for use in the diagnosis, cure, mitigation, treatment, or prevention of disease in man or other animals; and (C) articles (other than food) intended to affect the structure or any function of the body of man or other animals; and (D) articles intended for use as a component of any articles specified in clause (A), (B), or (C). A food or dietary supplement for which a claim, subject to sections 403(r)(1)(B) and 403(r)(3) or sections 403(r)(1)(B) and 403(r)(5)(D), is made in accordance with the requirements of section 403(r) is not a drug solely because the label or the labeling contains such a claim. A food, dietary ingredient, or dietary supplement for which a truthful and not misleading statement is made in accordance with section 403(r)(6) is not a drug under clause (C) solely because the label or the labeling contains such a statement
Ergogenic aids	Any external influences that can positively affect physical or mental performance. These include mechanical aids, pharmacological aids, physiological aids, nutritional aids, and psychological aids. They may directly influence the physiological capacity of a particular body system, thereby improving performance; remove psychological constraints that detract from performance; or increase the speed of recovery from training and competition
Food	The term *food* means (1) articles used for food or drink for man or other animals, (2) chewing gum,

	and (3) articles used for components of any such article
Food additive	Any substance the intended use of which results or may reasonably be expected to result—directly or indirectly—in its becoming a component or otherwise affecting the characteristics of any food. This definition includes any substance used in the production, processing, treatment, packaging, transportation, or storage of food
GLUT-4	An important factor in the regulation of blood glucose, and the primary glucose transporter in skeletal muscle
Hyperinsulinemic	A condition in which the level of insulin in the blood is higher than normal. Caused by overproduction of insulin by the body. Related to insulin resistance
Hypocaloric	A diet characterized by a low number of dietary calories, usually 1,000–1,200 kcal/day
MedWatch	The U.S. Food and Drug Administration (FDA) Medical Products Reporting Program is an initiative designed both to educate all health professionals about the critical importance of being aware of, monitoring for, and reporting adverse events and problems to the FDA and/or the manufacturer and to ensure that new safety information is rapidly communicated to the medical community, thereby improving patient care. The purpose of the MedWatch program is to enhance the effectiveness of postmarketing surveillance of medical products as they are used in clinical practice and to rapidly identify significant health hazards associated with these products
Obese	For adults, an individual with a body mass index (BMI) greater than or equal to 30.0 kg/m^2
Overweight	An individual with a BMI of 25.0 to 29.9 kg/m^2

Pharmacovigilance	The pharmacological science relating to the detection, assessment, understanding, and prevention of adverse effects, particularly long-term and short-term side effects of medicines. Generally speaking, pharmacovigilance is the science of collecting, monitoring, researching, assessing, and evaluating information from health care providers and patients on the adverse effects of medications, biological products, herbal products, and traditional medicines with a view to identifying new information about hazards associated with medicines and preventing harm to patients
Phytates	Compounds present in plant foods that bind iron and may prevent its absorption
Rangers	A specially trained elite unit of the United States Army
Special Forces	Special Forces are highly trained and organized elite groups of soldiers who take part in covert warfare, reconnaissance, counterterrorism, and other specialized and dangerous missions. They include U.S. Army Special Forces, Navy SEALs (Sea, Air, Land) and Special Warfare Combatant Craft Crewmen, Air Force Combat Controllers and Pararescuemen
Thermogenics	Supplements that induce the production of heat